Biomedicine

in an Unstable Place

EXPERIMENTAL FUTURES: TECHNOLOGICAL LIVES,

SCIENTIFIC ARTS, ANTHROPOLOGICAL VOICES

A series edited by Michael M. J. Fischer and Joseph Dumit

Biomedicine
in an Unstable Place

INFRASTRUCTURE AND PERSONHOOD

IN A PAPUA NEW GUINEAN HOSPITAL

ALICE STREET

Duke University Press ■ *Durham and London* ■ 2014

© 2014 Duke University Press

All rights reserved

Printed in the United States of

America on acid-free paper ∞

Typeset in Chaparral Pro by Westchester

Book Group

Library of Congress Cataloging-in-Publication Data

Street, Alice.

Biomedicine in an unstable place: infrastructure and

personhood in a Papua New Guinean hospital / Alice

Street.

pages cm—(Experimental futures : technological lives,

scientific arts, anthropological voices)

ISBN 978-0-8223-5761-2 (cloth : alk. paper)

ISBN 978-0-8223-5778-0 (pbk. : alk. paper)

1. Madong General Hospital. 2. Medical care—Papua

New Guinea. 3. Hospital patients—Papua New Guinea.

4. Hospitals—Medical staff—Papua New Guinea.

I. Title. II. Series: Experimental futures.

RA993.P26S77 2014

362.109953—dc23

2014000773

Cover art: Photographs by Alice Street.

FOR JAMIE

Acknowledgments, ix

Prologue, 1

PART I ▥ **PLACE**

1 Making a Place for Biomedicine, 11

2 Locating Disease, 39

3 Public Buildings, Building Publics, 59

PART II ▥ **TECHNOLOGY**

4 Doctors without Diagnosis, 89

5 The Waiting Place, 115

6 Technologies of Detachment, 143

PART III ▥ **INFRASTRUCTURE**

7 The Partnership Hospital, 169

8 Research in the Clinic, 194

Conclusion: Biomedicine in a Fragile State, 223

Notes, 237

Bibliography, 261

Index, 281

It is always difficult as an anthropologist to write critically about persons and practices in the places where we work. Navigating this politics of representation is particularly tricky in Papua New Guinea where, as this book describes, people are rightfully sensitive to their portrayal in international academic and media circuits. In 2006, while I was writing the doctoral thesis that provided one starting point for this book, I voiced some of these concerns about representation and audience at Cambridge's PhD writing-up seminar. With little hesitation the seminar convenor, Marilyn Strathern, stated that it was up to me to create my own readership. This book owes much to that advice, which has assisted me over the years in navigating the politics of research in Papua New Guinea's health sector and the politics of representation in the anthropology of Papua New Guinea. It is from a sense of obligation to the many doctors, nurses, and patients that I met who struggle to sustain life and lives under difficult conditions that I have sought to heed this advice and maintain a critical edge. Nonetheless I accept that there are many people who will not like what I have written.

First and foremost, I am grateful to the doctors, nurses, managers, administrative staff, and patients at Madang General Hospital who have accommodated me over the years with extraordinary patience, who have tolerated my many questions and taught me everything I know about biomedicine and hospitals in Papua New Guinea. I hope that those who read it find that the stories this book tells do justice to the hopes, frustrations, and experimentations that they conveyed to me as being at the heart of hospital life.

Also in Papua New Guinea, Greg Murphy has been an ongoing source of support, warmth, hospitality, and inspiring conversation. Without my frequent drop-ins to sit on his sofa during hospital breaks this book would never have been written. I am deeply grateful to Bryan Kramer for his friendship and assistance over the years. At Divine Word University, where I was a visiting fellow in 2010–11, I am thankful to Kichawen Chakumai for assistance navigating the Papua New Guinea (PNG) health system's bureaucracy, to Margaret Samei for important insights to hospital management, and to Leah Tuka for much valued research assistance.

The William Wyse Fund, the Bartle Frere Foundation, the Smuts Foundation, and St. John's College, Cambridge, provided funding for the initial doctoral research on which this book is partly based. The Economic and Social Research Council and the Nuffield Foundation provided the funds that enabled subsequent research and important changes of direction to take place.

There are many people who have influenced the ideas that have gone into this book. It was Marilyn Strathern's suggestion that I go to a hospital in Papua New Guinea, when I was still thinking about Papua New Guinean weather stations. James Leach provided important advice and guidance in all things Melanesian during the doctoral years. Adam Reed responded to early field reports and has been an important sounding board and critic both at a distance and personally. My peers at Cambridge provided much valued inspiration, and many of them continue to do so, most notably Ann Kelly, Jon Mair, and Jacob Copeman. Mario Biagioli pressed me to get the book written (much quicker than I have done so) and has been an important source of support for the project. At the University of Sussex and the Institute of Development Studies I would like to thank Simon Coleman and Melissa Leach for their mentoring and support and Rebecca Prentice and Dinah Rajak for keeping new ideas flowing. Hayley Macgregor has been a fountain of good sense and valuable criticism as well as a good friend. Two periods that I spent at the Research School of Asia and the Pacific at the Australia National University as a visiting fellow were crucial in forming my understanding of Melanesian anthropology and medical anthropology. I am grateful to Alan Rumsey, Francesca Merlan, Assa Doron, Margaret Jolly, Nicolas Peterson and Kathy Lepani in particular for their warm hospitality and intellectual generosity. Warwick Anderson has offered both criticism and encouragement in the manuscript's later stages. As the series editor Michael Fischer has read more versions of this manuscript than anyone would wish to and has greatly assisted in its improvement. My colleagues at the University of Edinburgh have been wonderfully supportive in the completion of the manuscript.

Earlier versions of parts of chapter 5 appeared in the article "Artefacts of Not-Knowing: The Medical Record, the Diagnosis and the Production of Uncertainty in Papua New Guinean Biomedicine," *Social Studies of Science* 41, no. 6 (December 2011): 815–34.

Joanna Lowry, Brian Street, and David Green first introduced me to anthropology, provided unending support through some very difficult years, and have donated ideas and sustenance in equal measures. Jamie Cross has taught me pretty much everything else and for his companionship in everything I do I am truly grateful.

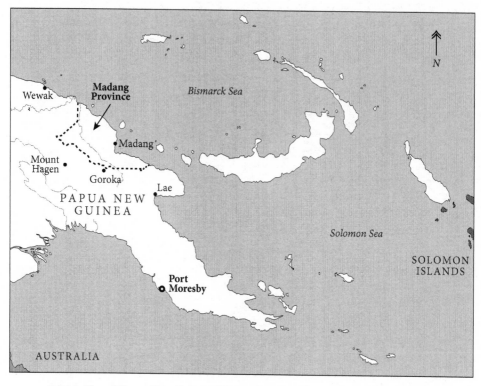

MAP 1. Map of Papua New Guinea, showing Madang Province and major urban centers. Based on an original map by Jamie Cross, © Daniel Dalet, d-maps.com.

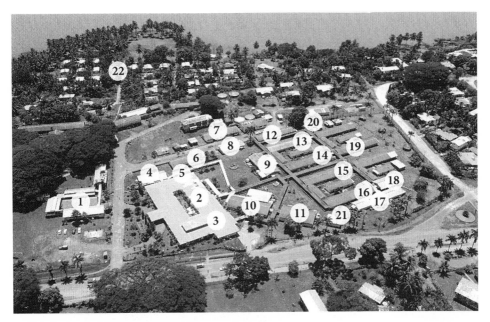

A.1. Photo of Madang Hospital and grounds.

Key for site of Madang Hospital

1	Administration Office	12	Ward Kitchen
2	Intermediate Ward	13	Pediatric Ward
3	Outpatient	14	Surgical Ward
4	Children's Clinic	15	Medical Ward
5	Dispensary	16	Obstetric Ward
6	Medical Store	17	Eye Ward
7	Laundry	18	Physiotherapy
8	Morgue	19	Disused Wards
9	Operating Theater	20	Biomedical Workshop
10	Maternity Ward	21	Red Cross Blood Donation Center
11	X-ray & Pathology	22	Workers' Compound

■ In the small, curtained cubicle at Outpatients, William Gambe lay long, thin, and silent on the bed. The young health extension officer (HEO) who saw him was shocked by the protruding swollen nodules that covered William's body. William, however, claimed his problem was not the skin nodules, which were not painful, but the severe back pain that had now been troubling him for two weeks. Unable to make any connection between the back pain and the skin disease, the medical student admitted that he could not make a diagnosis. Obligated to fill in the admissions form, he wrote only a "provisional diagnosis" of "syphilis" at the bottom of the page. He also noticed that William's skin was very pale, particularly around his fingernails and eyelids, and so he also wrote down "anemia" and ordered iron supplements for William.

The admissions form was placed in a yellow file with William's name and home village written at the top. This file would go to the ward with William and would continue to collect other pieces of paper as further examinations and investigations took place. Meanwhile, the student took a blood sample from William's arm and filled in the form requesting a full blood count, which he put in a tray to be carried to the laboratory by a nurse. He then filled in another form ordering a chest X-ray and an X-ray of William's back. The medical student helped William's wife and sister, who had brought him to the hospital, heave him from the examination bed on to a trolley. The yellow file and X-ray form were balanced on his chest, and his relatives wheeled him slowly along the uneven walkways to the X-ray unit.

At the medical ward, the registrar, Dr. Bosa, reviewed the blood tests, which showed a very low hemoglobin level of 5.6g/dL but little else. The X-ray was so blurred and unclear it was nearly impossible to read. According to the technicians, the fluids used in the machine had deteriorated in the heat and a new order was, as usual, yet to arrive. Despite the blurring the doctor thought he could detect some malformation of the lower vertebrae. The X-ray drew his attention away from the skin nodules and towards tuberculosis as a possible cause of spinal malformation. Tuberculosis, he noted, was also something they could treat for. He started William on the short course for treatment of tuberculosis but also sent a consultation form to the surgical team, who he hoped would shed some light on the strange skin condition.

Arriving at the medical ward, the surgical team found William weak and confined to the bed, barely able to communicate. His wife, a young, quiet woman, sat next to his bed, slowly weaving her string bag and staring at the floor. William's sister, Clare, who with his wife slept on the stained linoleum floor next to his bed, was more forthright and listened intently to what the surgeons had to say. It was Clare who mentioned that William had worked in a chemical factory in Lae, a city two hundred kilometers southeast of Madang, before he had become sick and returned to the village. The surgical consultant, an abrupt but efficient Polish doctor who had come to the hospital many years before with the Catholic Mission and was now the only European doctor in the hospital, was interested in the chemical factory. It was possible, he explained to Clare in Tok Pisin, that William could be suffering from some kind of chemical poisoning. Writing up the consultant report in the nurses' office after the examination, however, many possibilities were raised, including HIV (which coindicated a rare nodular skin disease, erythema elevatum diutinum), a bone marrow condition, cancer, tuberculosis, and tertiary syphilis. The truth was, the surgical doctor admitted, they really did not know what could be wrong with William. The only thing they could do was take a biopsy to send to the capital, Port Moresby, for analysis.

The difficulty was that William's hemoglobin count was too low to operate and the hospital blood bank was nearly empty. The surgical registrar returned to the ward to explain to the sister that she would need to get members of her family to come to the hospital to donate. Later that afternoon, William's wife returned to the village with the request for blood.

The next day, Clare's husband turned up at the hospital with a male cousin to donate blood. Clare's husband had other news. He told Clare that William's wife, Bertha, had returned to her own family in a nearby village and was not coming back. Clare was not surprised. Bertha and William had only been married a few months when William had left to find work in Lae. While he was away they heard many stories about his relations with other women. When he returned, sick, to the village, he had been angry and irritable with his wife, regularly beating her. Privately, Clare's husband also noted that the two women had not been getting on. On entering the hospital Clare had immediately taken up her position at the side of her brother's bed and set about giving Bertha orders for his care. Now she would be on her own.

Later, Clare and her husband waited quietly on the small bench outside the operating theater while inside the surgical registrar placed William under local anesthesia, sliced off two nodules from the skin's surface and placed them in a small labeled jar to send to Port Moresby Hospital. Clare placed much hope in the surgeon's proactive response to her brother's suffering. It suggested that his sickness had been recognized as treatable with hospital medicine (*sik bilong marasin*) and the surgeons' evident intention to cure him made it more likely the hospital medicines would work. Her own presence outside the operating theater and her good thoughts about her brother were also vital in making sure the surgeon's knife did not slip and the doctors were able to complete their work successfully. She had made sure she told William to close off all thoughts of his wife and the conflict between them when he entered the theater.

Inside the operating theater, meanwhile, the surgeons were busy discussing what little they could do for William. The test results would not arrive for up to a further eight weeks and he needed effective treatment quickly. The surgeons were clear, however, that his management was the medical doctor's responsibility, not their own. He had not been admitted to the surgical ward, and they had enough on their plate. After the operation, William was carried on a stretcher back to his bed. The surgeons returned to their own ward and their own patients.

The medical doctor was increasingly concerned about the possibility that William was HIV positive. But over the days and then weeks, multiple HIV screening tests came back from the laboratory with negative results. The problem was that it was difficult to trust the laboratory results. Frequent power cuts meant that the reagents were not always stored at the right temperature. In any case, antiretrovirals were not yet available in Papua New Guinea. With few other options, he continued to treat William for tuberculosis. There was nothing he could do but wait to see how William responded to the treatment. Dr. Bosa had not completed his medical training to become a consultant physician, but the hospital had been unable to recruit a specialist physician for months, meaning that he was solely responsible for all forty patients on the ward. With so few resources and so many patients, he knew that if William did not have a common disease that responded to available treatment, there was little he could do to make a diagnosis or treat him.

Clare began to have suspicions about the medical registrar, who she complained did not talk to her and had done nothing for William, in contrast to the surgeons who had come to see him, told her that his illness was caused by chemical poisoning, given him blood, and taken him into the operating theater. Clare wondered whether the doctor in the medical ward intended to cure William at all. She followed all his orders, making sure William took his medicine at the right times, but he still did not improve. At ward round, she noted that the doctor didn't look at William properly; he just talked to the nurses in English and moved onto the next bed. Perhaps, she conceded, this was because William was a difficult and irritable patient. But without the doctor's attention or good intentions, she feared that the hospital medicine would not work. Now the surgeons had disappeared, it seemed that William had become invisible. "Ol i no lukim mipela" (they don't see us), she complained.

Even more worrying, since the surgeon's suggestion of chemical poisoning, she had not heard any further mention of a "name." "At ward round they come, look at the picture [X-ray]. But they don't say anything to us. They look at the picture but they haven't found a name. I don't know. Have they found a name? They haven't said anything. Do you know?" she asked the anthropologist, who might or might not also be a doctor. Without a name, she feared that William might not be on the right medicine, or that he might not actually have the kind of sickness that could be treatable with "white people's medicine" at all.

William was deteriorating. He had also become troublesome on the ward, often shouting at his sister or the nurses. At other times he lay on his bed writhing and groaning with pain while the other patients looked on anxiously. He was moved into bed number two, closer to the nurses' office in order to receive twenty-four-hour nursing care. Patients placed in these beds were those that nurses described as being "bikpela sik" (severely sick). Nurses tried not to become too attached to those patients because they knew they could die at any time.

Clare wondered about the few people from the village who had come to donate blood or who brought gifts of garden food to supplement the hospital's meager fare of soggy white rice and watery grey tuna donated by the tuna factory along the coast from the town. Every week she instead made the trip to her village on the PMV bus, carrying back large string bags full of taro, yams, and bananas from her garden that strained on her head. The problem, Clare knew, was that William had many people who were angry with him and who could be causing his sickness. Even his broken relationship with his wife could be making him worry and stopping the hospital medicine from working.

Trying not to think about those social conflicts, or her own growing frustrations with her brother, Clare followed the nurses' advice and prayed to God. William had "sinned" in Lae, becoming a "bikhet" (big head), drinking and smoking marijuana and fighting with men from other places. It was up to "bikpela" (God) to make William better, and he would only do this if he saw that the family were *wanbel* (of one mind) with Him. The nurses told her that He would know this if they prayed and made sure William took his medicine, which was a "gift from God." After a while, she stopped watching for the doctor to walk past. He couldn't find William's sickness, but God could see everything.

William wasn't interested in praying to God. As his condition worsened he became more certain that sorcery had been committed against him. He had fought with some Tolai in Lae, a group from New Ireland who are renowned for their powers of sorcery. William was sure that the Tolai were to blame, claiming that they had hit him on the back, and that this was where his illness had first begun (*kamap*). Another patient in the ward, Anna, put Clare in touch with a *glasman* (medical diviner) who lived in New Town, a settlement on the edge of Madang town. He offered her his services for a fee of three hundred kina (about one hundred U.S. dollars), thirty times the ward fee Clare had paid to admit William to the hospital. Sneaking into the ward while the doctor was away, the glasman pulled off two of the nodules from William's upper thigh with his hands and then cupped his hands over the sores and "pulled out the poison," although Clare did not see what it looked like.

The nurses hid in the office, refusing to go into the ward while the glasman was there. Nurse Kanu leant low over the desk pretending to fill in a nursing report. She was sure she felt eyes boring into her head, even though no one could see her from the ward. She rang the doctor in the consultation clinic on the pretext of needing to find a file, but by the time he arrived, the glasman had left.

Following directions, Clare quietly put the skin nodules in a small white bowl with some water and placed it in a dark place beneath the ward's water storage tank. The next morning, she threw it away in the shrubs at the back of the hospital grounds.

William did not improve. Clare had used all her money, including donations from her husband's family, to pay the glasman. Now she asked the registrar for a medical certificate she could send to the chemical company in Lae in order to request William's unpaid wages. She would need the money to keep paying for travel back to the village and the extra food she often bought in town. She was also beginning to think about the money it would cost to transport William's body back to the village if he died. For ten kina Dr. Bosa wrote a letter stating William's diagnosis to be tuberculosis. He admitted he had no idea what William was actually suffering from, but he needed to write a clear diagnosis on the document, otherwise the company would not pay up.

Clare was tired of the hospital. The ward was hot and airless. The bathrooms were always dirty and no relatives who worked in town had visited or brought them soap for weeks. The water was making her skin itch and, like the other patients, she wondered whether it was safe to wash with it. To get clean water to drink she had to walk across the hospital grounds to a small single tap at the front gate. She had initially established relationships with some of the other patient guardians in the ward, sharing food, soap, and helping them collect food from the kitchen or to cook on the small wood fires at the back of the hospital grounds. But now many of the patients those guardians had cared for had died or left. She was increasingly aware of the exposure of the ward; all the strangers' eyes staring at her as she carried out her daily tasks.

When William was awake, which was more and more seldom, he was angry. Clare felt ashamed in front of the other patients and reluctant to look after her brother. To help her, her husband came to stay at the hospital. One day, he noticed that William began to "test" his sister, asking her to pull his fingers to relieve the pain, to bring him cold water, and wash his skin repeatedly. Angry and frustrated, Clare stormed out of the ward to sit outside on the grass with other patients, sharing her thoughts about difficulties of life in the hospital. Sitting next to the bed where William lay ailing, Clare's husband wondered to himself whether Clare's brother was dying and whether his persistent demands weren't a test to see if his sister was still wanbel with him. He didn't think it was good for Clare to have left.

Early the next morning, as the doctor did ward round, the room filled with Clare's wails of grief. The doctor was attending to another patient and did not respond. To do so when William had already died, he thought, would be pointless. "What is the one thing that is certain in life?" he asked the medical students later. He tried to stay away from relatives once a patient died. Things were in their hands now; there was nothing more he could do. The nurses quickly pulled an old tattered cloth screen around William's bed, leaving Clare inside still desperately calling out her brother's name. As the doctor continued on his ward round, the patients lay silent in their beds, the relatives quietly whispering to one another in the shade of the walkway outside. Later, Clare reflected on what had happened. She had not been wanbel with her brother, she knew, and he had been angry with her. She wondered if this was enough to make him die.

He tried not to show it to the patients, but William's death had also upset Dr. Bosa, for whom it compounded the difficulties and frequent impossibilities of saving lives in the hospital. Several days later Dr. Bosa sat musing over William's death certificate, which he needed to fill out in order for the family to gain access to William's wages and payout from the chemical company in Lae. Without that money he knew they would not have the means of transporting William's body, which was still in the morgue, to the village for burial. But Dr. Bosa didn't like filling in the death certificate. It made him feel personally responsible when he also knew there was nothing else he could have done. Eventually he pulled a pen out of his top pocket and wrote the cause of death as "tuberculosis" on the form. This was the best he could do he explained; this was the treatment regime William had been on.

Following its travels to the hospital records office, where it would be compiled into statistics and sent on to the Department of Health in Port Moresby, William Gambe's documented diagnosis would ultimately contribute to the disease incidence figures for tuberculosis in that year, 2003.

Six weeks after the death of William Gambe a histology report was received from Port Moresby. The opaque body that had lain in a bed on the ward, which was diseased but without a specific disease, was now replaced by a laboratory specimen, described in visual terms and microdetail, and which revealed to the laboratory technician's eye a unique pathology. "Rhabdomyosarcoma" the laboratory technician suggested. Cancer. Nonetheless, the report noted, it was unclear exactly what kind of tumor the specimen might be; this was still only a preliminary diagnosis, with several differential diagnoses also noted. "Correlate clinically" concluded the report.

PART I ■ PLACE

CHAPTER 1

Making a Place for Biomedicine

In Madang Hospital, Papua New Guinea, biomedical practitioners struggle amid severe resource shortages to make the diseased body visible.[1] Bodies like that of William Gambe, described in the prologue, rarely crystallize into clear biomedical objects. Here medical devices such as X-ray machines do not work well in the hot and humid climate, pathology machines are old and difficult to calibrate, and the reagents stored in fridges are rendered unreliable by the frequent power cuts. This is the murky world of biomedicine as it is practiced in the mundane places of poverty that traverse much of the globe. In such places, weak states, structural adjustment, and extractive capital have led to the degradation of public health infrastructure, and people must strive to make biomedicine work in conditions of institutional instability and medical uncertainty.

Opened in 1962 by the Australian colonial administration, Madang Hospital was intended to be a showcase for modern medicine and a catalyst for the construction of a modern independent Papua New Guinean nation-state. Situated in the third largest town in Papua New Guinea and serving as the referral hospital for a provincial population of more than 365,000 people, Madang Hospital today embodies a paradox that runs through the public health systems of many of the world's poorest countries.[2] On one hand, since the end of the Second World War public health professionals, policy analysts, government representatives, and development workers in Papua New Guinea have condemned the drift of health resources away from rural primary health care and toward urban centers and curative medicine. In a country where an estimated 87 percent of the population lives in rural areas that are frequently inaccessible by road,[3] and depends largely on subsistence livelihoods, the concentration of medical professionals, technologies, drugs, and infrastructures in urban hospitals seems unjustifiable and unsustainable.[4] On the other hand, hospitals in Papua New Guinea are derided for failing to provide the levels of care that might be expected of such "modern" institutions. Hospitals, political and media representations suggest, are simultaneously overfunded and underresourced. They divert attention and resources away from preventative and primary health care, and yet they fail to accomplish the technological feats associated with modern biomedicine. It turns out that hospitals are necessary after all and that, in Papua New Guinea, they do not do what people expect of them.

It is in institutions like Madang Hospital that most people in the world are likely to encounter biomedical doctors and specialist biomedical technologies. Here biomedicine does not follow a universal template that originated in Europe. Nor is this hospital a pale imitation of "proper" hospitals in Western countries (though this narrative is sometimes adopted by people in the institution). Rather, it is in institutions like Madang Hospital that twenty-first-century biomedicine, in constantly coming up against the limits of its own practices and technologies, is continually reinvented, imagined, and done. It is thus in these mundane spaces where funding and resources are scarce that we are most likely to gain insight into what biomedicine means for the people who create and engage with its practices, and what kinds of social and physical worlds it makes possible. To understand what hospitals are and the social relationships of contemporary biomedicine, it is to these "peripheral" institutions that we must turn.

If hospitals are places of biomedicine, however, they are never solely biomedical places. A central argument of this book is that once we take the *place* of biomedicine as our field of enquiry, this forces our attention toward the mutually constitutive relationships between scientific orderings of the world and other orderings, such as those entailed by kinship practices and projects of development or state building, that are crucial to the production of this place as a hospital and through which people attempt to transform and improve their lives and those of others.[5] It is hospitals' paradoxical capacity to be at once sites of "total" biopolitical management *and* places where alternative and transgressive social orders emerge and are contested that makes them crucial ethnographic sites for exploring relationships between science, society, and power.[6] The complexity of the relationships between biomedical and nonbiomedical orderings that make up hospital infrastructures becomes all the more apparent in a place like

Madang Hospital, where resource shortages make it difficult to map biomedical authority onto hospital space and where the successful execution of biomedical practices may in fact require doctors and nurses to harness the kinship relationships of staff or patients as a resource: for example, when patients' kin provide much needed in-hospital care, blood donations, food, and privately purchased pharmaceuticals.

The story of how bodies, persons, and diseases are made visible or invisible in Madang Hospital is not, therefore, only a story about biomedical work. It is a story about the history of hospital infrastructures as sites of colonial and postcolonial state building. It is a story about the coproduction of Papua New Guinea as a site of global infectious disease control, medical research, and public health. And it is a story about people's encounters with urban institutions and biomedical technologies and the bodily and personal transformations that this makes possible.

In Madang Hospital, this book shows, the struggle to render the biological body visible and knowable to the clinical gaze becomes entangled with attempts by doctors, nurses, and patients to make themselves visible to external others (to clinical experts, global scientists, politicians, and international development workers) as socially recognizable and valuable persons. Here the visual operations of modern biomedicine become intertwined with the visual politics of personhood in an unstable place where the infrastructures necessary for producing knowledge and governing populations are tenuous.

What is a hospital when its bodies remain blurry? When foreign donors and international organizations label the state as fragile and the health system as failing? When its nurses are regularly on strike against a state they accuse of neglect? When its doctors are frustrated by their inability to diagnose or treat people in the manner they have been trained? When its infrastructural poverty becomes a scientific resource and the basis for the construction of well-resourced research enclaves? When its patients are caught between kin who might have made them sick in the village and doctors who seem not to see them at all? On one hand, this book argues, such a hospital is a place of deep ontological uncertainty and instability, where knowledge of oneself and others cannot be taken for granted. On the other hand, it is a place of experimentation, where technological and bureaucratic apparatuses provide opportunities for making persons visible and knowable in new, unpredictable, and powerful ways. In a place where people predominantly imagine themselves to be invisible (to the state, to doctors, to a global scientific community) the hospital becomes an intense site of visibility work where bureaucratic and biomedical technologies are engaged with as relational technologies that can make the person visible in recognizable and affectively persuasive forms.[7]

The chapters that follow explore the everyday relationships between persons, bureaucracies, technologies, and spaces that transform the body and the person into recognizable entities. In doing so they attend to the spatial and temporal differences in the ways in which biomedicine is practiced and the kinds of bodies and persons it renders visible. Social science's temporal register for such "differences in medicine" takes its cue from Foucault's influential account of the historical disjuncture at the end of the eighteenth century that marked the birth of modern medicine.[8] Although the anthropology of biomedicine and hospital ethnography have in many ways departed from a Foucauldian approach in recent years, it is worth reviewing Foucault's conception of biomedical difference and its relation to the hospital as a site of visibility as a starting point for considering how such differences might also be attended to in the context of the global hospital today.

In *The Birth of the Clinic* Foucault described the coemergence of a new kind of institutional clinical space and new ways of seeing and knowing disease in the body. Between the investigations of doctors working in the mid eighteenth century who, for example, divided and weighed the different portions of the brain to classify its properties and those working at the beginning of the nineteenth who *saw* and *described* the brain's qualities in order to seek out new empirical truths about disease, Foucault identified differences that are "both tiny and total" (2003, xi). Up until the early nineteenth century disease was located in the limited two-dimensional space of the nosological table and was construed as external to the body in which it became manifest. The total range of possible permutations of disease was fixed by the limited classificatory series of the table and any variations were attributed to the body of the patient and construed as an external impingement on the natural course of the disease. With the emergence of pathological anatomy came a new kind of gaze that penetrated the body and saw into its depths. Disease became localizable in and specific to the individual body. It was now conceived as part of a dynamic and inchoate field of "life," which required management through both a clinical gaze and public health governance.

According to Foucault, modern medicine emerged out of the conjuncture of pathological anatomy with its internal geography of the body and the modern clinic as a space where vision and visibility become privileged as a basis for truth. The "careful gaze" of pathological anatomy restructured clinical practice so that bodies no longer needed to be opened up on the autopsy table for doctors to locate disease in their depths. Tapping, listening, prodding now all became techniques of vision that brought the dynamic geography of individual life into view. In this new "empire of the gaze" doctors "learned how to establish dossiers, systems of marking and classifying, the integrated accountancy of individual records" (Foucault 1980, 70), such as the individual case files that rendered the individuated body knowable, facilitated medical talk about the body, and made clinical intervention possible (Foucault 2003, 131–152).[9] What underpinned these shifts in the spatiality of medical knowledge, he argued, was a redistribution of the "visible and invisible" (Foucault 2003, xii) that represented "a whole new 'regime' in discourse and forms of knowledge . . . a modification in the rules of formation of statements which are accepted as scientifically true" (Foucault 1980, 112). It was with these transformations, Foucault argued, that the individual emerged as both the subject and object of knowledge and that the human sciences were born.

Foucault was peculiarly sensitive to medicine's historical epistemic breaks, perhaps even to the extent of overstating them,[10] nonetheless his account of the clinic ran pathology, clinical knowledge, and medical research together within a homogenous epistemic space.[11] This book, by contrast, pays attention to the ways in which differences in medical knowledge and practice are distributed across hospital, national, and global geographies. When we attend to medicine's social and geographic diversity we might find that pathology does not always and everywhere provide the dominant way of stabilizing disease. Instead the hospital is revealed as a space of sociomaterial complexity, where differences in biomedicine, disease, and biology might coexist through their distribution in space and time (Mol 2002). The kind of body that is made visible by medical practices in Madang Hospital's private wards is different from that made visible in the hospital's public wards. The kind of clinical knowledge produced in the medical ward differs from and frequently takes priority over the knowledge of pathology produced in the hospital's laboratory. Moreover, biomedical practices in these hospital spaces do not entail the diagnosis of an underlying disease through the exercise of an authoritative gaze so much as the development of pragmatic collaborations with medical devices, professionals, patients, and relatives and experimental "tinkering" with technologies, bodies, and everyday lives in order to create solutions that people can live with.[12]

When differences in knowledge practices, disease, and bodies are traced across global rather than institutional geographies more is at stake for everyone involved. Recent ethnographies of care in non-Western hospitals have emphasized the fluid, experimental, and improvised nature of biomedicine in contexts of institutional poverty. Oncology doctors in Botswana must "borrow, adjust, and even deny, but never simply import metropolitan knowledge," writes Julie Livingston, of their attempts to align their latest readings on advances in oncology care in wealthy countries with the possibilities of care in Botswana's cancer ward. "There are moments in the trajectories of cancer illnesses or survivorship where therapy becomes an experimental zone in which innovation and guesswork is dominant."[13] In such spaces, "resource" becomes a verb and doctors learn to "improvise new options from the resources available—material and social." This involves cobbling together "social networks, material goods, short-term opportunities and ideas to craft ad hoc solutions to the problems they faced" (Wendland 2010, 154).

That biomedicine generates its own contexts of uncertainty and improvisation is not unique to resource-poor institutions. As Atul Gawande, the American surgeon and popular medical writer has observed, hospitals are often bewildering spaces where "the gap between what we know and what we aim for persists. And this gap complicates everything we do" (2003, 3). This means, Gawande argues, that much of the biomedical work that is done in hospitals is pursued not through the rational application of available scientific knowledge to a particular case, but through "habit, intuition, and sometimes plain old guessing" (2003, 7). Such "complications" (Gawande 2003) of biomedicine may be universal, but they are also heightened in institutions like Madang Hospital.[14] Here murky biomedical knowledge rarely clears to reveal lucid etiologies or diagnoses. The adaptive and experimental qualities of biomedical "tinkering" in such places are vital to making sure that lives are saved.

This has implications for thinking about how the hospital, as a sociotechnical assemblage, travels and what matters to whom about differences in medicine when they are distributed across contexts of relative wealth and poverty.[15] As the acting CEO explained to me on my first day in Madang Hospital, "Here we don't have all the resources to make diagnoses on hand . . . final diagnoses are only made when the patient leaves." In Madang Hospital, as I describe in chapter 4, disease is not only enacted *differently* in different places; it frequently fails to appear at all. In Madang Hospital, I argue, patients' bodies are clearly diseased but do not always have specific diseases. Instead doctors must deal with bodies that they describe as "generally sick."

What kinds of capacities and futures do generally sick bodies and Papua New Guinean medical experts have? These questions are important because "improvisational medicine" (Livingston 2012) is not the only kind of biomedicine practiced in Madang Hospital. Papua New Guinea has been a site of intensive biomedical research interest since Robert Koch visited the Northeast Coast to carry out malaria research in 1901, but ongoing international investment in medical research through successive colonial and postcolonial governments has rarely overflowed into the public health system (as described in chapters 2 and 8 of this book). As global funding for infectious diseases has grown in tandem with pressures to meet the health-focused Millennium Development Goals, so do resource-poor clinical medicine and internationally funded medical research increasingly converge in Madang Hospital. Papua New Guinean doctors claim uncertainty as a locally appropriate biomedical resource in the hospital's public wards. Meanwhile foreign medical researchers' experimental apparatuses enable them to stabilize the individual diseased body as an object of knowledge, and in doing so raise questions about the validity and quality of Papua New Guinean doctors' management of "generally sick" bodies.[16]

In Papua New Guinea differences between the bodies, biologies, and expert persons produced within medical research and clinical medicine have a history as long as biomedicine itself. These are differences that are coproduced alongside racial and emerging class distinctions and that make different kinds of expertise and interventions possible. Here, this book argues, differences in medicine frequently coincide with the production of differences between persons. What kinds of biomedical objects can be made visible, by whom, and with what material and technical resources is a question that puts the global circulation of scientific expertise and infrastructure at the heart of the anthropology of personhood and the body.

BEYOND BIOMEDICINE

Hospitals are often portrayed as intensive sites of biopower where biological life is incorporated into a field of political calculation, governance, and management. But in Madang Hospital "life—or living—is not a matter of biology alone" (Marsland and Prince 2012, 463; Fassin 2009). In fact, as the story of William Gambe shows, the bodies that are made visible in this space are not necessarily biological bodies at all. Institutional poverty weakens the efficacy of bureaucratic and biomedical technologies. Diseased and laboring bodies confound institutional regimes of legibility; doctors struggle to make patient bodies visible to the medical gaze. Patients and their relatives struggle to make their bodies seen by medical experts. Relationships between persons, technologies, and buildings in such spaces cannot be seamlessly accommodated to the biomedical and bureaucratic agendas of the institution. Indeed, this is where hospital ethnography significantly departs from the anthropology of biomedicine and enables us to explore the complex institutional life of a simultaneously biomedical and nonbiomedical, contained and permeable, place (Street and Coleman 2012).[17]

In Madang Hospital, I argue, relationships are not dominated by the biomedical project of knowing disease. In fact, diseases often fail to be made visible at all. This intensifies uncertainty but also opens up opportunities for experimentation with bureaucratic and biomedical technologies and the generation of new kinds of knowledge and forms of personhood. Hospital technologies remain open to "interpretive flexibility" (Pinch and Bijker 1984) as people incorporate them into diverse projects of biological and relational transformation. The experimental quality of this place invites us to explore the effects and affects of different projects of transformation as they encounter one another, and the different bodies, persons, and biologies that they make visible.

Patients, this book shows, are as involved in projects of visibility and knowledge as are biomedical professionals and state actors. They scrutinize the body as an index of a person's relationships and social capacities.[18] Transforming the body through the elicitation of productive relationships with others necessitates transforming oneself into an object of the other's regard. With kin both in the village and the town this involves exchanges of money, food, and bodily substance. The trouble is that such relationships are difficult to engage in from the hospital bed. Instead patients worry that relatives have forgotten them, that they have become socially invisible, and that this is leading to the direct weakening and deterioration of their body. In chapter 5, I show how patients engage with biomedical practices and technologies as relational technologies that elicit relationships that will transform their body. Particular value is placed on imaging technologies such as the X-ray, which patients anticipate will visualize them in a form doctors will be compelled to treat. When diagnostic technologies fail and when doctors refuse to enter into interpersonal relationships with patients, this is again experienced as their own failure to make themselves visible to others in the appropriate form.

Madang Hospital is a place where new kinds of knowledge and the visualization of new kinds of persons are made possible, but where the stabilization of such reified forms is difficult. Uncertainty provokes improvisation and sustains hope in future well-being, personal transformation, and national development. But the hospital is also a place where failure is frequently experienced as the endpoint of hope, where people (doctors, nurses, patients, and relatives) discover they are socially invisible—unrecognized as a person in their relationships with doctors, kin, the state, or the networks of global science. As Susan Whyte has described, medical uncertainty can generate both doubt and hope, leading to a pragmatic process of "trying out." Crucially, this "process of questioning, doubting and trying out is about social relationships as well as individual disorders" (1997, 3). The ontological instabilities of Madang Hospital demonstrate the importance of an anthropological approach to postcolonial technoscience, which explores the ways in which scientific practices become involved in people's everyday efforts to improve their lives and build relationships with others in places of poverty and suffering.[19] Such a project extends the focus in science and technology studies (STS) on how scientific facts or technological assemblages travel to and become stabilized in different places in order to explore the historically specific relationships between multiple ontologies that constitute postcolonial places of science and medicine.[20]

POSTCOLONIAL INSTITUTIONS

The story about what or who is made biomedically visible or invisible in Papua New Guinea is also a story about the peculiar genealogy of the colonial and postcolonial hospital. In the Papua New Guinean hospital, this book shows, the collectivized, "generally sick" body has emerged historically out of the intersection of state power, race, and medicine.

The design and construction of public hospitals has been integral to the projects of modernization and social improvement pursued in the developing world. Between the seventeenth and twentieth centuries colonial hospitals became the "focus for the dissemination of Western Medicine" worldwide (Harrison 2009, 1). Moreover, it was in the colonies that many of the new experiments in hospital organization were taking place, and in postcolonial, usually low-income countries that the majority of the world's hospitals are located today.[21] It is therefore surprising that hospitals remain somewhat neglected sites for the study of colonial, postcolonial, and development relations in the social sciences.[22] In fact, historical accounts of the emergence of the modern hospital remain extraordinarily Eurocentric.

Colonialism made hospitals a major export of the Western world and an important part of the infrastructure of governance. In many colonized countries, biomedicine and its institutions were introduced as material signs of progress, rationality, and civilization that justified the colonial venture and operated as important tools in the shaping of colonial regimes, bodies, and subjectivities. European medical intervention "represented progress towards a more 'civilized' social and environmental order" (Arnold 1988, 3). Hospitals were spaces where colonial state authorities sought to impress the value of science and modernity on their colonial subjects at the same time as they transformed and improved their bodies. Yet the efficacy of those biopolitical regimes can also be overemphasized. In Papua New Guinea consecutive German, British, and Australian colonial states exerted limited influence over people's everyday lives, while persistent ill health and a rugged terrain constantly reminded colonial administrators of their precarious presence in the country. Here isolated hospitals, Foucault's "small scale, regional, dispersed panoptisms" (1980, 72) never extended into a generalized system of public health. Archipelagos of governance did not accumulate into territorial grids. Under these conditions, as I describe in chapters 2 and 3, hospitals became isolated sites of ongoing yet fragile state-building projects, constructed against a background of fears about the viability of the colonial enterprise.

In many postwar colonial and postcolonial regimes, hospitals gained new significance as monuments of nation building and modernity. Hospital-building programs were at the center of nationalist planning strategies for newly independent regimes across Africa and Asia. In Papua New Guinea, still administered by the Australian department for external territories up until 1975, hospitals in the postwar period nonetheless became important indicators of the colonial administration's commitment to the development and eventual independence of the territory and to the health of the Papua New Guinean (as opposed to solely European) population. Amidst concerns that a Papua New Guinean nation did not exist and that the state was perceived as a distant, foreign entity by the country's rural inhabitants, the hospital became a crucial site in which administrators hoped to nurture civic allegiances, construct new publics, and demonstrate the presence, power, and benevolence of the modern state.

Yet there were important continuities in the ways in which bodies were visualized and racialized in the early and late colonial hospital in Papua New Guinea. The "generally sick" body that is made visible in Madang Hospital today finds its antecedents in both the early colonial makeshift hospitals and the postwar nation-building hospitals that have defined twentieth-century state building in Papua New Guinea. In particular, the distinction between medical research and public health, which continues to generate diverse practices of care, biomedical trajectories, and experiences of social and biological legitimacy in the contemporary hospital, cuts across multiple colonial and postcolonial regimes and provides an ongoing motif for the institutional inequalities that lie at the heart of this book.

The forms of medical expertise and notions of health governance that were established within the walls of the Papua New Guinean hospital changed radically over the course of the twentieth century alongside shifting notions of tropical medicine, race, and disease. However, the hospital remained a crucial nexus within which different formulations of the state, person, and public were coproduced. Hospitals, this book argues, need to be explored ethnographically as historical as well as spatial infrastructures. As spaces of ongoing state building and monuments of modernity and progress, their material form carries the traces of past interventions, ideologies of race and development, and shifting biomedical terrains into the present. These remainders of colonial and postcolonial regimes continue to shape doctors,' nurses' and patients' living environment and reproduce differences in race, class, and scientific prestige.

DESIRING THE STATE

Twentieth-century dreams of nationwide networks of hospitals that would display the latest advances in technology and medicine and provide the same level of care to patients in Africa and Asia as those in the West were often short lived. Today the archetypal image of the crowded and dirty "third world" hospital circulates through the international media and development reports. In Papua New Guinea, as in many postcolonial countries, structural adjustment programs, neoliberal economic policies, and elite corruption led to the dilapidation of already inadequate colonial infrastructures. Today, as described in chapters 3 and 7, the "failed hospital" has become emblematic of the "fragile state."

For many of Papua New Guinea's donors of development aid, the rendering of William Gambe's body as invisible would be understood as a stereotypical story about the failure of modern institutions in a fragile state. Contrary to such accounts, which focus on the internal implosion of the Papua New Guinean state, this book traces the ways in which the hospital has been produced simultaneously as a site of invisibility and intense visibility work through international circuits of medical knowledge, bureaucracy, funding, and governance. The Papua New Guinean hospital has long been a site of experimental governance for foreign governments, agencies, and organizations. Through these interventions the hospital has not historically emerged as a technology of governance so much as the site of multiple ongoing, incomplete, and contested projects of state *building*. What those efforts have produced, this book shows, is a state that frequently fails to see, recognize, and care for its subjects. This book explores the ways in which those historical power relationships are materialized in hospital space and inflect Papua New Guineans' perceptions of and engagements with the institution. I therefore follow Mary-Jo Good and her colleagues in exploring the hospital as a site of "postcolonial disorder," where struggles to transform the sick body and personal experiences of suffering are inseparable from processes of political change and social transformation (Good et al. 2008).

Madang Hospital is a public hospital and people's experiences of the institution are fundamentally shaped by their perceptions of it as a place of government.[23] This is crucial for understanding the ways in which people engage with biomedical practices and respond to biomedical uncertainty. In a predominantly rural society with notoriously weak state infrastructure, the hospital is a crucial site of production for the everyday state, a place where people engage with, imagine, and contest forms of state power. This relationship between biomedicine and the state is all the more significant in a place where state systems of governance have been historically precarious and where depictions of state failure today dominate political discourse both inside and outside the country. In Papua New Guinea's public hospitals, the uncertainties generated by dilapidated state infrastructures and discourses of corruption collide with the uncertainties inherent to biomedical knowledge production. Here, the tropes of the failing state and the state that either cannot or refuses to see are central to people's experience of biomedical and bureaucratic technologies.

State power is not given in Papua New Guinea, but it is often desired.[24] Engagements with hospital technologies, attempts to forge relationships in the institution, and encounters with international medical research or donor infrastructure are all, I argue, mediated by attempts to elicit a desirable relationship with the state or with emerging statelike actors. What is at stake in these interactions is frequently not people's experience of governance by the state but their ability to *make the state see*. Patients, doctors, and nurses in Madang Hospital seek to make themselves into an object of the state's regard.

The hospital has become an archetypal site of visibility in the social sciences. There the biological body is opened up to an expert biomedical gaze, and the diseases located deep within its recesses are made visible and knowable.[25] Statistical data about biological life is collated, categorized, and standardized so as to make it available to a state that seeks to govern the health of its population.[26] Architecture and spatial organization are ordered so as to afford the observation and supervision of patients by staff and staff by one another.[27] Accounts of the modern hospital have therefore focused on the ways in which everyday technical and bureaucratic practices coalesce around the ordering, classification, and representation of bodies, persons, diseases, and things as recognizably distinct entities that afford intervention (Bowker and Star 2000).

Underpinning this understanding of the hospital as a site of visibility is the metaphoric association between visibility and knowledge that runs through Euro-American epistemology (Jay 1994). In recent commentaries on modern medicine and governance this association is inflected with the operations of power. For Foucault the modern clinic rendered the body an object of both a specific and generalized gaze. An understanding of biological life as a site of intervention and management became dominant among the medical profession and also came to structure ideas about how to govern the welfare of the population in general.[28] The clinic was a point of origin for a new conjuncture of power/knowledge that harnessed visibility as a precondition for new mechanisms of control. This was control that worked indirectly through the internalization of the medical/institutional/policing gaze and its norms for healthy living rather than the exercise of external force.[29]

This relationship between knowledge, visibility, and power has today become central to anthropological and sociological approaches to personhood, power, and subjectivity. Statistical techniques that differentiate populations according to their genetic makeup or risky lifestyles and new therapeutic interventions for knowing and healing individual psychologies and biologies are shown to generate new possibilities for imagining and relating to the self and others, either as experts or biological subjects (Rabinow and Rose 2006). Biomedical, numerical, and bureaucratic technologies for categorizing persons, it is argued, bring those "kinds" of persons into being (Hacking 2007). Bringing these relationships between technologies of visibility and processes of person-making to the fore, for example, Rayna Rapp describes how the widespread use of ultrasound scanning during pregnancy in American hospitals leads some women to internalize new disease possibilities and medicalized imaginings of risks at the same time as such practices both personify and gender the fetus (Rapp 2007).[30] As the language and technological practices of oncology are translated for Botswana patients, and cancer becomes ontologically stable as a disease object within patient lifeworlds, describes Livingston, so do those patients learn to understand their bodies, experience temporality, fear death, and invest hope in technology in new ways (Livingston 2012). According to Hacking, the diseases that technologies such as the ultrasound or new psychotherapeutic interventions make thinkable, affect the "outer reaches of your space as an individual" (Hacking 2007, 156). The processes of normalization through which particular versions of disease and the body become materially and discursively stabilized affect the very core of our being. As the activist Adam Levin pointed out in relation to the widespread discursive penetration of AIDS: "The world has AIDS" (quoted in Comaroff 2007, 198).

What about a place where such objects are not stabilized? Where the technologies of visibility associated with modern medicine and modern governance cannot be taken for granted? Where doctors struggle to locate disease? Where hospital statistics are considered unreliable as a basis for policy and intervention? Where patients experience themselves as invisible to both medical practitioners and the state? Visibility is often associated with power insofar as processes of reification, which reduce complexity and render persons and things in discrete, recognizable, and legible forms, also facilitate practices of governance and control. Where those practices of governance and control are not taken for granted, however, this book shows people actively seeking to make themselves visible (reify themselves) as particular kinds of bodies or persons in the expectation of eliciting a productive relationship.

In places where access to medical services and vital lifesaving drugs is scarce, relationships between technology, knowledge, and personhood are refracted through people's desires and demands to be seen by medical authorities, the state, development organizations, or pharmaceutical companies who increasingly take on statelike roles of welfare provision. In countries with fragile public health infrastructures, state and nonstate supported technologies and resources have proliferated around "crisis" diseases, such as HIV in South Africa and Brazil (Robins 2006; Biehl 2007), or radiation sickness in the Chernobyl fallout zone in the Ukraine (Petryna 2002). In such places, biomedical conceptions of the self and knowledge of one's disease are not only imposed from above by medical authorities, but are often formed from below as the basis for making citizenship claims on elusive statelike actors whose benevolent gaze is biologically selective (Rose 2007, 133).

The value placed on visibility in the new public health politics has an analogue, I would like to suggest, in anthropological writings about Melanesian exchange practices, which might help us understand what kinds of power are being put into effect by such visibility work. Euro-American knowledge practices, Strathern points out, explicitly attempt to *reify* and define relationships between external, innately differentiated "things" in order to build up an understanding of "the world": "By reification I simply intend to point to the manner in which entities are made into objects when they are seen to assume a particular form ('gift,'—'exchange'). This form in turn indicates the properties by which they are known and, in being rendered knowable or graspable through such properties, entities appear (in Euro-American idiom) as 'things'" (Strathern 1999, 13).

In Euro-American biomedicine, for example, the uniqueness and particularity of the sick body is given in nature; the objective is to visualize it as "disease" in such a way that its unique complexity is reduced and rendered legible to science. Conversely, Strathern argues that Melanesian knowledge practices explicitly *personify*, that is, they use transactions to distinguish between innately similar persons and relationships (Strathern 1988, 180). While biomedical knowledge practices concentrate on finding the appropriate way to conceptualize, classify, and categorize things so as to understand their natural properties, Melanesian practices of personification, by contrast, must "make the form [of things or persons] appear" in the appropriate way (1988, 180). They take the conventions (e.g., gender and disease) for reifying persons for granted but do not know whether they will be able to convincingly realize those conventions in any given instance. Institutional anxiety follows from uncertainty over whether they will be able to appear in the appropriate form and sufficiently affect and move their audience to respond.[31]

It is in the processes by which aesthetic conventions are determined and normalized that anthropologists tend to locate power relations. Uncovering power is a process of uncovering the artifice that goes into the construction of our conceptual categories; hence Foucault's exploration of what "governs statements, and the way in which they govern each other so as to constitute a set of propositions which are scientifically acceptable, and hence capable of being verified or falsified by scientific procedures" (2003, 112). By contrast, Strathern argues that Melanesians take the norms that govern reification, the "conventionalised assumptions through which revelation works" (1988, 176), for granted.[32] Effort is focused instead on the capacity to realize that form in a particular, unique, and powerful way that elicits a response from others and mobilizes future relationships. By contrast with the penetrating, universalizing, and constant gaze of biomedicine, this often involves the secreting away of persons and things in order for their aesthetic qualities to register in the eyes of onlookers when they are revealed (Strathern 1988; Biersack 1982; Leach 2002). Moreover what is revealed in the moment of display is not a person's essential, individual qualities but his or her capacity for mobilizing the relationships that have transformed him/her (and the things attached to him/her) into a powerful form. Knowledge of persons' individuated capacities is here less an effect of constructing representations of an external reality than the disruptive effect of engaging in that world through the elicitation of other people's actions, thereby producing knowledge of one's own and others' relationships and relational capacities.

Although Strathern herself does not go down this route, we might think of Melanesian personification as a mode of power that complements and reveals the underside of Foucauldian theories of knowledge/power. If Foucault invites us to understand the "intellectual Euro-American obsession with how we come to know and describe things" (Strathern 1999, 251) as a basis for modern modes of power as control, then Strathern invites us to understand people's attempts to reify themselves for others' consumption as the basis for relational effects.[33] A "form is put before the viewer, and thus forced on an audience, (the coercive metaphor is appropriate) for the audience to confront. . . . The dance decorations mean nothing without the viewer's, the participant observer's, absorption of the effect which the dancer's person makes" (1999, 260). Here power inheres in the affective "persuasiveness of form, the elicitation of a sense of appropriateness" (2004, 10) that occurs when a successful display takes place and viewers must occupy a vantage point on the person displayed. The "disclosure of persons in locally relevant forms," as Hirsch puts it, "is intended to persuade others of the appropriateness of their appearance and of the capacities thereby displayed" (Hirsch 2001, 22–23). To appear efficacious also performs efficacy by compelling the viewers to respond.

As Brighenti argues in relation to dominant understandings of visibility as something that is done *to* people: "We should not be misled into believing that being watched is a passive behavior. . . . I would venture to say that not only is there a form of seeing, but also a form of *being seen*. . . . Often the relationship of visibility is controlled not by the one who looks, but by the one who is looked at" (Brighenti 2007, 330). In a related vein Martin Jay points out that Foucault's influential analysis of visibility in the clinic's "empire of the gaze" as a disciplinary trap (Jay 1994, xx; cf. Foucault 2003) reinforced a trend of antiocularcentrism in twentieth-century French intellectual thought by focusing on visibility's disempowering effects. Together, growing networks of health activism and Melanesian "persuasive forms" provide a crucial antidote to such thought by pointing toward the potentially empowering, even coercive, effects of making oneself visible (reifying oneself) for others' consumption.

In Madang Hospital, where the ability of modern knowledge practices of governance and medicine to make bodies, persons, and diseases visible and knowable cannot be taken for granted, and where lives are at stake, visibility takes on new kinds of value that are not related to knowledge but to effect. The engagements of doctors, nurses, and patients with biomedical and bureaucratic technologies, this book shows, are directed toward the transformation and revelation of their bodies in affective forms, which will compel medical practitioners, politicians, and foreign scientists to recognize a relationship and respond to their needs. Indeed such activities give Strathern's notion of "institutional anxiety" new force: the question that hangs over people's everyday activities in the hospital is whether they will have the capacity to make themselves an object of another's regard.[34]

MAKING UP PERSONS

As an anthropologist, however, I cannot escape a disciplinary interest in processes of reification. If power inheres in the capacity of people to make themselves into an object of another's regard, what implicit conventions govern the aesthetics of recognition in Papua New Guinea's hospitals? What kinds of persons and bodies are rendered visible by engagements with biomedical technologies and other objects of exchange in this institutional space? Are new "human kinds" made up and new subjectivities formed? What aesthetic criteria determine recognition of these "human kinds"? And what kinds of knowledge practices, or what kinds of relationships between persons and things, are entailed in this revelatory process? If biomedical practices are seldom able to reveal bodies in a recognizable form in this space, what about the kinship practices of patients, or their engagements with hospital technologies and staff? These are questions that still need to be asked by the anthropologist, even if we resist imputing them to our informants.

We might infer from a large body of anthropological writing that persons are predominantly "made up" in Papua New Guinea in a relational form. Indeed Strathern's comparison between personhood in Melanesia and Euro-America was intended to highlight the possibility of alternative ways of conceiving of personhood and agency that do not take the biological individual as the ontological ground for socialization. In their given state, Strathern argued, Melanesian persons do not exist as biologically differentiated and gendered individuals but as microcosms of the multiple relationships that have conceived and grown them. It is only when a person engages in acts of exchange and elicits a response from other persons that their other relationships are eclipsed, and they are revealed as a particular kind of (gendered) person within that singular relationship. These are the conventional forms of personhood that she argues Melanesians take for granted.

Strathern's Melanesia/Euro-America axis of comparison is most commonly understood as a negative strategy that reveals the limited ability of conceptual frameworks such as that of the "individual" or "society" to travel and that compels anthropologists to extend or develop new concepts.[35] But Strathern and other recent anthropologists of Melanesia have equally employed the comparative method as a technique of positive analogy that turns the concepts we develop to analyze others back on ourselves, for example, in order to understand the latent centrality of personification and relational personhood to "Euro-American" cultural practices (Strathern 2009; Gell 1988; Leach 2005; Reed 2011b). Both personification and reification are crucial components of all symbolic action: the issue is where we locate our efforts and what we take to be the ground for our action (see also Wagner 1975; Weiner 2003).

Such positive analogies have had particular purchase in social studies of science and medicine. As Warwick Anderson observed in his historical account of the scientific institutions that grew up around kuru, a neurodegenerative disease, in Papua New Guinea in the mid twentieth century, the circulations of body parts and other artifacts are just as crucial in the formation of scientists' personhood as they are in Papua New Guinean kinship practices (Anderson 2009). In cutting across clear distinctions between Euro-American and Melanesian domains of symbolic action, Anderson's study of the relationships between the persons, places, and things that made up the world of kuru, takes us beyond negative strategies to explore the possible positive strategies that can be derived from using the tools for studying personhood and agency that have developed in more traditional anthropological studies of Melanesian kinship to explore the social dynamics of postcolonial technoscience in the region.

Strathern's comparison of Euro-America and Melanesia rested on the intentional reification of both as a convenient "fiction" (1988, 7). When "binary division" is "the moment at which a distinction between terms could lead analysis down different routes" (Strathern 2011) it clearly has value. As critics of Strathern's work have pointed out, however, such intentional reification also entails dangers. Critics have argued that Strathern's comparative approach essentializes cultural difference, negates the shared social and cultural arenas in which so-called "Melanesians" and "Euro-Americans" commune, and conceals the historical power relationships that have helped to generate differences between their worlds.[36] The shift from productive reification to dangerous essentialization, in other words, entails precisely the kind of operation that Strathern implores us to resist: the lazy application of conceptual frameworks across materials that might entail tiny but significant differences. Such slippage is a risk that Strathern herself is particularly careful about, but that anthropologists of Melanesia still need to be sensitive to, especially as they increasingly move away from traditional "village ethnography" to explore urban and institutional social forms.

The danger is that, as anthropologists employ concepts of relational personhood in multiple contexts in Papua New Guinea, it ceases to operate as a means of contesting and extending dominant conceptions of the person in anthropology and instead becomes a dominant and mobile framework itself. Bifurcation is useful when it opens up conceptual difference but is dangerous when it collectivizes or homogenizes ethnographic materials. It is tempting, for example, to argue that the "context" people in Papua New Guinea "make for their own actions" is never the same as the context that anthropologists, capitalists, and governments make for them (cf. Englund and Leach 2000). And yet some anthropologists are also showing that in urban and institutional environments conventions are emerging for imagining personhood in new formations (Foster 1995c; Reed 1999; Rollason 2011).

The radical position of what has become known as New Melanesian Ethnography was to recognize that individualism is not enacted everywhere in the world.[37] This book starts from the analogous position that we cannot assume that relational, "dividual" persons are enacted always and everywhere in Melanesia.[38] We cannot assume that persons and bodies are made up in a certain way because they are located in Melanesia, just as we cannot presume they are made up in a certain way because they are in a hospital. To do so would depend on an erroneous understanding of the continuing stability of their relations of enactment.[39] As this book argues, the relationships through which persons are conventionally established as either "dividuals" in Melanesian kinship or biological "things" in Euroamerican biomedicine remain inherently *unstable* in Madang Hospital.

The power of the ethnographic method lies in its capacity to locate universalizing projects such as biomedicine within their situated practices and to provide detailed assessments of how health identities are formed and constrained in relation to local histories and cultural forms (Whyte 2009). It is in the spirit of this ethnographic commitment to registering unpredictability and surprise that this book proceeds. This means being open to the possibility that people in Papua New Guinea might begin to countenance new conventions for "making persons up" (Hirsch 2001). Indeed one of this book's key arguments is that patients presume that white people (and by extension doctors who have been educated in white people's ways) have different conventions for making persons appear. They are ignorant of these conventions, which exist in parallel to their own, but might tap into their power through engagements with their biomedical technologies. As I argue in chapter 6, this has significant implications for the ways in which anthropologists often read transformations in subjectivity into the adoption of new forms.

In Madang Hospital, the historical emergence of weak state infrastructures and unstable technologies has generated conditions of ontological uncertainty for those who inhabit the hospital. Here biomedicine, the archetypal Euro-American knowledge practice, does not exert a consistent hegemonic hold over the institution. Biomedical objects are unstable. But these sociomaterial conditions make the anthropologist's commitment to the ethnographic ethic of surprise all the more vital. In this clinical space of invisibility neither "Melanesia" nor "Euro-America" can be taken for granted as the context for people's actions. People in the hospital do not know what kind of a person they will become or what kinds of capacities they will be revealed to have through their everyday engagements with X-rays, food, bureaucratic forms, hospital buildings, or international medical research. Here maintaining an ethnographic open-mindedness about what is made knowable and who is made visible is crucial for understanding the "uneven seepages" (Rapp 1999, 303) of science and its transformative possibilities into everyday lives in Papua New Guinea.

This book therefore intends to move us away from the abstract delineation of Melanesian or Euro-American models of personhood and agency. Stories of everyday engagements with biomedical practices, state institutions, and techno-scientific projects of improvement instead focus attention on the kinds of knowledge, bodies, and persons it is *possible* to make visible in a public hospital, and asks what the implications are for social and biological survival in contemporary Papua New Guinea.

ANTHROPOLOGICAL TECHNIQUES

Notions of failure and experiences of social invisibility also framed the ways in which I was able to conduct my research, generating both ethnographic opportunities and ethical dilemmas. When I first arrived at Madang Hospital in 2003 I was surprised by the level of access I was granted. In the medical ward, where I carried out the majority of my research, I joined doctors as they carried out ward rounds and consultation clinics and nurses as they carried out observations, distributed medicines, and tended to patients in their beds. I followed the movement of patients, beds, medicines, bodily tissues, and documents to and from consultation clinics, the pathology laboratory, the operating theater, the Outpatients Department, and other hospital wards. I carried out interviews with staff in five-minute breaks between tasks, in lunch hours, and in their homes. The welcome reception that I received in all of these spaces, despite my intrusive questions and the potential for interference in tricky procedures or sensitive situations, was, I soon realized, due largely to people's supposition that I was there to witness the impossibility of doing their jobs effectively given the severe shortages of staff, drugs, and equipment that they faced on an everyday basis.

I would, I told people, be writing about the real conditions inside Papua New Guinea's hospitals and the everyday lives of the people who worked there. People's willingness to share their experiences, including practices that they knew would not meet international biomedical standards, needs to be understood in relation to people's dominant sense that those experiences and stories went largely unnoticed by those outside the hospital. My anthropological work, hospital staff hoped, would help make their clinical work more visible to people in the Papua New Guinean government and other countries, forcing them to recognize and respond to their predicament.

Similar expectations accompanied the development of relationships with patients and their relatives. I spent hours sitting on patient beds, talking about the events that had led to their arrival in the hospital and their life inside and outside the institution. At other times I would sit in the shady walkways outside, talking with the patients' guardians, or helping them cook in the small fireside shelters erected at the back of the hospital grounds.

Those that I came to know well, I gradually came to realize, forged links to me in part because of my apparent connection to the hospital establishment and therefore the possibility that our relationship might help them to attract the attention of the hospital staff and expedite their treatment. As I describe in chapter 5, fears that they had not been seen or recognized by the doctor as a treatable person dominated patients' thoughts. The realization that they saw me as another instrument of visibility, akin to hospital technologies such as X-ray machines, that could induce the doctor to see and treat them was socially disconcerting and ethically troublesome. Things became even more tricky when new patients regularly mistook me for a doctor. Despite my protestations to the contrary, it was difficult to persuade patients that I did not have access to "white people's knowledge" about medicine, development, or money, which they might expect to be revealed in exchange for their stories. Explaining exactly what my work entailed and why I was doing it was a daily task that involved listening, empathy, and negotiation rather than a one off moment of "informed consent."

Patients' interest in me as another "hospital technology" also provided important insights into patients' fundamentally pragmatic approach to medical knowledge. Papua New Guinea is well known in medical anthropology for people's apparently pluralist orientations towards Western medicine. People are willing, it is argued, to accept multiple explanations for sickness, including both traditional notions of causation by social conflict or sorcery and Western notions of biological disease. But while patients in the hospital rapidly alternated between notions of *sik bilong ples* (village sickness) and *sik bilong marasin* (sickness pertaining to Western medicine) in our discussions, it soon became apparent that explanation was less significant in those conversations than the relationships the terms evoked and the actions they motivated.

By telling me they had sik bilong marasin or *sik i kamap nating* (sickness without social cause) patients clearly hoped that I would recognize a relationship with them and use my "white people's knowledge" to assist them. Referring to sik bilong marasin neither required them to develop a clear account of what this term meant (in fact most patients insisted they were entirely ignorant about sik bilong marasin), nor precluded the necessity of engaging in relationships with relatives outside the hospital, which could equally be affecting their body and which required immediate action to ameliorate. Patients' medical pluralism, in other words, was relational and pragmatic rather than geared toward explanation.

I did often find myself mediating relationships between patients and doctors. I would sometimes ask doctors to take a second look at someone, or pass on comments that one doctor made on ward round to another. On numerous occasions I pointed out that a patient's catheter was full, drip had run dry, that a doctor had forgotten to send a patient for an X-ray, or that relatives had already donated blood for a patient whom hospital staff had presumed was still waiting for donation before a transfusion could take place. The fact that I am not medically trained and that I was a guest of the medical and nursing staff on the ward only added to the discomfort that accompanied patients' expectations that I could assist them. However, the fact that, in a few cases, I did participate in the process by which bodies were made biomedically visible in the hospital also made the arbitrary and fragile nature of this process, for both hospital staff and patients, strikingly apparent.

My attempts to do "fieldwork," to use interviewing and participant observation to build up a picture of the conventions by which people in the hospital engaged with and produced institutional life, was inherently at odds with their attempts to "invent" me (Wagner 1975, 20) through relationships that they anticipated would lead to bodily and personal transformation. This is not only a distinction between Euro-American and Melanesian knowledge practices. The difference between my own anthropological knowledge practices and the biomedical knowledge practices of doctors was equally significant. As I argue in chapter 4, Papua New Guinean doctors' knowledge practices are as pragmatic in orientation as are patients.' They are more concerned with multiplying pathways for action than diagnosing and categorizing disease, just as patients multiply the relationships they anticipate will transform their bodies rather than multiply explanatory models of sickness causation. While doctors, nurses, and patients were involved in the production of hospital life and the improvised creation of well bodies and persons, I was absorbed in the description and analysis of those processes.

These are different kinds of projects of visualization. While they were busy producing persons I was busy representing those "aesthetic" conventions of personhood. That difference raised people's expectations about my role in their bodily or professional transformation and made it frustratingly impossible for me to meet them. Nonetheless, good description is not inert. It motivates people to interpret, adapt, and appropriate it for their own transformative projects. The hallmark of an engaged and reflexive anthropology is that it brings a place to life, describes the struggles encountered within it, and seeks to understand those struggles in the terms of those who are caught up in them. It is a fundamentally affective project that seeks to move its readers and open up new windows for understanding. It may even be appropriated by nonanthropologists in their attempts to transform those places through activism or public policy. I therefore hope that the stories that are told in the pages that follow are able to convey something of the intensity with which the Papua New Guinean hospital operates as a place of both hope and failure for those who work within it, that I do justice to the inequalities and impossibilities of hospital life and at the same time challenge bland clichés about the "third world hospital." To produce good description in this way is to go some way toward the development of an anthropology that "participates *in* reality" (Mol 2002, 153) by revealing ways in which that reality could be made better.

A further note is also necessary on the use of the past and present tense in the text. New Melanesian Ethnography has conventionally been less concerned with contextualizing Papua New Guineans' experiences in a historical narrative than with "trans-temporal comparison" (Holbraad and Pedersen 2010, 384) between different knowledge practices. From this perspective, an "ethnographic moment" first recorded in the Papua New Guinean Highlands four decades ago can continue to provide surprising insights into the legal frameworks that are still emerging around genetic technologies in present-day Britain (Strathern 1999; Holbraad and Pedersen 2010). But this is not only a book about comparative knowledge practices and different ways of making things and persons knowable. It is a book about the historical conditions in which people are able to make themselves recognizable to others and the implications of this for relationships of inequality and survival. In a resource-poor public health institution, where one's interlocutors are constantly striving to draw one into their own struggles for personal transformation and survival, "trans-temporal comparison" is impossible. How the conditions of possibility for transforming bodies and persons changes historically alongside shifting relationships between governance regimes and medical technologies is central to the story. For example, as I describe in chapter 4, the roll out of antiretroviral therapy (ARVs) and the highly centralized response to the HIV crisis in Papua New Guinea, which only began after my first period of fieldwork was completed in 2004, had a significant impact on the ways in which bodies were differentiated and treated in the medical ward of the hospital. For this reason, whenever I have used specific ethnographic examples or referred to particular events in the hospital, I have always put them in the past tense.

However, I returned to Madang Hospital to conduct three further months of fieldwork in 2009 and made a third six-month visit to Madang Province in 2010–11, which included follow-up research on patient trajectories from the village to the hospital, and finally returned for one month in 2013. Over this ten-year period, I have observed peoples' enduring experience of the hospital as a place of social invisibility. In making general and analytic remarks about hospital relationships I therefore often revert to the present tense. This "present" should nonetheless be judged in relation to the book's publication date.

THE STRUCTURE OF THE BOOK

The book is organized into three parts: "Place," "Technology," and "Infrastructure." Part I describes the historical emergence of Madang Hospital in relation to nation- and state-building projects in Papua New Guinea. How do bodies like that of William Gambe (described in the Prologue) come to be made invisible to kin, to doctors and to the state? The production of "generally sick" bodies in the medical ward of Madang Hospital, bodies that slowly deteriorate without ever receiving a single diagnosis, I argue, has a long colonial and postcolonial history. In this opening section of the book I explore the historical production of the patient body in tandem with the construction of the colonial and postcolonial hospital and the building of the Papua New Guinean state. Chapter 2, "Locating Disease," examines the prewar colonial hospital in Papua New Guinea as a lens onto the dynamics of visibility and invisibility that characterized these spaces and the production of racialized, individual, and collective bodies within them. It pays particular attention to the early interest that the region around Madang held for medical scientists and the emergence of a mutually constitutive relationship between the colonial hospital and tropical medicine at the same time as those relationships forged infrastructural inequalities between research and public health in German- and Australian-governed New Guinea. Chapter 3, "Public Buildings, Building Publics," examines the continuities and discontinuities in these contours of invisibility within the postwar hospital, when the "publics" of public health were being imagined in new ways, and when the hospital became perceived as central to the manufacture of a developed nation-state and national consciousness. This chapter shows that, despite the new focus on indigenous health and development, the design and organization of hospital space and relationships continued to fundamentally reference the idiom of race, and created the conditions for variability in biomedical visibility across different kinds of racialized bodies. In many ways, the kinds of Papua New Guinean bodies that were made visible in the new "modern" hospitals of the postwar era resembled those of the ramshackle "native" hospitals they were intended to replace. These two historical chapters show the long-standing dominance of hospital infrastructures in Papua New Guinea's public health system, its role in the ongoing work of state building in the country, and the historical foundations that colonial hospital forms laid for the reproduction of inequalities between biomedical research and public health, public and private health care, and the visibility afforded "white" and "black" bodies in the present.

Part II explores the politics of biomedical knowledge production and engagements with biomedical technologies in Madang Hospital under conditions of profound biomedical uncertainty. Chapter 4 explores how biomedicine is done amid a fragile diagnostic infrastructure. Where anthropological and scientific studies of biomedical work have tended to presume that inconsistencies and lacunas in diagnostic knowledge production are fundamentally problematic for biomedical practitioners, chapter 4 describes a situation where diagnostic uncertainty is not rendered problematic and where the open-endedness of the diagnostic process gives rise to new forms of medical expertise and practice. Where diseased bodies fail to be made visible in this place, "generally sick" bodies, which are more susceptible to medical intervention in this particular hospital, are. This expertise is precarious; the anticipated gaze of foreign doctors and medical researchers continually impinges on doctors' capacities for not-knowing, and threatens to devalue their locally derived expertise.

How is biomedical uncertainty negotiated by the hospital's patients? Chapter 5, "The Waiting Place," brings us back to the questions raised in the book's Prologue and what is at stake for those who subject themselves to a biomedical gaze in the hospital. It follows the experience of one patient as he moves through the hospital and describes his experience of the institution as a place of invisibility where he is caught between the social worlds of kinship and biomedicine, village and town. His inability to operate in either is experienced in the material deterioration of his body. While doctors employ biomedical technologies to build up knowledge about and intervene in the biological body, patients engage in processes such as X-rays or ultrasound as "relational technologies" that mediate white people's power and agency. In a reversal of Foucauldian critiques of biomedical technologies, the chapter describes how patients perceive such processes as crucial means by which they might make themselves visible and recognizable to doctors as treatable subjects.

Chapter 6, "Technologies of Detachment," explores the national and international circulation of things that constitute the doctor as an expert person in Papua New Guinea. Scientific personhood, like Melanesian personhood, it argues, depends on the generation of external recognition. But where doctors are already embedded in relationships with their rural kin and where relationships with patients can potentially proliferate out of control doctors frequently find they are unable to exercise the modes of either detachment or attachment on which external recognition from an international medical community depends.

How is it possible that a place envisaged as a monument of development and progress becomes experienced by hospital workers and patients as a place of invisibility and failure? Part III examines the transformation of Madang Hospital into a "partnership hospital" modeled on international collaborations with NGOs, development agencies, research consortiums, politicians, and business. Chapter 7 describes the ceremonial gifting of infrastructure (such as vehicles, buildings, and machines) to the hospital by politicians and aid agencies. These ceremonies are experienced as moments of recognition and social visibility by hospital staff. But as those infrastructures deteriorate, hospital workers realize that their exchanges with politicians and bureaucrats are supports for the latter's relationships with foreign actors; they have never become an object of political regard themselves. Instead, the chapter describes how nurses turn to the law as an alternative technique of visibility and harness it to extraordinary effect.

Chapter 8, "Research in the Clinic," explores the growing importance of Madang Hospital for global medical research and the ways in which a scientific infrastructure is reconfiguring the hospital landscape. It traces the interrelationships between the assemblage of persons, pills, machines, and buildings that makes up the hospital as a place of research and of clinical practice to show how technological infrastructures that afford the capacity of some persons and knowledges to be both embedded in the hospital and to travel elsewhere simultaneously confine other persons and knowledges to a hospital that is resolutely "local."

The concluding chapter "Biomedicine in a Fragile State" brings together the preceding ethnographic chapters to argue that contemporary technological and managerial trends in public health reform are contributing to the creation of spaces of omission, forgetting, and failure at the heart of state institutions. These mirror the spaces of exclusion that social scientists have identified at the margins of the state. As a space of invisibility, I argue that the public hospital becomes a space of friction between sociomaterial projects that seek social improvement, survival, state building, and self-transformation. Inside Papua New Guinea's hospitals, which are both public institutions and containers of invisible bodies, new kinds of relationships between science, technology, and society are being formed.

CHAPTER 2

Locating Disease

■ On November 6, 1885, two foresters, a gardener, a retired officer, and a naturalist employed by the German Neuguinea Compagnie arrived by boat at Finschafen on the Northeast Coast of what is now Papua New Guinea. They were soon followed by thirty-seven Malays recruited from Java "who were to be employed in carrying out the heavier work, as the natives could not be relied upon."[1] In May of that year, the company had been granted a charter from the Imperial government in Germany to establish the colony of Kaiser Wilhelmshafen on the northeast of the island. The company had a purely economic interest in the territory, driven by fantasies of a plantation and trading economy to parallel that of Dutch East Indies, and they quickly established stations along the coastal strip, from which they planned to acquire land from the indigenous inhabitants for copra, cotton, and tobacco plantations. By 1887 they had acquired, through dubious means, fifty thousand hectares of land, and between 1887 and 1903 it is estimated that twenty-six thousand indentured laborers were shipped in from Singapore, China, and other Melanesian islands to work on these plantations (Firth 1982, 41).[2]

The company had been given sole rights to acquire and dispose of land on the condition that it also would establish a working government in the colony. Very soon they discovered that safeguarding the health of their employees would be a major challenge in the pursuit of economic success. By June 1887 the company doctor, Dr. Schellong, reported that every European and 86 percent of Melanesians at the station were suffering from malaria. At the time there were thirty-two Europeans, twenty-five "Malays," and ten Chinese at Finschafen alongside laborers brought in from the Gazelle Peninsular and the Solomon Islands. During the twenty-six months that Dr. Schellong spent at Finschafen he estimated that he treated 1,402 cases of malaria (Ewers 1972, 5). In 1891, following an epidemic that killed a third of the Europeans at the station in the space of three months, Finschafen was abandoned. But the scourge of malaria was to follow the hopeful colonialists, first to the new station at Stephansort, an area of intense plantation development further west along the coast, and again ten months later when they relocated the administrative center to the harbor at Friedrich Wilhelmshafen, known today as Madang Town.

At Friedrich Wilhelmshafen, conditions improved slightly. But between 1893 and 1896 the company doctor, Dr. Dempwolff, recorded 225 cases of malaria for 57 Europeans while imported laborers also suffered greatly (Ewers 1972, 10). Of 306 recruits from islands off the coast of the New Guinea mainland who were brought to Kaiser Wilhelmshafen in June 1894, half were in hospital with malaria by November (Firth 1982, 38). Between August 1891 and February 1892, 1,699 coolies arrived to work on the plantations at Friedrich Wilhelmshafen, of whom 60 percent were said to have died, most probably from disease (Sinclair 2005, 49). The persistent problem of malaria was compounded by frequent outbreaks of dysentery among the laborers, thought to have been imported with coolies from Malaysia or China. Dreams of a plantation utopia were rapidly fading.

This chapter explores relationships between state, territory and person, tropical medicine and public health as they played out in the hospitals built in the region surrounding Madang over the first half of the twentieth century. During this period, which traverses both German and Australian colonial administrations, associations between race, environment, and tropical disease led directly to the development of a hospital-centered public health policy. Colonial anxieties coalesced around the threat of malaria, and the hospital emerged as a vital space of scientific research and intervention that reproduced and entrenched notions of racial difference. Yet such institutions did not operate as an efficient machinery of modern scientific governance, and a scientific focus on tropical diseases did not translate into biomedical resources for diagnosing and treating disease within the individual body. A focus on the material infrastructure of the hospital shows that early colonial hospitals were underfunded and transitory institutions that frequently failed to make the bodies they contained visible to a coherent state gaze. They were designed primarily to protect the white colonial enclave from the untamed, racialized tropics outside rather than train a disciplinary gaze on the bodies within. These colonial hospitals, then, are better thought of as spaces of state building than as sites of operation for preformed state power.

Between the 1880s and 1940s, hospitals were at the heart of colonial activities and investments in health and medicine. But in their rationale and organization these spaces could not be said to correspond to a wider system of public health governance. Instead this chapter argues that they were constructed as frontier spaces that would protect a European population from an external threatening environment of diseased people and places. Hospitals were necessary because the continuing existence of the colonial state was always uncertain.

FAVORABLE LATITUDES

In German New Guinea the spread of disease was quickly recognized to be a threat to the colony's economic viability. Health conditions, the annual report for 1890–91 stated, "are of paramount importance in maintaining [the efficiency of] the workforce and [of] the Europeans directing it." They were, in this regard, crucial to the "realization of the objectives of the whole [imperial] enterprise."[3] The decisions to employ a doctor and to construct hospitals at the Finschafen site were not only taken "for humanitarian reasons" but also "in the financial interests of the company, which are better served by keeping the laborers in good health than by saving a doctor's salary."[4] Accordingly, the health of the European and colored laborer population was monitored and measured in terms of economic losses. The number of malaria cases was documented in company records as the number of sick days taken off work as a proportion of the total number of persons in residence.

These concerns about health and economy were framed by emerging European ideas about "the tropics" as both a climatic region and a cultural repository for uncivilized customs, relationships, and bodies (Livingstone 2002; Arnold 1996). Scientific research was at the time deeply imbued with racial ideas about bodily difference. Tropical places were closely associated with tropical bodies, cultures, and moralities which were considered to determine one's susceptibility to disease.[5] Earlier conquests by European powers in Africa had raised serious questions about the suitability of tropical environments for habitation by white men.[6] Doctors debated whether the inherited physical constitution of Europeans prohibited tropical acclimatization in Papua New Guinea, while the indigenous population was held to have inherent racial characteristics that made them relatively immune to the native afflictions of the land, but simultaneously more vulnerable to diseases of European origin such as tuberculosis (Eves 2005).

The fear that the tropical climate could jeopardize the entire commercial venture in German New Guinea was most evident from the protestations of early annual report writers that the climate was *not* the cause of poor health in the colony. Climate provided the conceptual framework for monitoring and interpreting health conditions, but early reports were largely optimistic. The annual report for 1886–87, for example, declared that "natural conditions favor plant and animal life. They are also generally favorable to human life and permanent residence. The Administrator has on occasion expressed the opinion that there are few, if any, tropical regions in the same latitudes with a climate as pleasant as that at Finschafen. . . . The Europeans living at Finschafen, apart from those affected by malaria, suffer no loss of either physical or mental powers."[7]

A preoccupation with the effect of the environment on health and economy was intensified by miasmic theories of tropical diseases. Prior to the 1890s, malaria was considered to be caused by poisonous particles in the soil becoming airborne. In German New Guinea this notion of "bad air" became associated not with the intractable tropical climate, which it was argued played a "subsidiary role" in the causation of malaria, but with the hygienic habits and living conditions of the native inhabitants and imported laborers. The cause, the company doctor claimed, could be found "in the processes of decomposition active in the vicinity of the dwellings, in swampy ground or rotting wood and other vegetable refuse, in the lack of adequate ventilation and in confined living quarters, and last but not least in the lack of cleanliness frequently associated with crowded conditions."[8] These were conditions that, it was hoped, would radically improve "as the foundations of colonialism strengthened."

This optimistic tone shifted following the disastrous malaria outbreak of 1891. From this time on, concerns about the effect of the climate on both disease incidence and the physical and mental constitution of the Europeans and the laborers became an increasingly frequent topic of government reports. The annual report for 1891–92, for example, alluded to both physical and moral disadvantages of climate when it complained that fresh arrivals of colored laborers who were not yet accustomed to the climate and diet were "prevented from working in the wet season due to illness, or still have to be trained or taught to work."[9] Meanwhile, problems in the recruitment of European employees was blamed both on people's "strong inclination for good living which goes hand in hand with a disinclination for strenuous work" and "the effect—often underestimated—of the tropical climate on physical health and will-power."[10]

This association of climate, disease, and race demanded segregated living conditions and health services. The hospital, like the jail and the army, was an important institutional site for the discursive and material articulation of racial difference (Arnold 2004, 263). From the very beginning the company built separate hospitals for "Europeans" and "natives." What to do with the "colored" laborers from other Pacific Islands, Malaysia, and Indonesia was a more difficult question. They were soon discovered to be more susceptible to local diseases, especially malaria. They also brought new diseases, such as dysentery, into the territory, presenting a threat to the local population labor force. Local depopulation became a persistent theme of the annual reports and a major concern for the future economic viability of the colony. Eventually, a quarantine unit was established on an island off the coast at Stephansort, where colored bodies could be "acclimatized" before they mixed with black bodies in the labor compounds and native hospitals. Associations between race, climate, and disease led to the development of hospitals that primarily served the purpose of segregating and isolating racially distinct bodies. With only one company doctor in the territory for much of the time, native hospitals were little more than containers for sick bodies, built to keep them out of labor camps and away from Europeans.

PROTECTING THE ENCLAVE

In Europe the emergence of the modern hospital in the early nineteenth century is generally understood to have coincided with the emergence of public health as a new mode of governance. The expert gaze that was trained on individual bodies within the clinic had its counterpart in the emergence of a network of public health authorities and inspectors "whose intersecting gazes form a network and exercise at every point in space, and at every moment in time, a constant, mobile, differentiated supervision" (Foucault 2003, 35). A new spatialization of governance created "*both* a diffuse medicalized social geography, an unspecific medical gaze casting its eye over the whole social realm, *and* a much more antisocial medical geography, an intrusive gaze facilitated in key sites (the reinvented hospitals) of clinical and teaching practice" (Philo 2000, 17). Hospitals, Foucault argued, were "small scale, regional, dispersed panoptisms" (1980, 72) that connected up with new institutions for policing social space to generate a diffuse and generalized "grid" of surveillance (2003).

In German New Guinea the inward-facing gaze of the colonial hospital was not complimented with the external gaze of public health. As Denoon has argued, the colonial administration's preoccupation with tropical disease and hospital medicine essentially confined the operations of colonial medicine to those protected institutional spaces (Denoon 1989, 25–33). The concentration of the German administrations on hospitals was coupled with only limited extension of German colonial power beyond the administrative centers. In the Madang area, the German administration explored very little of the interior. Early expeditions were aborted due to the rough terrain and sickness. Two scientific expeditions were made down the Ramu River, and punitive expeditions were made following uprisings in 1904 and 1907 and again by the newly established native expeditionary force following skirmishes between bird of paradise hunters and villagers along the Ramu River in 1912. But colonial influence beyond the coastal strip was modest.

As Denoon describes, the rural indigenous population were largely excluded from the problematization of and strategic interventions in early colonial public health, which prioritized the health of its own administrators and officers. Some attempts at health extension were made by the administration. By 1907, it had established a system of local leadership, comprising headmen, called Luluais, and their assistants, Tultuls, in patrolled villages. A head tax was introduced in 1905 and extended in 1910 to cover the costs of hospitals and the medical services. Training of selected villagers in basic first aid and hygiene began on the German administered island of New Ireland in 1909 and was closely followed in 1911 with the introduction of hospital training programs for local medical orderlies. This policy was rapidly adopted across the territory and the administration began to send some of the trained assistants back to the villages to become medical tultuls, who were expected to treat minor conditions and report outbreaks of epidemics. This model of public health extension closely modeled that of Germany, where health officers were at the time being appointed to record, count, and observe incidences of disease in order to prevent the spread of epidemics such as cholera (Porter 1999, 104–110). The German Annual Reports also record increasingly frequent vaccinations of villagers following outbreaks of smallpox and dysentery along the coast, and some attempts to improve access to clean water through the building of wells in nearby villages.[11]

Nonetheless these extension activities were confined to those villages close to the colonial settlements and plantations. Vaccinations of "free natives," for example, responded to the fear that epidemics among the labor force at the stations would be impossible to control once they spread to nearby villages. Very few activities extended more than a few kilometers inland. Hospitals continued to eat up the larger portion of the administration's budget and rural health services for "free" natives were largely left to the growing number of missionary groups, who had been allowed to enter the colony since 1886.[12]

No diffuse, multiperceptual medical gaze extended across the colonial territory of German New Guinea. Hospitals did not aggregate into a territorywide grid of medical surveillance but were defensive infrastructures built against the dangerous tropics imagined to exist outside the enclave. The topology of medical governance was better imagined as a patchwork of enclaves rather than a network of surveillance.

THE ARRIVAL OF THE MICROSCOPE

As the German Neuguinea Compagnie struggled to establish itself on the North Coast, scientific ideas about tropical disease were in fact undergoing a shift away from an emphasis on their causation by climatic conditions and toward bacterial, germ-based and parasitical theories of disease. By the late 1880s it was known that malaria was caused by parasites rather than miasma, and in 1887 Ronald Ross had identified malaria parasites in the stomach wall of the *anopheles* mosquito. And yet the introduction of bacterial and parasitical theories of disease did not put an immediate end to colonial anxieties about relationships between diseased environments and diseased natives (Worboys 1996). The association between the tropical climate, disease, and the racially differentiated body was in fact reinforced in German New Guinea by the malaria research carried out at Stephansort by the famous bacteriologist, Robert Koch, in 1901. Koch's research practices and findings also further reinforced the importance of the hospital as the prime means of addressing the colony's health problems.

Koch sought to confirm Ross's mosquito theory and research appropriate treatment regimes. He identified Stephansort, with its plantation laborer population of six hundred and native hospital, as an ideal research station for this purpose. Koch carried out an extensive survey of laborers and local villagers, using a microscope to count the malaria parasites in their blood. It has become local legend that he paid villagers for a vial of their blood with a stick of tobacco. He provided evidence that people growing up in areas of endemic malaria had an acquired immunity and that imported laborers were more vulnerable to the disease. By studying the distribution of malaria cases across local villagers and foreign laborers, who had spent a variable number of years on the mainland, Koch was able to map the distribution of endemic malaria across the region.

Koch was interested in acquired immunity, but this concept was regularly conflated with race in the colonial imaginary. In 1899, for example, the annual report declared it "notable" that two white women who had spent several years in the territory "are seldom troubled by Malaria" while on the other hand "half-blood women and girls suffer from it to a greater degree."[13] This distinction between the susceptibility to disease of the "pure white" and the "half-blood" body resonated with the associations that scientists and medical writers working elsewhere in the colonial south had formed between notions of racial weakness and the tropical climates in which they resided (Arnold 2004).

Today these scientific discoveries are seen as "the origin of the worst disaster to befall Melanesians" (Denoon 2002, 20). As Denoon has shown, the status given to doctors and scientists and the excitement surrounding laboratory discoveries led to the development of colonial public health policies that emphasized cure rather than prevention. The lessons learned by European governments in the nineteenth century, who had found that investments in public works such as improved housing and sewerage could have a more substantial impact on public health than curative medicine were lost on administrators in Papua and New Guinea, where many of the medical positions were filled by doctors. "The scientific discoveries about mosquito behavior might have led to intense field-work: in practice they gave rise to laboratory-based experiments, more likely to seek out cures than to prevent infection. A disaster for public health in the colony" (Denoon 2002, 20).

In 1901 Koch remained entirely focused on quinine as a tool for managing malaria and entirely ignored the habitat and behavior of the mosquito. This approach was not preordained. While Koch sat in the small adjunct laboratory at Finschafen hospital, Sir Ronald Ross was busy advocating a very different method of malaria control in the tropical colonies, one that focused on the mosquito rather than the malarial parasite. This was a method that harnessed colonial manpower to the task of larval control by seeking to eradicate larval breeding grounds (Ross 1910; Spielman and D'Antonio 2001). As Kelly and Beisel point out, this approach to disease control enacted a different kind of malaria from that focused on eradication of the parasite in the human blood (a version of the disease which they argue continues to be neglected amidst the war metaphors employed by global funding regimes today) and a pragmatic approach to colonial administration, "that did not rule with the iron first but rather as decentralized management to local bodies composed of willing participants" (Kelly and Beisel 2011, 75).[14]

In southern Italy, meanwhile, Celli was expanding the parameters of malaria control even further. If Koch focused on the parasite, Ross on pragmatic strategies for larval control that related mosquito/parasite relations to conditions of colonial living, then Celli was concerned with the social and economic conditions of agricultural feudalism in Italy under which the possibilities for malaria transmission became possible. "The elimination of Malaria, in short, required social reform and effective agrarian development" (Packard 2007, 112). Nonetheless, like Koch, Celli remained focused on quinine as the best control measure (Cueto 2013).

In German New Guinea Koch's focus on quinine limited the spatial parameters for governance and intervention to the hospital rather than extending it to the living rural environment. Although one might also conjecture that Koch's field station, embedded as it was within the available hospital infrastructure, lent itself to the development of hospital-focused solutions. He carried out extensive tests on the efficacy of quinine as a prophylaxis and treatment and helped develop strict rules for the medical regulation of the labor force. A year after his return from Stephansort, Koch was to come to international fame for his quick response to a cholera outbreak in Hamburg. There he relied on early bacteriological detection, isolation, and treatment for preventing the spread of the disease. In German New Guinea in 1901 he took a similar approach based on hospital-based pathological identification, treatment, and containment to the problem of malaria (Jackman 1990). There was no other way to defeat malaria, he argued, than through the periodic testing and treatment of all suspect cases. Specialist doctors, a microscope, regular supplies of quinine and a good isolation hospital were the required tools: "The mosquitoes play no part in the regimen which I prescribe: indeed, they are disregarded. . . . Measures such as pouring petrol on water where the insects breed, using repellents and mosquito-proof dwellings, have but a limited effect and, in general, are not used in the fight against malaria" (Koch quoted in Jackman 1990, 136). With the addition of a microscope and a bacteriologist the native hospital was transformed into a makeshift laboratory.

Research carried out in colonial hospitals in Papua New Guinea contributed to the emerging discipline of tropical medicine and reinforced its foundational differentiations of climates and peoples.[15] The disease-specific focus of this particular version of tropical medicine furthered the need for colonial hospitals as spaces for the application of new curative medicines and for research on tropical peoples. In lieu of any comprehensive surveillance of wider territorial space, New Guinea hospitals became key sites for measuring disease incidence. These statistics were gathered in separate charts for the "European," "colored," and "native" populations, further facilitating scientific comparison between racially distinct bodies.[16]

It was against this background that the decidedly hospital-centered policy of consecutive administrations in German New Guinea developed. On the one hand, the hospital enabled the isolation and subjection of dangerous, diseased bodies to medical expertise. On the other hand, the racially segregated hospital protected white bodies from black (and vice versa) and protected precarious colonial enclaves from the threatening, ungoverned and unknown, tropical environment beyond.

MAKESHIFT INFRASTRUCTURES

The health policy of German New Guinea was hospital centered, but the individuation of disease that took place under Koch's trained eye and microscope in his small adjunct laboratory did not extend to the public wards. In fact hospital infrastructure had little to differentiate it from other company or domestic buildings. Both European and native hospitals were makeshift, temporary structures. From 1985 to 1986 the company doctor at Finschafen treated his patients from a canvas tent. In 1887 materials were shipped over from Europe and Australia to erect sixteen new buildings at the station, including a much needed hospital for "coloreds" and a house that was to be used as a hospital for the European employees. The colored hospital provided free treatment to company employees, but was overcrowded and understaffed. The two other hospitals, at Hatzfeldthafen and Herbertshohe, were each looked after by a German medical orderly as there was only one doctor in the territory.

At Friedrich Wilhelmshafen (now Madang Town) two racially segregated hospitals and a quarantine hospital were built on different islands in the harbor soon after the administrative headquarters were moved there in 1891. These were constructed using local timber and covered with corrugated iron roofing. The native hospital was little more than a long open-walled shed lined with rows of patients. Meanwhile, the European hospital on Biliau Island often doubled up as a hotel for visitors and was presumably a little more salubrious (Sinclair 2005, 42). A persistent shortage of staff meant that patients at either establishment would have received very little attention from the doctor. At Friedrich Wilhelmshafen, the administration employed one doctor and two nurses, who arrived in 1891, to serve the two hospitals and the doctor would travel between the two hospitals by boat. In general one qualified European nurse served up to five Europeans but "only one European medical orderly and two 'colored' helpers for 40 to 50 'coloreds'" (Jackman 1990, 129).

The excitement surrounding Koch's research and his specifications for malaria treatment did not translate into increased resources or numbers of doctors to carry out the tasks of surveillance, microscopy, and treatment that he recommended. Mark Harrison has pointed out that many colonial hospitals had "an ephemeral existence. Many were flimsy structures and liable to collapse under heavy rains or high winds, and they frequently shifted from site to site." The lack of infrastructure and investment meant that the hospitals built in German New Guinea were probably of a lower standard than those built in other colonies at the same time. Indeed, Harrison suggests that the Germans invested far more in their African hospitals than their Pacific counterparts (Harrison 2009, 15). Apart from their sporadic participation in international medical research, hospital inhabitants in German New Guinea were rarely subjected to an authoritative medical gaze that sought to diagnose and treat their individual disease. The everyday hospital in German New Guinea was a place where sick bodies were isolated and racially segregated to ensure the continued existence of a precarious colony outside, rather than a place where daily observations and treatment regimes penetrated and discovered new truths about the biological body. Scientific tropical medicine might have been disease focused, resulting in hospital-centered public health governance, but this is not to say that the biomedicine practiced in those hospitals correlated individual bodies with individual diseases. The black bodies populating the native hospitals were considered generally diseased, but the medical practices of the day frequently left them without specific diagnoses of disease. The practice of tropical medicine informed but remained significantly different from tropical medical science.

THE MANDATE LABORATORY

The complex interface between scientific research and public health in New Guinea's colonial hospitals continued following the defeat of Germany's meager army by Australian troops in 1914. At this time New Guinea came under Australian military rule and in 1919 was formally transferred to Australian administration under a League of Nations Mandate. The mandate system was developed as a solution to the confiscation of the axis powers' colonies following the Great War. For the Allied Powers to annex those territories themselves was considered contrary to the principles of democracy and freedom for which the war had been fought. The mandate system was therefore established in explicit contradistinction to colonialism (Anghie 2002). Mandated territories were not governed by European powers for the purposes of exploitation but for those of protecting backward people and assisting their development towards self-government.

The mandate system helped establish a new international order in which an international bureaucratic apparatus would provide surveillance over mandatory rulers, such as Australia for New Guinea, who were expected to report annually on the progress of their mandates to the League of Nations. With its goals of welfare, progress, and self-government, the mandate system can thus be considered a nascent prefiguring of the international development discourse that emerged after the Second World War (Elyachar 2012, 115). The League of Nations graded mandated territories "A," "B," or "C," according to their position on a linear trajectory from "backwardness" to "self-government." New Guinea was graded C. This meant that Australia was given extensive powers in its governance that were, in practice, coextensive with those of annexation, although Australia was under pressure to contribute to social progress in the territory in a way that differed from its administration of the southern part of the island, Papua, as a colony.

The mandate system created an ambiguous form of colonial governance in New Guinea that rested on the unspecified future anticipation of the territory's sovereignty (Anghie 2002). The territory was not a colony, and Australia was supposed to be assisting its social progress, but on the other hand its peoples were considered so backward that self-rule could not be imagined within any formal time frame. In Australia this ambiguity played out against Australia's own dominion status, concerns about its future viability as a white nation, and its place in a new international order. The ways in which health would be governed in Papua New Guinea would play a significant role in the Australian formulation of these problems.

Papua New Guinea was mandated to Australia at the height of the White Nation policy in Australia and at a point when tropical medicine was playing an increasingly important role in those debates. The establishment of the Townsville Institute of Tropical Medicine in 1911 was intended to ascertain the adaptability of the white body to tropical conditions and the feasibility of settler colonialism in northern Australia through medical research focused on the productivity, health, and hygiene of the white body (Anderson 2005, 117). While indigenous peoples were widely expected to die out, the ability of a "working white race" to survive and reproduce in the intrinsically unhealthy climate of tropical Australia was considered doubtful (Harloe 1991). At the formal opening of the institute in 1913, William MacGregor, the previous governor of British New Guinea, emphasized the contribution of the institute to those debates when he stated its importance for "reserving Tropical Australia as a home for a white race" (quoted in Anderson 2005, 108).

In 1910 Anton Breinl arrived from Britain to take up the position of director of the new institute and to begin studying the diseases of northern Australia. Breinl had been trained at the Liverpool school of tropical medicine under tutelage of Ronald Ross and shared the latter's focus on public health and preventative medicine, but he was to find this approach had no place in an institute closely governed by authorities obsessed with the question of White Australia. Brienl was able to carry out some surveys in Papua but was forbidden from carrying out more extensive research on the health of the indigenous population in New Guinea or Papua out of concern that this would distract from the main focus of the institute on the survival of the white working class body in tropical climes (Harloe 1991).

As research by Brienl and his team, supported by advocates of northern settlement such as Cumpston, the director of the newly established Commonwealth Department of Health, established that the physiology of the white body in the tropics did not differ from that in temperate climates, the focus of Australian tropical medicine shifted away from white physiology and onto the threat posed by tropical flora and fauna, including that of the black indigenous body as a carrier for disease (Anderson 2005, 117). At the same time growing anxiety about maritime commerce and the movement of disease between Pacific Islands and Australia connected the governance of public health in the two locations. Even the decline of the indigenous population in New Guinea due to the introduction of new diseases, which had also greatly concerned the German administration who had feared its effects on the labor pool, was construed in terms of Australian national security. Indigenous population decline, it was feared, would lead to the eventual populating of the country by Asiatic coolies and could lead to possible future conflicts with Australia (Cameron-Smith 2010, 62). By the 1920s therefore, the duty to "uplift" the indigenous peoples of New Guinea increasingly dovetailed with the administrative concern to safeguard the health of White Australia.

In the 1920s and 1930s Australian Tropical Medicine simultaneously constructed the black New Guinean body as a site of imperial responsibility and a threat to the viability of the Australian nation. On the one hand the mandate system made Australia responsible for extending public health to New Guineans. On the other hand, tropical medicine construed the black population as a reservoir for disease, and it was imagined that they would need to be excluded or segregated for the white population to survive. "White cleanliness and purity and self-control—the constituents of White Australia—were naturally positioned against colored disease agency and danger and promiscuity" (Anderson 2005, 124). As climate became less of an issue, race became more of a danger.

This ambiguity, the product of a deeply entrenched paradigm of racial difference, significantly shaped the administration of Public Health in Papua New Guinea. It was an ambiguity that was embodied in the figure of Raphael Cilento who worked for the Australian Army Medical Crops in Papua New Guinea in the First World War, took over from Breinl as director of the Townsville Institute on his return to Australia in 1922, and was seconded to Papua New Guinea as the director of public health between 1924 and 1928. Raphael Cilento played a particularly important role in translating ideas about racial difference into public health policy. Indeed, he was a staunch nationalist and white supremacist, committed to the duty of populating and developing the "Australian tropics" (Yarwood 1991, 47). He was especially concerned about the "inelasticity" of the "native races," their weakness in the face of common diseases such as influenza and their inability to adapt to the changing colonial environment (Cameron-Smith 2010, 62). For Cilento tropical disease was tied to race and hereditary predisposition.

And yet the League of Nations Mandate also made Australia responsible for the improvement of the health and welfare of the indigenous population. The way Cilento squared this apparent contradiction was through exactly the kind of imperial ambitions that the mandated system was intended to contrast with. By the time Cilento arrived in New Guinea, there was growing confidence about the ability of the white body to adjust to and master their tropical environment and Australian tropical medicine was becoming more outward looking. In fact scientists at the Townsville Institute argued that colonialism should be an experimental venture with new settlements including trained scientists who could study settler populations from the beginning as part of a natural experiment. Papua and New Guinea were now construed as experimental spaces where Australia could test and demonstrate its own capacities to extend its territorial powers. At the same time the governance of indigenous health in the territories enabled Australia to exercise its own regional imperial influence and assert its significance as a regional power in the new international order. The Townsville Institute and the Commonwealth Laboratory it established in Rabaul in Papua in the 1920s became a crucial node in these regional networks of medical research and health governance. Medical policy in New Guinea and Papua circulated through the institute through the training of doctors to serve in the dependencies, and through research collaborations (Denoon 1991, 15). Indeed Cameron-Smith has argued that the brief attempt in the late 1920s to establish the Townsville Institute as a center to which imperial administrators in the Pacific would look for training, epidemiological research, and technical information, revealed imperial ambitions to mark out an "Austral-Pacific" region of influence (Cameron-Smith 2010). "In place of formal empire" he argues, "government doctors worked to extend an informal authority over the Pacific Islands by establishing Australian pre-eminence in the knowledge and practice of tropical medicine and the government of Indigenous people" (Cameron-Smith 2010, 70). If Australia had hitherto been perceived by Britain as a natural experiment in settler colonialism and racial viability and was perceived "as little more than a willing repository of scientific raw material" (Brasier 2010), Australia could now demonstrate its own preeminence through the establishment of New Guinea and Papua as equivalent laboratory domains. Indeed, while historiography of science and medicine in Australia has tended to emphasize isolation, the links between Australian medical research and global biomedical advances are gaining increasing attention: "Despite their profound geographic remoteness, practitioners working in this mandated territory remained closely linked—via training, correspondence, publications, and travel—to wider networks of imperial medicine" (Hobbins and Hillier 2010; Anderson 2009). For Australian administrators such as Cilento, therefore, the League of Nations mandate importantly identified Australia as an imperial power independent of homeland Britain. This vision of Australian dominance over a region never quite happened, but as a Mandated Territory, New Guinea became one space where Australian influence was paramount. For Cilento, his efforts in New Guinea were driven by Australian nationalist and imperialist ambitions rather than concerns about indigenous health. Nonetheless, during his brief period in New Guinea he was to have a significant and lasting impact on the shape of the territory's health institutions.

Under Cilento's directorship the military style of health administration that had been established under military administration during the First World War was continued. Rigorous military discipline was imposed in hospitals, hygiene conditions on plantations were closely regulated, and quarantine regulations were strictly imposed (Butler 1938). For him tropical medicine was imbued with the "language of military and political conquest" and the "imagery of armed struggle" (MacLeod and Lewis 1988, 6–7). He also presided over a series of public health campaigns for hookworm and yaws treatment. Cilento saw the extension of health services to the rural population as a key way to command their respect and admiration. During the 1920s and 1930s growing numbers of native hospitals were built with state funds, the medical tultul system was reestablished after a brief period of inactivity under the military administration, and the number of medical personnel was increased (Denoon 1991; 2002, 48). Attempts were also made to extend the influence of the colonial state over inland areas through exploratory patrols into the highlands, often accompanying commercial prospectors for minerals, once they were opened up in the 1930s.

Nonetheless, the pattern of health administration over this period manifested in medical infrastructures that looked in practice very similar to those of the German colonial administration. Rural health extension and campaigns against specific diseases did not extend far beyond administrative or commercial centers, and rural health continued to be left largely to the missions. Most significantly, the growing interest of the Australian administration in public health as a means of extending the visibility and influence of the colonial state, and the pressure that the League of Nations Mandate placed on the Australian administration to extend health services to the indigenous population did not lead to a demise of the hospital as the centerpiece of health policy in the territory. Health policy remained oriented primarily to the protection of the European population and their native or immigrant employees; and this meant hospitals. Moreover, as race grew in significance as a framework for health governance the hospital became increasingly valuable as a tool of racial segregation.

As Cilento stated, "One of the main principles of all health work in a tropical native country is the segregation in separate areas of racial units and national groups having different standards of living and varying rates of morbidity. In fact, many authors regard it as the first essential in public health work in the tropics, and undoubtedly such a policy means a great saving in sickness rates, especially among the European community" (quoted in Denoon 2002, 86). Hospitalization, racial segregation, and quarantine continued to lie at the heart of colonial public health. This entailed the variable allocation of medical resources to those distinct populations, with the continued prioritization of the European population. Specialist medical care in native hospitals was limited and strict rules for how the medical staff should interact with the native patients focused on the control and confinement of those bodies rather than their disciplining or moral improvement (Denoon 2002, 45). Medical education in the territory also stalled. Cilento barred the sending of New Guineans to train as native medical practitioners in the newly established medical school in Suva on account of their intellectual backwardness.

Despite continued interest in PNG as a site of medical research, this did not translate into therapeutic standardization and efficacy. Hobbins and Hillier argue that medical practice "as applied to Aboriginal and other Indigenous peoples across Australia's protectorates was regularly characterized by a worrisome absence of empirical data" (Hobbins and Hillier 2010, 6). As in Australia, so in New Guinea, the benefits of tropical medicine "flowed onto the indigenous people only if the means of production were endangered, or their diseases were likely to infect the colonizer" (Harloe 1991, 45).

In Australia in the 1920s and 1930s, as in Europe and the United States, hospitals were undergoing an architectural and technological revolution driven by shared visions of modern technological medicine (Logan and Willis 2010). In New Guinea, meanwhile, the hospitals built by the Australian administration differed little from their German predecessors. As I go on to discuss below, this would be the cause of numerous problems in the aftermath of the Second World War when the shift of the territory from a Mandate to a UN Trusteeship increased pressure on the Australian government to improve services. In the 1920s and 1930s, however, little scrutiny was given to the state of the native or European hospitals, and there was certainly no sense that they should be keeping pace with corresponding institutions on the Australian mainland.

In Madang, a new European Hospital was built in 1933. This hospital was located in the center of the town, near the main businesses and colonial residential areas. The hospital was a white timber bungalow built on a small hill at the furthest point of the town's peninsular. A veranda spanned the length of the building where male patients could catch the sea breeze and look out at the volcanic islands that dotted the Madang coastline, while the female patients would sit inside beneath the slow turning fans. The native

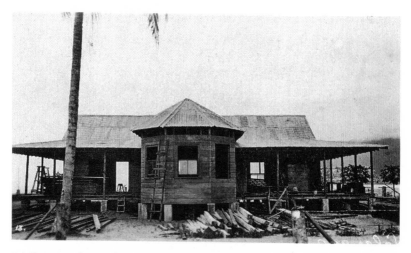

2.1. European hospital in course of construction at Salamaua, Morobe Province, New Guinea, circa 1928. This design was typical of prewar European hospital design. National Archives of Australia, A6510, 1645.

hospital, however, continued to operate out of the building built during the German administration, on an island in the harbor, and the government doctor took a boat out to it when he needed to do a medical round. In fact the native hospitals of the Australian administration differed little in architecture and resources from the German establishments they succeeded. They were staffed by nurses and locally trained orderlies, with doctors only attending sporadically. The native hospitals were little more than sheds with rows of planks for beds. The European hospitals had to survive without fully qualified doctors or technically advanced facilities such as X-ray machines or equipped operating theaters. The frequent absence of a doctor and the lack of medical equipment in Madang, for example, meant that the European hospital was run largely as a space of nursing, while any serious cases were quickly shipped back to Australia. As in the previous regime, these hospitals were imagined as spaces of containment in regard of natives and convalescence in regard of Europeans.

The segregation of hospitals was mirrored in the racial segregation of the towns themselves. These administrative and commercial centers were increasingly being serviced by an indigenous labor force, who were housed in dormitory-style labor compounds on the outskirts of the town. Men were not allowed to bring their families to the town and they were also given a strict curfew (Connell and Lea 1995). The town was still very much a white public space and sick black bodies were discreetly shipped to the native hospital via boat from the labor compounds, plantations, or neighboring villages.

CONCLUSION

Denoon lays the blame for the continuing sidelining of public health in New Guinea over this period squarely at the door of Australian tropical medicine: "How is it that such criminal neglect persisted for fifty years? It is hard to escape the judgment that it was the evolution of Tropical Medicine, and its transmission through Townsville and the new Commonwealth Department of Health, which was chiefly responsible" (1991, 22).[17]

A regular stream of medical researchers indeed flowed into the territory via the Commonwealth Laboratory in Rabaul and utilized the administration's hospitals and patients as a valuable scientific resource. These visitors contributed to the hospital's value to the colonial administration, but the latest advances in tropical medicine were not practiced within them. If, as Denoon argues, rural public health was neglected during these years in favor of a disease-focused tropical medicine, the latter existed only in the laboratories of Townsville and Rabaul and not in the public wards of the native hospitals, which often remained as neglected as the villages from which their patients were recruited.

A chronic shortage of resources in the territory's hospitals was coupled with the targeted distribution of those resources along racial lines. Clearly, the priority of both German and Australian administrations in prewar New Guinea was to protect the colony's seemingly precarious capitalist enclaves and immigrant populations (Denoon 2002, 83) rather than to extend state power (and services) across the territory. Over the course of German, Australian military, and Australian civilian administrations in New Guinea, the hospital remained central to this protectionist public health policy. While the emergence of public health institutions and public hospitals were reconfiguring relationships between the state and its citizens in Europe, hospitals in Papua New Guinea served a different kind of state-building function. I suggest that the hospitals that were built over this period might be best understood as frontier hospitals. Rather than centers of calculation, the nodes of an extensive network of health governance, they were isolated institutions built in defense against an encroaching disease-ridden tropical environment imagined to exist beyond the colonial enclave.[18] The emergent discipline of tropical medicine "gave scientific credence to the idea of a tropical world as a primitive and dangerous environment in contradistinction to an increasingly safe and sanitised temperate world" (MacLeod and Lewis 1988, 7). Hospitals represented a frontier between the emerging discipline of tropical medicine with its myopic focus on individual "tropical" diseases, and an external tropical environment that threatened the very possibility of colonial endeavor in the territory. They were designed as enclosed spaces of colonial governance and medical knowledge production that pushed the state's frontier against the tropical environment but did not penetrate or transform it. As the next chapter describes, following the Second World War, hospitals in Papua New Guinea shifted from being inward to outward looking institutions, intended to serve a Papua New Guinean population and instill a modern consciousness in the individuals who encountered them. Nonetheless, continuities in the organization of space and the kinds of racialized visibility that space afforded persisted.

CHAPTER 3

Public Buildings, Building Publics

■ On April 7, 1961, Paul Hasluck, the Australian minister for territories, stood up from the padded swivel office chair that had been placed on the concrete walkway outside Madang's newly built public hospital and took his place underneath an Australian flag on the podium. Behind Mr. Hasluck was the hospital's main block, its white weatherboard cladding shining in the sun. In front of him more than one hundred Australian expatriates, leaders from local churches, and newly elected "native" politicians were seated in rows on metal foldable chairs, which had been placed neatly on the mown and watered lawn and shaded by a canvas canopy extending out from the main building. Standing beyond them in crisp white uniforms and nurses' caps were the hospital's Papua New Guinean employees. This was the new public for whom the hospital had been built.

After the ceremonial opening, village groups from nearby districts performed dances and songs in their traditional costume, and the local expatriate and indigenous communities were invited to take the opportunity to look around their new public hospital. At the end of the day Paul Hasluck and the Australian director of public health in PNG, Roy Scragg, were given a guard of honor by hospital orderlies and infant, child, and maternal health nurses, and they chatted between themselves as they sauntered down the line, shaking hands jauntily as they went (see figure 3.1). The opening of Madang's new hospital was filmed by ABC television in Australia and the event was later given wide coverage in the Australian and regional Pacific Press.

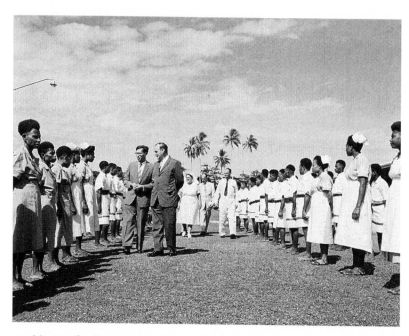

3.1. Minister for the territories, Mr. Paul Hasluck, had a guard of honor of hospital orderlies and infant child and maternal health nurses when he arrived to open the Madang General Hospital, New Guinea, on April 7, 1961. National Archives of Australia, A1200, L38803.

This ceremonial opening was not an isolated occurrence. The building of Madang Hospital represented the most recent stage of an ambitious postwar hospital-building program that extended across the Australian governed territory of Papua New Guinea and included plans to build eighty-six new institutions. Madang Hospital cost the Australian government £662,000, with over £7,000,000 pledged for the building of new hospitals across the country. These new modern buildings were to replace war damaged and rotting "native" and "European" hospitals made from bush materials and old army barracks, dotted sporadically across dispersed administrative centers, which had in recent years become an embarrassment to an Australian administration keen to demonstrate its commitment to economic and social development in the protectorate.

Where the health policy of prewar colonial administrations had focused on the European population and rarely touched areas beyond urban administrative and commercial enclaves, the postwar administration sought to extend a uniform health service across the territory and saw its primary obligations as being to the indigenous population. This was an era when the establishment of the World Health Organization (WHO) and the push toward decolonization by the UN were helping to forge new connections between health and development. The notion of primary health care was rising up the international agenda and the development of culturally appropriate and accessible rural health services was seen as a key responsibility of colonial and newly independent states in the developing world.

The emphasis was on rural outreach, public health, and preventative medicine rather than the highly specialized services of technologically advanced medicine, which were perceived to benefit urban elites and exacerbate health inequalities at the expense of the rural majority. And yet the fixed-facility hospital in Papua New Guinea, as in many colonial and newly independent states, remained a surprisingly central tenet of postwar health policy and infrastructure development. The director of public health in the immediate postwar period, Dr. John Gunther, was clear that the construction of well-equipped "world standard" hospitals was central to the development of a modern health system fit for a future independent nation. It was impossible to imagine a modern nation without furnishing it with modern hospitals along the lines of those that were simultaneously being constructed as part of the postwar welfare state in Australia and Europe.

The hospitals that were envisaged and built by the postwar Australian administration were very different from those that populated the early colonial urban landscape. Their physical design summoned different publics, incorporated new kinds of medical knowledges and technologies, and spatialized new kinds of state-citizen relationships. Yet despite historical variation in the colonial experience in Papua New Guinea, a country that saw eight different colonial administrations over the course of ninety years, the hospital remained a central fixture of public health policy throughout the colonial period. The unswerving commitment to the general hospital in Papua New Guinean colonial medicine highlights the significance of this institution as a locus for state and nation-building efforts.

In the late colonial period hospitals were reimagined as spaces that would shape and serve Papua New Guinean citizens as a new public body. But there was in fact intense ambiguity about what kinds of (racial) bodies constituted those publics, which were played out in debates over the material form and design of the institutions themselves. Racially distinct bodies continued to be categorized and medically scrutinized within the hospital. However, these activities took place against a backdrop of anxieties about the very viability of the nation-state.

In the postindependence era the hospital became a prime site of state building for foreign organizations and bilateral agencies, which carried out their hospital intervention in the name of "development." As this chapter describes, Papua New Guinea's hospitals, and Madang in particular, now became emblematic of postcolonial decline rather than beacons of a future modernity, and were primed for further development interventions. In fact what these interventions demonstrate is the ongoing significance of the hospital as a site of state building (rather than an efficient technology of governance) on the one hand, and historical continuity in the racial differentiation of space and bodies on the other. To tell the story of how government hospitals became "public," and what this means today, is to tell a story about changing relationships between institutional and territorial space and about the kinds of bodies and persons that are made visible in those relationships.

THE NEW AUSTRALIAN PUBLIC

The hospital-building program of the 1950s was designed and approved under very different political conditions from the hospital-building activities of the prewar era. Pressure on Australia to move toward decolonization was intensifying and health was becoming aligned internationally with development in new ways. During the war the territories of Papua and New Guinea had been administered by a single military administration and this was now mirrored in the establishment of a new Australian administration to govern the whole territory. Where prior to the war self-government had seemed an unachievable and possibly unnecessary goal, it was now presumed (by the UN at least) that, in the foreseeable future, this new territory would follow recently independent African and Asian countries in becoming an independent nation. The newly conjoined territory of Papua New Guinea was governed by Australia as a UN trusteeship, and this entailed great surveillance by the international bureaucracy and greater pressures on the Australian administration to contribute to the territory's social and economic development.

In Australia, the contribution made by Papua New Guineans to the Pacific War effort had made their neglect by prewar public health policies politically unpalatable.[1] The notion that widespread surveillance, recording, and regulation of the health of a population could be a force for social and economic improvement and the strengthening of the state, which had been floated by prewar administrations but never effectively put into practice, now became imperative. The new colonial state was deemed to be responsible for the welfare of the Papua New Guinean population and for their ability to achieve a level of economic development that would enable independence in the near future.

Amidst local concerns that Papua New Guinea lacked a manufacturing industry or any prospects for economic development other than small-scale horticulture and cash crops, health (along with education) was seen as key to the emergence of a physically and intellectually equipped population for whom political independence would be a realistic possibility. Across Asia and Africa colonial and newly independent governments were aligning science and development in the construction of ambitious irrigation, resettlement, and agricultural planting programs.[2] In Papua New Guinea at the same time the rapid construction of rural and urban health infrastructure in the immediate postwar era was the most visible manifestation of the Australian state's new commitment to "development" and "modernization" in the territory. These measures were thus both deemed "humane" and vital for economic progress.

At the forefront of health reform in the territory was John Gunther, a young visionary and notoriously stubborn Australian doctor who was appointed as the director of public health in 1946. Gunther's directorship was characterized by an endless haranguing of the Canberra administration to free up resources to allow for greater numbers of medical patrols, the recruitment of European refugee doctors who could not be legally employed in Australia, retention of ex-army medics as medical assistants, the education of native medical officers and the monitoring of village hygiene. Gunther also took full advantage of the new array of antibiotics and other drugs that became affordable and accessible in this period, and coordinated numerous campaigns against malaria, leprosy, tuberculosis, pneumonia, diarrhea, polio, and yaws. This was paternalist medicine at its heights. Gunther's establishment of an effective centralized health administration, his contribution to the creation of an indigenous medical workforce, and his heroic medical campaigns have received much attention in the history of tropical medicine in Papua New Guinea (Denoon 1989; Anderson 2009; Burton-Bradley 1990). The centrality of the hospital to Gunther's vision has been less widely noted.

Gunther considered the hospital a crucial tool in the development of a modern Papua New Guinean nation. As soon as he entered office, he began lobbying Canberra to fund a universal "world standard" hospital-building program. In 1950, he established a "Hospital Committee," composed of himself and two other medical officers, and embarked on a territorywide survey of current hospital infrastructure, resources, and geographic distribution.

Gunther envisaged that the "world standard" modern hospitals built as part of his planned construction program would have powerful affects on their new Papua New Guinean publics, actively interpolating them as national subjects, instilling hope, and mobilizing them as a force for development. The physical appearance of the hospitals was as crucial in this regard as the technological processes that took place within them. The hospitals that Gunther imagined to be capable of effecting such wider social transformations and of propelling Papua New Guinea into a new era of modernization and development would be specialized medical spaces equipped with the latest medical technologies and fully trained medical experts. They would be removed from everyday social life, bounded by an exclusive medical expertise and authority, yet placed in prominent urban locations. These would not be simple timber bungalows, furnished with beds and inhabited by nurses and an occasional doctor, but buildings designed and constructed specifically for the purpose of medical practice and training and to house the latest medical equipment such as X-ray machines or laboratory services. They would be equivalent to the new centers for scientific medical expertise that were simultaneously springing up across the Western world.

Gunther was acutely sensitive to the aesthetics of these spaces.[3] In its report to Canberra, his Hospital Committee emphasized that the new native hospitals should not be built from "bush materials," but should be clearly differentiated in materials and design from the style of native houses. It was envisaged that the difference in appearance would prove instructive for the native population and demonstrate the superiority of Western medical knowledge. The hospitals should be "built in such a way that they offer an inducement not found by the native in a hut of his own making" and that will encourage them to "seek more and more the medical aid offered."[4] The report proposed that the new buildings be of "nissen hut style" with aluminum used for the more important buildings. The modern style would clearly identify those buildings as "public" spaces built and provided by the state, as opposed to temporary structures that might be construed on a continuum with the native hut. The hospital was therefore envisaged as instrumental for instilling in the indigenous mind a distinction between "tradition" and "modernity," which was considered vital to the emergence of a modern consciousness and the creation of individual desire for national development.

Gunther was interested in the hospital patient as an active but impressionable subject who could be shaped by his surroundings. He decided it was

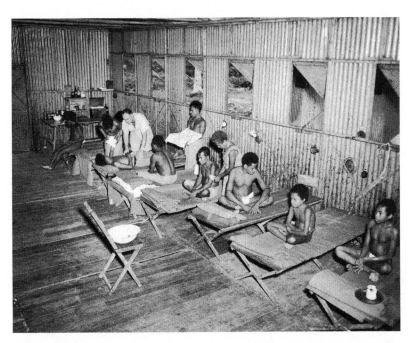

3.2. Patients in a village hospital, circa 1950. National Archives of Australia, A1200, L9942.

vital, therefore, that the hospital architecture should enable patients to see. His attention to detail even extended to the type of wall openings on the hospital: "The native hospital wards at Kavieng, Sohano, and Madang have the fixed Army 'Eyebrow' type of wall opening. This suffers certain innate disabilities in that patients cannot see outside the building."[5]

Gunther envisioned a health service that would be run by as well as for indigenous Papua New Guineas and under his guidance the health service became a key institutional space where administrators sought to engineer a national consciousness and civic ethic. To this end, the construction of modern hospitals was also a crucial component in the development of national training programs for Papua New Guinean nurses, doctors, and health extension officers (Gunther 1990; see also chapter 6). Moreover, the appearance of the modern hospital would itself act as an inducement to Papua New Guineans to want to study medicine or nursing and to serve their fellow nationals. Gunther was concerned that colonialism had taught Papua New Guineans to perceive hospitalization and treatment with modern medicine as an obligation rather than a blessing. The visible superiority of the modern hospital building would inspire them to access those services

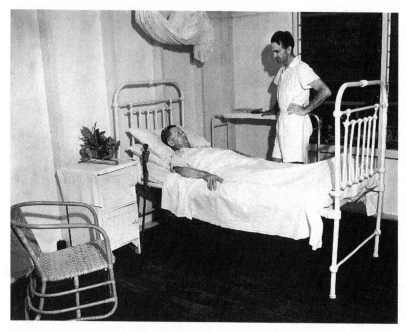

3.3. One of the single bed wards in the European hospital at Kavieng, 1950. National Archives of Australia, A6510, 1647.

more readily and to want to be involved in their development and provision at a national level.

The role of the hospital as a technology of progress was particularly important in a place where the existence of neither a governing state nor its publics could be taken for granted. Where the prewar hospital had been crucial in assuaging anxieties about the biological viability of the white colonial state, the postwar hospital addressed concerns that an independent state was unviable because of a lack of national consciousness among the indigenous population. In Papua New Guinea the reach of the state and the extent of national consciousness were of major concern for the postwar Australian administration. From 1951, the minister for territories, Paul Hasluck had followed a policy of "gradualism" based on the notion that development would occur organically given the right conditions, and the belief that the entire population needed to be lifted onto a higher plane of health and education before independence could be considered possible. At the same time, however, Australia was coming under pressure from the United Nations to achieve more rapid transformation and move swiftly toward decolonization. Debates over a timetable for independence questioned whether a nation-state could be sustained by an elite minority of educated nationals while the rural majority continued their lives largely unaffected by the benefits of modernity, and with little sense of allegiance to a nation or state. In this political context the hospital became a vehicle for social improvement.

In contrast to the authoritarian, prisonlike spaces of prewar hospitals, the new "modern" hospitals were designed to mobilize Papua New Guineans as active national subjects, people who would not be forced to enter the hospital but who would actively seek its modern services. The space of the hospital now corresponded in the political imaginary to a wider territorial field. Early colonial hospitals were not part of planned territorywide networks but were established on an impromptu basis. They were built where and as they were needed or when their construction and administration became feasible: when a new administrative center was established, when a new medical officer was recruited, or when an epidemic of malaria or dysentery necessitated an immediate response. By contrast, the postwar hospital-building project established an interconnected network of public health institutions that demarcated and served the territory as a single cohesive entity. The new hospitals were not envisaged as fortresses against an uncontrolled tropical environment and peoples, but as planned interventions designed to comprehensively traverse and transform the territory's physical and social landscape. They were outward- rather than inward-looking institutions.[6] As part of a territorywide health system, the hospitals would materialize a new relationship between the colonial state, its publics, and national space.

HOSPITAL TOURS

Native hospitals had previously been inward-looking containers, invisible to the European population. But as they become more important to the colonial state, they were opened up to a new kind of public gaze and moral scrutiny. In 1950, the Hospital Committee visited Madang in order to inspect the hospital facilities and report on its construction needs. The committee decided that the native hospital, which had been relocated from an island in the harbor to a labor compound serving a small port on the outskirts of town in 1949 by the Australian medical officer, Dr. Jackson, and was built from war surplus and temporary materials, needed eventual replacement but was "adequate" and a "suitable structure" for the time being. Only a few years later, however, the native hospital was to become the site of civil activism focused on the unfair treatment of the indigenous population. The Hospital Committee discovered that they were not the only people in the territory with an interest in public hospitals. Hospital campaigners had very different views on what kind of place a Papua New Guinean hospital should be.

On February 18, 1956, Dr. Knowles, the Australian doctor posted to the hospital, wrote to the director of public health in Port Moresby drawing his attention to "the most shocking state of dilapidation, filth and stench in this hospital . . . 13 out of 24 ward rainwater tanks are faulty, leaking or disintegrated; that patients cannot be washed and are coated with filth. Several of the ward floors are broken and pitted so that puddles and dirt accumulate, and roofs are rusted through. In view of these foul conditions, I have asked that all elective surgery be discontinued here until improvements are obtained."[7]

Dr. May, who was briefly acting as director of public health in Dr. Gunther's absence, visited Madang where he told Dr. Knowles to stop complaining, remarking that he thought the doctor lacked "pioneer spirit" and that he should leave if he was unhappy. Mr. Knowles subsequently decided to do this and wrote that he would return to Australia: "I will not conclude without commenting that I would never have believed that any civilized government could permit such shameful conditions, which are an insult and disgrace to humanity. It is hard to believe that the Commonwealth Government and the Department of Territories can be satisfied with the way in which the Dept. of Public Health in Port Moresby administers its hospitals here."[8]

Shortly after Dr. Knowles's departure, the minister for territories received a letter from the Pan Pacific and Southeast Asian Women's Society based on reports they had heard about the state of the native hospital in Madang: "The hospital itself is said to be in very bad condition, the wards were dark, with everywhere a pervading stench." A Missionary has stated that on his first visit to this hospital "the horror and the stench made him vomit."[9]

They had heard that there was no running water for the patient washhouses and most of the water tanks out of use. There was only one copper wash boiler suitable for domestic use and incapable of dealing with laundry from 150 to 200 patients. Patients were being given blankets that had not been washed after use by several previous inhabitants. In the same month, the secretary for territories received a letter from David Hodgkin, secretary of the World Council of Churches referring to complaints made by Dr. Knowles. Mr. Hodgkin pointed out that "we understand that one cannot think of New Guinean Native hospitals in the same terms as one would of Australian hospitals. . . . We are however disturbed by the specific matters raised, these being matters which would seem to need rectifying in the most primitive of hospitals."[10]

While native patients might not be expected to require the same quality of health care as the expatriate population, concern about their welfare had nonetheless become a public issue. Most irritatingly for the administration, these hospitals had also become a sightseeing stop on the colonial tourism itineraries of concerned Australian citizens. In December 1954, the secretary for the Department for External Territories received a telephone call from a Mr. H. T. M. Middleton from Toowong who had recently returned from a tour in Papua New Guinea. Mr. Middleton said that several people from Toowong had gone on a trip to Port Moresby and had made an excursion to the native hospital there. The secretary reported to the minister for external territories that "they said the condition of the Native Hospital is appalling, it is nothing but large open sheds, one of which has the posts set in barrels of concrete, and another of such shed goes right down to the muddy foreshore, and bandaged natives can be seen lolling about anywhere. The whole set up appears to be most unhygienic. Walking along the street some of them commented on the state of affairs—and men working there (quite evidently NOT liberals) remarked to them on hearing their comments 'well, that is all the Menzies Government can give the natives!' Etc. and suchlike remarks"[11]

The state of native hospitals in the 1950s was certainly no worse (and may indeed have been better) than that of native hospitals in the prewar period, yet they had not previously been a cause for widespread public campaigning and complaints to senior administrative officers. Isolated and temporary structures, they had been designed to render visible and act on the bodies they contained but had not been objects of visibility themselves. The outrage among Australian public servants and charitable institutions concerning the state of the hospital shows that those institutions were now objects of interest for and open to the scrutiny of a discerning and critical Australian public in a way they had not been prior to the war.

In the midst of this public outrage, however, the relative silences on and omissions of matters of racial inequality and segregation are notable. While the quality of native hospitals was a cause for concern, their separation from European hospitals was not. Meanwhile, there was no suggestion among complainants that native hospitals should be resourced to an equivalent standard with those institutions serving Europeans. It is also significant that there are no records of complaints from literate Papua New Guineans on the subject of health services. If these hospitals were now public in a new way, then their public was still clearly divided: between the dark bodies, imagined as passive victims and colonial subjects, and the active, campaigning Australian publics who observed and pitied them.[12] In fact, the continuing dominance of race as a paradigm for framing public health policy and organizing medical space was striking throughout the preindependence era.

WHITE PUBLICS

For many Australians living in Papua New Guinea, the state of the European hospitals was an even more urgent issue than the deteriorating native hospitals. The small, poorly resourced European hospitals in the territory compared poorly with the new citadels of medical science that were emerging with the postwar economic boom in Australia. In the prewar period, conditions in administrative centers in Papua New Guinea had not been radically different from those found in the administrative outposts of Australian states like Queensland. But public infrastructure in Australia was now undergoing a rapid transformation. A trip to Papua New Guinea suddenly seemed less like a hop across the water to another Australian territory and more like a journey back in time to the pioneering colonial days of the late nineteenth and early twentieth centuries.

In Madang, the European Hospital was one of the few buildings in the town to have survived the Second World War relatively unscathed. Most other buildings in the town were entirely demolished by allied bombardments of the Japanese. When the acting minister for external territories, Cyril Chambers, visited the hospital on a tour of the territory in May 1949, however, he was not impressed. He immediately wrote a report to the administrator of Papua New Guinea complaining that the hospital was in a bad state of repair with no surgical facilities and an X-ray machine but no electric power. He stated that at the time of his trip, the medical officer, Dr. Woods, was treating a patient for appendicitis who could require surgery at any moment, and yet the hospital did not have the facilities for this procedure.

The presence of an established Chinese population in the town, who ran many of the business establishments, challenged the long-standing racial order of the hospitals.[13] The Chinese were considered more educated and civilized than the native Papua New Guineans and thus might rightly expect more comfortable surroundings than that provided by the native hospitals. Nonetheless, the European expatriates were not expected to share an open hospital ward with them and, in a striking continuation with the nineteenth-century German colonialists, the need for racial isolation was conflated with the need for the isolation of infectious diseases: "At the present time there is no provision for the isolation of infectious cases and no provision had been made for the local Chinese population to be treated at the hospital. For this reason [Dr. Woods] had been compelled to conduct obstetric operations on Chinese women at 'Chinatown.'"[14]

Throughout the 1950s dissatisfaction with the government medical services grew among the European residents in the town. The perceived superiority of church-provided medical services played a significant role in these appraisals. At the time when the colonial authorities were building urban hospitals primarily to quarantine sick patrol officers and administrators from the perceived dangers of indigenous New Guineans and their tropical diseases (Denoon 1989), many early missionaries in the Madang area established rural health services for the indigenous population (see, e.g., Frerichs and Frerichs 1957, 93–104). For many people in the Madang area, their first interaction with biomedicine was thus mediated by the moral teachings of the Lutheran and Catholic churches. The missions were also the first authorities to provide medical and nursing training to local Papua New Guineans, and the Lutheran-founded hospital at Amele in Madang began training "native medical orderlies" as early as the 1930s.

Following the Second World War, the well-established Lutheran and Catholic health services continued to predominate in rural areas. In the postwar context of inclusive "primary health care," their aid posts and health centers played an increasingly important role in the health system. In 1949 the Lutheran Mission had opened up a new hospital at Yagaum, seventeen kilometers outside of Madang Town. The hospital was founded and run by Dr. Braun, an American Lutheran doctor who had worked in the Madang area of Papua New Guinea since 1934, originally setting up a hospital at Amele, which had been destroyed by the Japanese during the war.

The Yagaum hospital consisted of rehabilitated army barracks, which were shipped and then carried from an army base at Finschafen 150 miles away. The buildings were basic; long metal sheds with doors at either end. But the hospital was well resourced by donations from American Lutheran churches and had X-ray equipment, a well-equipped operating theater, a nursing school and separate wings for European, Asian, and native patients. At the time, Yagaum hospital was considered the best-resourced hospital in the territory. The European residents of Madang Town complained that the missions were providing better services than the government, and many residents chose to make the trip out to Yagaum to see Dr. Braun rather than use the Government "hospital on the hill." This involved a long drive through the villages along muddy unsealed roads and a ferryboat across the impassable Goum River where an ambulance would meet them on the opposite side. The missionary doctors at Yagaum, who considered their primary responsibility to be the local population, were not particularly pleased about the influx of European patients. But as many of them also socialized together in Madang's expatriate clubs, at social or charity events, they did not turn the European patients away (Guntner 2006, 18).

Papua New Guinean hospitals had now become public spaces in a new sense; they were exposed to the critical gaze of an Australian public who saw the provision of medical services, both for themselves and the native population, as a basic obligation of a state to whom they paid their taxes. Civil servants serving in the territory expected to receive basic health services equivalent to those they had experienced in postwar Australia.

This was all rather tiresome for the administrators in Papua New Guinea, who were busy struggling to establish a new comprehensive health service with extremely limited funds. Although the Department for Territories in Canberra frequently responded to civilian complaints with the demand that Port Moresby make a full investigation, the Papua New Guinean–based administrators also noticed the reluctance of Canberra to actually release any of the funds for public health that they frequently promised.[15] It was felt that Australians in Papua New Guinea had unrealistic expectations of the services that could be provided in an external territory. While social and economic development was important, it was perceived as clearly ridiculous to expect the same conditions in Papua New Guinea as one might find in Australia. The administrator, Donald Cleland, for example, did not consider poor Dr. Knowles to be cut out for colonial service: He blames "everyone and everything but his own shortcomings for his inability to meet the situation" and has "no knowledge of how to understand native people."[16] Clearly the postwar colonial character lacked the "pioneer spirit" of earlier decades. In 1953 Gunther complained to the Legislative Council that the visibility of the urban medical services and the relative invisibility of the rural village were leading to public pressure to invest in urban services at the expense of rural areas.[17]

By the 1960s it was clear to the government in Canberra that something had to be done about the state of its protectorate's hospitals. The pressure to do so came from multiple directions—Australian indigenous rights activists, Australian expatriates in PNG, and those who subscribed to Gunther's vision of an independent and healthy nation. The "deplorable" condition of hospital buildings, which had "been the subject of severe criticism of public bodies and visiting members of parliament" was cited as a key reason for the cabinet's approval of Gunther's large-scale hospital-building program.[18] Perhaps the most important factor, however, was the scrutiny that the UN afforded their governance of the trusteeship and the questions that were beginning to be asked about Australia's progress toward self-government in the territory. In a cold war climate the ability of Australia to properly secure "development" in the trusteeship, of the kind that was being put into practice elsewhere under the provision of the Marshall Plan, was significant for Australia's relationships with its allies and its standing in the international community.

MATERIALIZING THE STATE

For the Australian government to build new public hospitals that could produce new modern subjects it had to abolish what had become one of their defining characteristics. The racial segregation of hospitals had been integral to their role as enclaves of protection and isolation since the erection of the first institutions by the German and British administrations in the late nineteenth century. The new hospitals would now serve a collective of Europeans and natives who had never previously congregated as a public around one place. The hospital opening in Madang therefore inaugurated both a new building and, built into that material structure, a new configuration of social relations.

European and native patients would now reside on the same compound and share the same medical infrastructure; female European nurses would now administer to male native patients where such mixing had previously been strictly prohibited, and for the first time hospitals would also be staffed by female European doctors. However, the justification for this move away from racially segregated hospitals was not based on a changing notion of what was socially or humanely acceptable but economic calculation. For the new "world standard" hospitals to be provided to both native and European communities and remain affordable, the administration argued, the construction of racially segregated institutions was no longer sustainable.[19]

Prewar European and native hospitals had been entirely separate institutions, often located several miles apart from one another. Now they would be combined in the same compound. The move was not quite as radical as it might at first seem. They were still in many respects separate hospitals. As the Hospital Committee report noted:

Where both European and Native Hospitals are to be provided at any place, the committee, as a general policy considers that these should be combined sufficiently to allow common use of such services as operating theatre, x-ray, laboratory and, in some instances, kitchens. It would be quite uneconomical to duplicate such facilities in each case. The committee, however, considers it essential to separate European and Native accommodation sufficiently to avoid objections as to proximity and intermingling. Layouts at Port Moresby and Lae have been arranged as to achieve this, and yet retain types of ward handy to the above mentioned services. It is recommended that this general policy be followed in arranging layout of Regional Hospitals also.[20]

The new General Hospital at Madang covered a substantial area on the site of an old German plantation near what now served as the town's native labor compound. The site stretched between the ocean on one side and the main road leading into the town center on the other. Up on the hill overlooking the sea was the "European Hospital," which was also described in public documents as the "paying ward." With long verandas, rooms for 16 in-patients and views of the ocean, the European Hospital was an elegant colonial building and received the best of the sea breeze in the stifling tropical town. The European wing was smaller but more spacious than the native wing, allowing greater isolation of patients in private or semiprivate rooms in line with emerging medical concerns about patient-to-patient contagion and the need for space and the flow of air between patients (see figure 3.4).

The "native hospital" was built on the flat next to the road, and in the following months there would be much campaigning by the hospital workers to the Advisory Town Council for the road surface to be sealed owing to the substantial amounts of dust that was being thrown up into the wards (Sinclair 2005, 227). The eight public wards housed 320 beds and were divided according to disciplinary distinctions between pediatrics, surgical, internal medicine, and obstetrics and maternity. The wards were of the nineteenth-century "nightingale style." They consisted of long sheds, made of weatherboard and gauze, with doors at each end. The beds were carefully spaced and small windows allowed airflow between them, while fans were suspended above. Each ward was divided in half by a nurses' office, from where an observation window allowed the nurses to supervise the patients.

Between the "native" and "European" blocks were administrative buildings and a laboratory and general service blocks that were shared by the two hospital wings. Although racially distinct substances could intermingle in

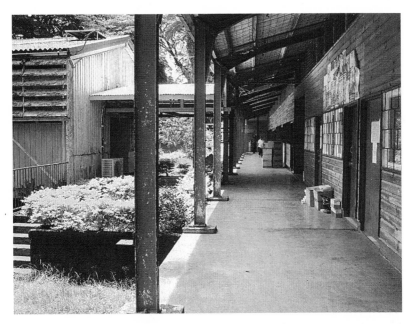

3.4. The European Hospital in Madang, now used to house the Provincial Department of Health. The patient wards are on the right of the corridor, the operating theater on the left.

the laboratory, the European wing had its own operating theater to prevent different colored bodies coming into contact with one another while unconscious. The European and native wings each also had their own kitchen providing "Western-style" and "local" fare respectively. The hospital was staffed by two Australian doctors, two Australian trained medical assistants, eleven Australian nurses and forty-six "native hospital workers," the latter based in the native wards. The European staff were shared between the two wings and had to run up and down the hill to and from the European section. Behind the hospital a compound had been built for the hospital staff, including small two-room houses or single dormitories for native staff and larger detached houses for the European staff.

Where tower-block hospitals were emerging in the 1950s and 1960s in Europe, America, and Australia, the need for centralized administration and specialist services and the racial segregation of wings meant that hospitals in Papua New Guinea continued to be of an older "pavilion" style, comprising several separate buildings with different functions, connected by covered walkways or corridors. The European Hospital was designed according to new medical theories of contagion and new requirements for patient privacy. However, this design coincidently solved a perpetual problem facing the racially segregated hospitals of the past; the question of where to treat Madang's substantial population of people of Asian origin. It was considered that the relatively developed and civilized "Asians" could not be treated in the native hospitals, but equally the European population objected to their sharing the open European wards of the old European Hospital. The isolated rooms of the new European Hospital were important insofar as they allowed Asian patients to be accommodated on a par with the European community, but to be kept spatially distinct.

Meanwhile, the native hospital continued to be designed in line with the medical knowledge of a previous era, when the ability to observe and treat large numbers of patients at once took primacy over privacy, and the flow of air between beds was intended to provide protection against free floating miasma rather than infectious microbes carried by other bodies (Prior 1988; Porter 2002). The native population now had newly discovered "rights to health," but the differentiated designs of the European and native hospitals suggest that these rights were attached to different kinds of person: individuated and collectivized. Differences between the European and native wings suggest that their design cannot only be read as a discursive expression of the medical knowledge of the day (Prior 1988) and that the layering of discursive space was implicated in the production of racially differentiated publics.

The construction of the hospital as a spatial device for rendering the state visible to its potential publics coincided with its reproduction as a technology for knowing, differentiating, and acting on those publics. The Australian administration's ongoing colonial paternalism reproduced the racial segregation and accompanying fears of the prewar era. Madang Hospital was not simply "a" public hospital, but was in fact two hospitals designed for two distinct publics: the "European" and the "native." These publics required different kinds of buildings, food, staffing, and medical resources. Different modes of medical visibility and corresponding practices of care were built into the "world standard" hospital at Madang from its beginning.

Questions were raised about the standards of Papua New Guinea's new hospitals from the start. In 1959, only two years after the Lae hospital was built in the neighboring province of Morobe, complaints were raised at the Provincial District Advisory Council that the hospital's equipment was poor, the hospital was full of flies, and the pillowslips were patched.[21] The *New Guinea Times Courier* ran a story with the lead line, "Lae has a modern hospital which is not being run on modern lines."[22] In 1961, at the time of

Madang Hospital's opening, Lae Hospital ran out of food and patients had to be sent home.[23] Meanwhile a report by the Royal Australian College of Surgeons on the newly opened Port Moresby General Hospital in 1959 reported overcrowding, inadequate staffing, and poor building construction in the native wing of the hospital.[24] The dream of the modern Papua New Guinean hospital was unraveling as quickly as the blueprints were being turned into timber frames and concrete blocks.

These early criticisms would be forgotten in a later era, when the failure of Papua New Guinea's hospitals was reconceived as a reflection of postcolonial decline. As I argue below, these contemporary narratives do not capture the *longue durée* of ruination; inequality, depravation, and dilapidation were built into the new hospitals from the start (Stoler 2008).

THE HOSPITAL IN DEVELOPMENT

By the time another open day was held at the hospital on September 13, 2003, the state of the hospital infrastructure was no cause for celebration. The purpose of the open day, the hospital board argued, was to show the public the "hardships" the hospital was facing.[25] Hospital staff were told they should not try to glamorize the hospital, but should present the difficulties they faced in order to persuade the local community and donors to help. In contrast to 1961, this open day was not organized to show off the hospital's "world-class" facilities. The hospital was not presented as a physical manifestation of a new, modern nation-state. Instead, when the hospital chairman stated that "the hospital development reflects the development of the nation" it was to emphasize that "like the nation the hospital has a long way to go to fulfill its potential and maturity and to serve the community." By 2003 the "failing hospital" in Papua New Guinea, of which Madang Hospital was held to be a prime example, had become an emblem for wider frustrations about the decline of public services, growing inequalities, and large-scale corruption among the political elite.

This discourse of failure resonated with the dominant tropes of the "fragile" or "failed" state that circulated through international development organizations at the time. Papua New Guinea had long been perceived in Australia as a space of weak government, but the language of state failure both intensified and became increasingly technocratic in the aftermath of 9/11, when development became aligned with security in new ways and a political discourse of "state building" emerged, which merged the "security concerns of metropolitan states . . . with the social concerns of aid agencies" (Duffield

2002, 1067). In Australia, PNG's closest neighbor and ex-colonial power, right wing political, academic, and media rhetoric had come to present Papua New Guinea as a problem space where aid money, good intentions, and modern institutions are sucked into a vortex of violence, traditional culture, and corruption. Papua New Guinea, Australian political right wing commentators argued, is a place "on the brink" of state and societal collapse.[26] Like other countries such as Haiti, Somalia, or Afghanistan, Papua New Guinea has become emblematic of what the Comaroffs call a "metaphysics of disorder" that began to color the social imagination at the dawn of the twenty-first century. In this ideological framework, postcolonial nations such as PNG are viewed as Hobbesian spaces of lawlessness and social disorder.

Such views continue to extend deep into the government departments responsible for engagement with Papua New Guinea. In 2009 I spent two months interviewing AusAID workers in Canberra. They strove to distance themselves from right wing rhetoric but nonetheless frequently sought to impress on me that PNG is a "special case" where all attempts at modernization and development fail. "PNG is worse than Afghanistan" was a popular refrain of AusAID workers who had worked there.

Alongside the law-and-order challenges that grabbed headlines abroad, politicians, policymakers, and journalists in Australia and PNG focus on the incapacity of the state to provide basic services, including health care, to its citizens as an important effect of state fragility and a possible further destabilizing factor. That "bare nutrition, no schools or health services, are leading to the spread of malaria, tuberculosis and HIV/AIDS" is listed alongside unemployment as a factor leading to "deep dissatisfaction" which has erupted "in a culture of arms and violence" (Hughes 2003, 2). Health is added to a long list of failures, including the stagnating economy, the lack of transport, and poor access to education, which indicate that "Papua New Guinea is struggling to survive as a viable nation" (Hughes 2003, 2). Health infrastructures such as that of hospitals provide particularly powerful imagery lending communicative force to these ideas. In the reports written by development consultants and the newspaper articles published in the Australian print media a stateless Papua New Guinean landscape is frequently conveyed to readers through the imagery of dilapidated hospitals or rural clinics. These are places, it is implied, where the state is absent and a notion of the public good has collapsed.

Discourses of state failure, originating from academic and political circles in the United States, portray the decline of colonial state institutions such as hospitals to be a function of internal implosion rather than a layered history of colonial and postcolonial intervention. In Papua New Guinea it is argued that a mismatch between traditional political culture and modern political systems and bureaucratic institutions have led to the failure of the latter to function (e.g., Fukuyama 2006, 2007; Reilly 2004), explanations which are also given for state failure more generally (Fukuyama 2004; Rotberg 2004). The ethnic and linguistic diversity of the country, alongside the rough, inhospitable terrain, are routinely invoked as major obstacles to the effective consolidation of the nation-state. Meanwhile the redistribution of resources through loose kinship networks, by which people maintain relationships, alliances, and prestige (dubbed the "wantok system"), is cited as the prime inducement to corruption and inefficiency in the public sector. If the health system established by the Australian colonial state has fallen apart, it goes without saying that this occurred after, and possibly even because of, the departure of the Australian administration.

The failings of Papua New Guinea's hospitals are presented as recent, the result of poor postcolonial governance, and as an imperative for development intervention (as described further in chapter 7).

As Sinclair Dinnen has argued of "failed state" narratives in general, the portrayal of the dilapidated infrastructure of Papua New Guinea's Hospitals to be an effect of state implosion obscures the role of foreign organizations and governments in the restructuring of the health system and the reshaping of hospital infrastructure throughout the postcolonial period. Generic presentations of the hospital as a space of failure also gloss over significant continuities in the kinds of infrastructural inequalities that have been built into hospital space throughout the colonial and postcolonial periods.

At Papua New Guinea's independence in 1975, health was recognized to be crucial to a national agenda for development that emphasized self-reliance and economic autonomy. Development, politicians asserted, should be achieved universally rather than in a piecemeal fashion. A combination of localism and egalitarianism characterized the political rhetoric of the day.[27] Reflecting such values, the 1974 National Health Plan focused on universal access and primary health care while the health workforce was rapidly nationalized.[28] In line with the ideological thrust of independence the highly centralized health system was decentralized and responsibility for rural health care devolved to provincial governments, while hospitals remained directly under the authority of the Ministry of Health.

In fact "self-reliance" amounted to little more than political rhetoric (Amarshi et al. 1979). The Papua New Guinean economy remained highly dependent on foreign investment, foreign-owned businesses, and the export of primary products such as agricultural cash crops and mineral resources. The groundwork for an economic policy based on economic growth rather than fair distribution had been laid out in 1965 by a World Bank mission to the country. In contrast to the policy of "even development" promoted by the Australian administration of the time, the mission report argued that in order "to obtain the maximum benefit from the development effort, expenditures and manpower should be concentrated in areas and on activities where the prospective return is highest." These were to be in the "large areas of good land which are relatively accessible and where development is relatively easy" (Overseas Development Group 1973, 35–36). The same report noted that investments in services such as health were startlingly high and would need to be reined in. It was noted that Papua New Guinean hospitals had more in common "with those found in some countries of Europe than with those found in the less developed countries" (Overseas Development Group 1973). This was seen to be a problem rather than an achievement, and it was stated that standards should be lowered to meet "local conditions." "Uneven development" (Connell 1997), whether manifest in differences between European and Papua New Guinean hospitals or the contrast between urban infrastructure and rural isolation, was construed as the necessary cost of economic growth, now imagined to be the primary aim and purpose of the state.

By the mid-1980s world commodity prices were falling and an economy built on agricultural exports was faltering. In 1989 disaster struck when the Australian-backed gold and copper Panguna mine on Bougainville was closed following sabotage by local landowners and growing conflict in the province. At the time, the mine was providing 40 percent of the country's exports and 17 percent of national revenue. As Bougainville descended into civil war, the costs to the economy in expensive military operations and lost investment fuelled an economic crisis. In 1990, facing a balance of payments shortfall of 75 million Australian dollars, the government was forced to negotiate an emergency "rescue package" with the World Bank and IMF. This first structural adjustment program imposed a K100 million cut (given in the Kina, the PNG currency) in government spending over two years, a 10 percent devaluation of the kina, and substantial cuts in wages.[29] Such policies conformed to the line on deregulation, privatization, and trade liberalization that the World Bank was simultaneously pursuing in other low-income countries. In the Papua New Guinean health sector it meant a substantial cut in human resources and recurrent funding.

Despite some economic growth in the early 1990s following the opening of new mineral resource projects at Ok Tedi, Kutubu, and Misima, unemployment remained high, imports of foreign goods were expensive, and government departments became unable to meet expenditure commitments. By 1994 they had run out of foreign exchange reserves, which prompted a further devaluation of the Kina and a freeze on all public expenditure. The government was forced to turn again to the World Bank and the IMF, who provided another A$550 million loan—and accompanying structural adjustment program.[30]

Curiously, the 1995 loan agreement demanded that the government *increase* spending on health, which, along with education, was seen as a major impediment to economic growth (World Bank 1995, 5). Yet, contradicting this demand, the loan conditions also required reform of the public sector, including substantial cuts in human resources and government "consumption" (recurrent expenditure). The public service was depicted as overblown and inefficient. "Good" investment in health was therefore restricted to infrastructure projects and, in practice, this meant an increase in the local politician "slush funds" through which such projects were funded, at the expense of recurrent health budgets (Curtin 2000). Two hundred jobs in the Department of Health were cut, mostly in drug procurement, and strict ceilings were placed on recurrent spending. In 1973 there were close to six thousand centrally funded health officers. By 1998 there were only 4,453. At the same time the population requiring health services was growing and hospital usage was increasing.[31] In 1999 recurrent spending was limited to K2.57 million, and the World Bank set the goal for health spending at 8 percent of this figure (Curtin 2000, 9). Rural areas took the brunt of these reforms, but hospital budgets were also cut and the supply of drugs affected.

These changes in health financing had a profound effect on the spatial organization of hospital infrastructure and the kinds of publics these infrastructures were imagined to serve. This was nowhere more clear than in the emergence of the Papua New Guinean consumer of hospital medicine. By the 1990s hospitals, whose administration under the system of decentralization was entirely isolated from the provincial rural health services, were being restructured in line with models of marketization and a shift in responsibility for services from the government to users.[32] The World Bank recommended "cost recovery" through the imposition of user fees,[33] which were introduced in the 1991–95 National Health Plan (NDOH 1991).[34] Meanwhile, the 1994 Public Hospitals Act transformed the structure of the institution in line with managerial models from business and enterprise. Medical directors were replaced with management trained chief executive officers, and the hospital executives were overseen by a Hospital Board, made up of prominent local business people and community leaders. To inspire economic efficiency and interinstitution competition, hospitals were encouraged to raise their own revenue through user-fees and donor funding.[35]

The new infrastructural inequalities that accompanied this reimagining of the public hospital were made vividly apparent at the 2003 open day. At this event the staff who provided the open day tours to members of the public illustrated their own sense of hardship and state-neglect through the staging of a stark contrast between the hospital's private and public wards. The hospital's private ward is part of a new concrete building, established in 1995 with funds from the Japanese government. The ward was mapped directly onto the site of the old European ward, which had been moved down the hill to the main block in the late 1960s, when the separation of the European and native wings had become politically unsustainable. This was still where the expatriate residents in the town came for their medical care, but most of the patients were now Papua New Guineans who worked in the public service or local businesses. The ward was air-conditioned, and the cool air immediately hit you as you walked in from the humid corridor outside. Patients usually had a room to themselves, but if the ward was full, each bed had a curtain rail around their bed that carved a large private space out of the room for their own use. The ward was decorated with a shiny light beige floor, glossy painted white walls, Formica surfaces, patterned soft furnishings and fresh flowers. Here, as in the European ward of the postwar hospital, the organization of space afforded individual care.

"This is where you come if you have money" announced the medical student as he guided the public tour into the room. "A lot of money," said the nurse on duty and everyone laughed. The medical student showed the visitors the sliding doors that separate the ward into four separate rooms, enabling the nurses to quarantine patients or separate out male and female patients. "Here," he explains "the patients stay on their own [*stap wan wan*]." One member of the audience asked how much it cost and was told 200 Kina (around US$80) for the first three days and 60 kina a day after this. Several of the visitors gasped and exhaled loudly. The nurses nodded dramatically in sympathy.

The tour continued from the private ward to the public wards at the back of the hospital. These had changed little since the hospital had opened in 1961. They consisted of long timber sheds with the walls above shoulder height covered in gauze to facilitate air flow. Shielded from the sea breeze by a small incline, the wards were hot and stifling. Dust and noise from the road swept straight into the buildings and few of the fans in any of the wards were working. The wards were connected by covered concrete walkways. Here in the shade sat patients and relatives finding respite from the heat of the wards, sometimes talking to one another, more often sitting in silence as they watched the doctors and nurses walking backward and forward between the wards.

The tour group walked along the corridor and was guided by the medical student into the wards themselves. The walls of the wards were lined by a long row of beds, each with a number hanging above it. The beds were old rusted steel contraptions, most with plastic mattresses placed on top. As the tour was guided down the aisle, the audience members stared silently at the patients receiving care in their beds. This, not the private ward, was the place they knew they would come to should they get sick.

The nurses' portrayal of hospital infrastructure as a register for state failure departed in significant ways from the development discourse of postcolonial decline. Madang Hospital has never been one place; neither the care administered in it nor the bodies made visible through its practice have ever been of a single kind. Even when, in the postwar era, native and European hospitals were supposedly combined into a single public hospital, they in fact retained different wards with different resources, and that made different kinds of bodies visible. The differences that nurses highlighted between the private and public wards in Madang Hospital illustrate the continued significance of those architectural and administrative divisions in the present day. This was emphasized, for example, when, following the tour of the public and private wards the guides pointed out the old European hospital building, now the provincial health administration, to their groups and explained the old divisions that existed between the care provided for "whites" and that for "natives" (see Street 2012).

In Madang Hospital's private ward no doctor has privileged authority, and the hospital's consultants must collaborate with one another in the management of an individual body. A diabetic patient with an infected sore on their foot will, for example, be seen by doctors on both the surgical and medical ward rounds after they have finished the round in their respective wards. The doctors will need to communicate in person, or through the patient chart, on the treatment decisions made about the patient's care: for example, whether surgical intervention will be needed, how frequently the blood sugar should be measured, and what medications should be given. In the private ward a single patient is a point of focus for multiple experts.

In the public wards, by contrast, the ratio of patients to doctors is reversed. In the medical ward in 2003, for example, forty patients were cared for by a single doctor, who was not yet qualified as a consulting physician. The medical doctor might invite the consultant surgeon to look at a diabetic patient's sore, but they would not automatically be seen by a variety of specialists. In fact doctors are hesitant and often unwilling to look at patients in other wards for fear they might accrue responsibility for patients they consider lost causes. The private ward was organized according to divisions between individuals rather than professional specialisms. In the public wards, meanwhile, to be sent to the wrong ward on admission, a not infrequent mistake, could be potentially life threatening. In these spaces, as I describe in chapter 4, the ability to differentiate individual bodies and diseases is severely hampered by the resources available, and a different kind of biomedical practice becomes necessary; one focused on the "generally sick" rather than the individually diseased body.

CONCLUSION

This chapter has explored the connections between the construction of specialized medical institutions and the reorganization of "social space" by examining the different kinds of state-society relations that were envisaged and built into the emerging country's medical infrastructure alongside new kinds of medical objects. Hospitals in colonial and postcolonial Papua New Guinea consistently remained at the center of public health policies and I have suggested that this is in part because of their powerful role as spatial technologies for reconfiguring relationships between state, society, and territory.

In a place where the existence and the efficacy of the state has never been taken for granted, hospitals have been vital technologies by which the state was made visible to others and thus by which the public and the state have been brought into relationship to one another. For colonial administrators, hospitals were crucial spaces in which new Papua New Guinean publics would be summoned into being. As manifestations of state power and beneficence and demonstrations of modernity and progress, the planned hospitals were to interpolate Papua New Guineans into a new state-society relationship that would bind them to the development of a wider social collective and transform them into modern citizens. The hospital network would simultaneously establish a statewide medical system and create the public that it was to service and govern. The anticipated transformative capacities of the hospital were directed outward to the creation of a new territorial space inhabited by a new "developing" Papua New Guinean public, rather than inward toward the medical governance of individual diseased bodies. Just as hospitals were icons of state visibility for a newly politicized postwar Australian public, so they were significant for their demonstration of state and medical powers to, as opposed to their governance of, the public they were intended to interpolate.

By contrast with their design by Australia's colonial visionaries and bureaucrats, contemporary political discourse identifies hospitals as spaces of failure and postcolonial decline, places where state-society relations have dissolved and where the lives of Papua New Guinean subjects are needlessly lost. Such narratives of decline nostalgically presume that a perfect and ideal modern state was in place at the time of independence (Dinnen 2004; see also Morgan and McLeod, 2006). They paper over the questions that were raised about the adequacy of Papua New Guinea's colonial hospitals long before independence in 1975 and render invisible the ongoing, successive interventions of foreign agencies and governments, which have continued to shape state institutions such as hospitals ever since. Instead public sector failure is presented as a Papua New Guinean trait to which ongoing development interventions are external (see also Ferguson 1990). By contrast with the discourse of decline and state failure, this chapter has outlined a very different dynamic of institutional ruination. The state is not so much absent from the hospital, rather the hospital is a crucial space where the state has been reimagined and institutionally reconfigured in the course of rapid political and economic upheaval and change (Greenhouse 2002).

A focus on hospital building as state building attends to the public futures that are anticipated through such building projects and the centrality of hospitals to the development of state systems of governance, as opposed to the reading of hospital spaces as material condensations of a state power that is already given (Carroll 2006). To examine the ongoing role of hospitals in state building complicates descriptions of colonial medicine that depict medical institutions as having contributed to effective colonial governance in Papua New Guinea and elsewhere and draws attention to the incompleteness of the state-building project in Papua New Guinea and other places of development.

The kinds of nation-state that are being built in these hospitals, and the kinds of publics that they are imagined to serve, also delimit the kinds of bodies that can be made visible within them. In the postwar hospital building, the "development" of the minds and bodies of the Papua New Guinean population became inextricable from the etching of new medical technologies and monumental public buildings onto the Papua New

Guinean landscape. Here, the project of building the state by rendering it visible became entwined with the colonial state's project of visualizing and regulating its subjects. Nonetheless, the subjects that were made visible to a state and medical gaze in this institution differed little from those of the earlier colonial period. Ideas about racial difference and the need for segregation continued to provide a framework for hospital design. The public wards where new Papua New Guinean subjects lay may have had greater resources and more doctors than the prewar establishments, but their spatial organization was very similar.

Throughout Madang Hospital's history, we can apprehend spaces of individualized care on the one hand, and spaces of generalized care on the other, spaces where the individual body and its diseases are made visible, and spaces where the resources to diagnose and attend to the individual diseased body are not available. Where these differences were once produced through the idiom of race, in the new corporate hospital they are reproduced through the mapping of emerging class relations onto public and private space. The three chapters in the next section examine the experience of this space and the biomedical uncertainty produced within it by doctors and patients in the hospital as they strive to engage productively with its biomedical technologies and transform themselves into new kinds of person.

PART II ■ TECHNOLOGY

CHAPTER 4

Doctors without Diagnosis

■ In the medical ward Dr. Bosa was looking at a new admission, Daniel, who had arrived from the Rai Coast, a remote part of the province only accessible by boat. Daniel had been ill for several weeks, but it had taken a long time for the family to raise the money to transport him to the hospital. Like many patients from remote parts of the province, by the time Daniel arrived at the hospital his condition was severe. The outpatient notes stated that on admission Daniel was confused, had abdominal edema, a swollen spleen, and signs of anemia and fever. There was no diagnosis, only several differential diagnoses of severe malaria, meningitis, rheumatic heart disease, and, even less specifically, "infection." Dr. Bosa told Daniel to lie down and began a physical examination, looking under the eyelids for signs of anemia, listening to the chest with his stethoscope, palpating his abdomen. The patient is clearly "very sick" he told me solemnly, "but at this point it is difficult to say exactly what he has." Because severe malaria is so common in the province, Daniel was put on antimalarials straightaway at the Outpatients Department. In addition Dr. Bosa now ordered a blood transfusion. Without a clear diagnosis, he would have to watch carefully over the next few days to see whether Daniel improved or whether further interventions were necessary. He passed by the nurses' office on the way out to tell the officer in charge that Daniel was on hourly observations.

Later, I talked to the registrar in the surgical ward, Dr. Kalim, about why he had abandoned internal medicine as a specialism: "I don't find internal medicine satisfying because it is so difficult to make a diagnosis. Patients stay in the ward for a long time. There is no quick treatment and discharge, and so often your patients die. There is no completion. It is depressing because people are often generally sick with a lot of things—you can't just treat a specific problem and they will get better. The difference between those who want to be surgeons and those who want to be physicians is between those who get a kick out of treating a patient and watching them get better and leave, and those who get a kick out of the diagnostic process itself."

The representation of biomedicine as an essentially diagnostic endeavor, one based on the pursuit of scientific truth, is also widespread in the social sciences. It underpins Foucault's account of pathological anatomy and the locus of disease in the body's invisible interior. It also runs through the distinctions that anthropologists draw between the practices of "traditional medicine" and those of "biomedicine," where the latter is defined by its orientation toward the creation of classificatory knowledge as opposed to healthy persons.[1] In both professional and social scientific representations, internal medicine is understood to be primarily about making disease visible.

So what happens when disease is not made visible and knowable? When bodies like Daniel's remain opaque and their invisible interiors are not made visible to the expert eye? By contrast with representations of internal medicine as a quest for epistemological certainty, this chapter describes the routinization of uncertainty in the medical ward of Madang Hospital and the ways in which the kinds of knowledge practices that emerge in the institution destabilize associations between knowledge, disease, and diagnosis.

In the medical ward, doctors struggle to make opaque bodies visible and knowable with inadequate resources. Here, I argue, biomedical knowledge practices, and ancillary modes of relating to diagnostic technologies, do not bring about diagnostic closure. Instead a very different temporal dynamic of knowledge emerges that entails a different relationship to technology and the enactment (Mol 2002) of a different kind of biological body. In this clinical space, the contingency of medical fact becomes a productive end in itself and the open-endedness of the diagnostic process gives rise to more pragmatic forms of medical practice and more modest modes of expert personhood. Within Madang Hospital doctors claim this kind of medicine is superior to that found in Western textbooks. But they must also accommodate themselves to the fact that beyond Madang Hospital this kind of medicine has no legitimacy or authority at all; their Papua New Guinean expertise is entirely confined to place.

In the corner of the outpatients courtyard the hospital clerk, Fran, sat behind a small metal-barred window. In 2003 it was to Fran that patients were to pay their fees and give their clinic books before being seen by a doctor. There was no formal triage system, but Fran liked to take a good look at the patients' pallor and demeanor as they lined up and arranged the pile of clinic books accordingly. Here bureaucratic expertise segued into biomedical assessment.

The prospective patients were sent to sit on the long wooden benches in the courtyard. From here they could see through louvered windows into the small cubicles that had been built into the adjacent corridor and could hear snippets of conversation as other patients were examined. When a cubicle became free Fran called out the name on the next clinic book in her pile. There was much movement and bustle as patients crowded around the window and strained to hear what she was saying. There was often some confusion as to which name had been called and waiting patients were anxious they would miss their turn. Sometimes fights broke out. At other times patients were caught sneaking through the heavy sprung door next to the clerk's window trying to get ahead of the queue.

Inside the crowded cubicle Harry, a white-coated health extension officer in his early twenties, met the patient and their relatives.[2] The patient was invited to sit on a small plastic stool while Harry read their referral letter and the clinic book entry from the health center where they were originally seen. The questions he put to them would already be familiar from that first biomedical encounter and the answers had an abrupt, rehearsed, feel to them. "How long have you been sick?" "What are your symptoms?" The replies: "Two weeks." "Short of breath."

The medical history was a rushed affair; Harry could see the waiting patients peering and chattering through the louvers outside. Besides, he complained, new patients, especially if they have traveled from remote villages, are intimidated by the institutional environment and scared about what will happen to them there. One-word answers are whispered onto the floor. Even if he had time, he explained, he would never be able to elicit a proper personal and family medical history here.

The medical history might have little epistemological value but Harry used the opportunity to observe the patient's pallor, how well they could sit on the stool or whether they must lie on the plastic bench squeezed into the side of the cubicle, whether they could speak for themselves or must have a relative to speak for them, how comfortable they looked, and whether they had any visible symptoms or physical disfigurement. "Look at the hands and eyes to see if they are yellow, at the skin to see if it is hydrated." In many cases it was on the basis of these general observations that Harry must decide whether to admit the patient.

Once he had decided to make an admission Harry reached for a yellow cardboard admissions folder and fixed a piece of plain paper inside. He did not want to waste paper on a patient who would not be admitted. In that case they would simply write a summary of the examination in the clinic book and send the patient home after treatment. If the clinic book records the individual's trajectory through rural and urban medical institutions and charts those patient-clinic encounters against their personal biography, the writing of the patient's name on the front of the medical chart marks the start of their institutional biography. Harry hurriedly wrote up a summary of the history he had taken so far and attached the paper with the referral letter, if there was one, to the chart.

He asked the patient to lie down flat on the bed. The hospital did not have any prewritten admission forms for Harry to fill in, but he had memorized the international standard for writing up an examination, which he now replicated in tiny handwriting on a single piece of the hospital's scrap paper, folded into four to save space. First Harry checked the "vitals": the temperature, blood pressure, pulse, and respiratory rate. Then he checked the central nervous system: Is the patient dizzy? Conscious? Alert? Next he checked the cardiovascular system. He looked at the patients' fingertips to see if they had become clubbed, he checked for swelling in the legs and arms, and listened to their heart sounds with a stethoscope. Then the respiratory system. He used the stethoscope to listen for crepitation in the chest. He palpated the patient's abdomen, feeling for an enlargement of the liver, kidneys or spleen, watching for any "guarding" by the patient, a sure sign of pain. He listened for bowel movement with the stethoscope and looked for distension. He checked the musculoskeletal system by flexing the limbs and he asked the patient to push against his palm to check for resistance. This standardized process of looking, feeling, and writing reproduces a textbook "anatomical geography . . . that fleshes out a map to the terrain that is hidden under the skin" (Berg and Bowker 1997, 518). If necessary small diagrams were made inside the admissions folder—for example, where crepitations were heard in the chest, or a mass was felt in the abdomen. Sometimes, however, much to the frustration of ward doctors who would later read the chart, Harry forgot important categories or observations were missed out. In Madang Hospital the anatomical body is peppered with holes.

At the bottom of the page, Harry wrote a list of further investigations to be carried out, such as laboratory tests and X-rays. Underneath these was written a preliminary diagnosis. Very often this was not known and instead Harry wrote a series of two or three differential diagnoses. Sometimes he wrote several preliminary diagnoses and several differential diagnoses. This is a crucial moment in the patient's trajectory through the hospital for it is on this basis that the patient is allocated to a ward. When a patient is sent to the medical ward or surgical ward this determines the kind of biomedical gaze he will be subjected to and the kinds of interventions that are possible. Sometimes doctors later realize that a patient has been sent to the wrong ward; that they would, for example, be better off in surgery. But once they have been admitted, patients seldom move between wards. Chronic bed shortages mean doctors are reluctant to take on extra patients who have already been placed, particularly patients with hazy diagnoses for whom it seems little can be done. Patients who are sent to the "wrong" ward frequently fall through the gaps of professional specialization (Gibson 2004).

THE PATHOLOGY SHED

From the cubicle, the patient moves to the main Accident and Emergency room where a nurse sticks various needles in their arms, extracts fluids, bottles them, labels them with the patient name and ward number, and sends them via a student to the laboratory. In the laboratory, a small prefabricated shed in the middle of the hospital grounds, the technicians begin to work their way through the pile of sample bottles and test forms that rapidly build up through the course of the morning in the hope of getting through the load before lunch. Sometimes those tests that are not finished before lunch will not be completed until the next day.

In 2003, at one end of the room, where a neat space on the worktop had been cleared for a microscope and log book, Ann, the provincial microscopist sat with her head down, peering through the viewfinder at a blood slide. Each slide is stained with a blue Giemsa stain that makes the malaria parasites visible to the human eye when placed under the microscope. The microscope lens has a grid with a hundred fields engraved onto it. Ann's job was to identify the kind and number of parasites visible per a hundred fields. The trouble, she explained, is sometimes parasites are present in the blood but not in the small sample visible in her grid. Parasites outside the grid are not seen or counted. Sometimes patients had already received treatment, which had broken up some of the parasites so they were no longer visible, but they had not been completely eliminated from the blood. Given the chances of a false negative result, Ann was aware that the doctors might ignore the results altogether.

Ann had worked as an assistant on a medical research project run by an Australian scientist, who had taught her a different algorithm for counting the malaria parasites, which was meant to be more effective, and was now being recommended by the WHO. In the new system they did not count the number of parasites per field but the number of parasites for every two hundred white blood cells viewed. The research scientists had taught her how to use a mathematical formula to work out the number of parasites per deciliter. But this technique took up to five minutes longer per slide. As the only malaria microscopist for the entire hospital Ann would simply fail to get through her workload if she used this technique for her public patients (Ann usually needed to get through around seventy blood slides a day). She was thinking of just counting the number of parasites per two hundred white blood cells without the mathematical formula. Even this would take longer, though. After counting the parasites the usual way, Ann filled in her log book, copied the entry onto the test request form and sent it to the ward.

GENERALLY SICK

From Accident and Emergency the patient is wheeled by his relatives along the hospital's covered concrete walkways, past green lawns where patients dry their laundry, and into the medical ward. Their relatives carry string bags full of clothes, bedding, and cooking equipment. As the patient leaves behind the blazing sun and enters the dark enclosure of the ward building the other patients and relatives sitting on the closely aligned beds fall silent. They watch as the patient is wheeled down the aisle to the nurses' office, which lies between the acute and chronic sides of the ward.

Here a nurse glances over the admission file and allocates the patient to a bed, where the patient will wait for the doctor to see them. Which bed they are allocated will determine how much nursing care they will receive and how closely they will be observed. Beds 1–3, which are directly in front of the window onto the nurses' office are for "full nursing care" and are given to the "very sick ones." As the numbers trace the distance from the nurses' office the nurses' assessment of the patient's condition recedes from "very sick" to "a little sick." Those who are placed on the other side of the ward, in beds 11–20, are not thought by the nurses to be at immediate risk of dying. They are on their way out, either toward the chronic ward or discharge. As the doctor is usually absent at admission, the nurse makes her own assessment on where to place the patient, based on what she reads in the medical chart and "how sick the patient looks."

After lunch the doctor comes to check for new admissions. It is in this moment, in the slow haze of the afternoon, that the hospital's equipment and expertise becomes most clearly focused on the patient body as a site of potential diagnosis. The doctor reads through the admission notes, often muttering about their incomprehensibility or the mistakes that have been made in the write up. Now he takes out a fresh piece of paper and begins again. He asks the same questions for the medical history and progresses through the same series of bodily systems for the physical examination. Again the patient's answers take a rehearsed tone. But more time is given to the examination here than in the admissions cubicle. Now the doctor is also able to look at the X-ray and the laboratory results if they have arrived. Sometimes the clinical, pathological, and imaging diagnostic findings back each other up. They are aligned in a single diagnosis (Mol 2002, 57) and "jointly enact a common object" (Mol 2002, 61). Sometimes, for example, a patient's medical history of rapid weight loss and cough and the crepitation the doctor hears in the lungs with the aid of his stethoscope are aligned with the tuberculosis revealed in small white spots on the X-ray image of the patient's lungs and a sputum sample examined under a microscope. In a case like this, clinical, pathological, and radiographic versions of disease are aligned, making tuberculosis visible and stabilizing it as a disease object. The doctors like these patients. They allow for clear, focused, intervention: intervention that corresponded to a diagnosis.

But many patient bodies fail to present with such clarity. Imaging technologies in Madang Hospital do not always provide a clear visualization of internal disease. The blurred images produced by the hospital's X-ray machine are often intensely frustrating. Doctors and visiting medical students from Australia complained about X-ray images being distorted or damaged by the use of poor quality film or the lack of chemicals to use in the film's development. "You might think this is miliary TB because there are white dots covering the lungs" Dr. Masib told me, "but in fact that is from the chemicals they are using. It is a bad picture. You can tell because the white flecks are also outside the body. I asked the technician what was wrong and he was told it was short of chemicals." "I can't see anything in them," said the Australian medical student visiting for his elective. "The problem with medical students is that they cannot distinguish between the patient's condition and the quality of the film. There is no radiologist here—that is a real problem."

Ultrasound scanning is accompanied by similar problems. In 2003, Dr. Bosa struggled to read scans of livers and other organs. "I have no experience. I can't tell whether it is part of the liver I am looking at or just an effect of the machine." Doctors are often unable to affect a penetrative expert gaze. The internal states of patient bodies remain invisible. Even when internal organs and cavities are exposed in X-ray images or ultrasound scans, the effects of disease are indistinguishable from that of the technology itself (cf. Akrich 1994, 218). Knowledge cannot be disaggregated from its process of production. Here diagnostic facts remain unstable and unbracketed.[3]

Over the course of my relationship with Madang Hospital it has been the inability of the laboratory to carry out basic tests, more than anything else, that doctors have said makes it impossible to diagnose patients. Doctors cannot trust laboratory results because they are not sure the machines have been properly calibrated or that the reagents have been kept at the correct temperatures amidst the frequent black outs. When they do manage to get a sample and test request form to the laboratory, they are often sent back because the reagents that the technicians needed are delayed somewhere in the medical supply chain. The laboratory technicians, who are overworked and have few promotional opportunities, are slow to carry out urgent tests. Doctors have to be especially persuasive and attentive if they wanted a particular test to get done quickly. Sometimes they have to improvise (Wendland 2010; Livingston 2012) and take on the role of the laboratory technician themselves. In one case in 2004, when the laboratory claimed they were unable to carry out a test for cryptococcal (fungal) meningitis because they did not have the correct dye, Dr. Bosa walked into town to the local stationary shop to buy some calligraphy ink and carried out the test in the ward office himself.

Sometimes the test results from the laboratory fail to arrive in time for the ward admission. Maybe the laboratory technician hasn't got to that sample yet. Maybe he is still frustrated with the way the medical doctor spoke to him last week and is leaving that ward's tests until last. Maybe he is still at lunch break. In those cases diagnostic resources are temporally and spatially misaligned. The doctor can only look at the test results on ward round the next day, but then he will have far less time to consider how they align with his clinical knowledge. The work of laboratory pathology in Madang Hospital does not provide a more fundamental medical knowledge than clinical work; its results are not apprehended as closer to the truth of disease and frequently produce uncertainty and unclear bodies.

The bodies can also themselves be obstructive to the biomedical gaze. Doctors complain that many patients who arrive at the hospital are already so sick they have generalized symptoms. Some are febrile, some are vomiting, some are comatose. This was how Dr. Bosa described Daniel. He was not sure what exactly was wrong with Daniel. The investigations that were made on Daniel's admission showed that Daniel was severely anemic. The malaria test was positive, but the parasites were not at a high density. Moreover, malaria is so endemic this does not exclude the possibility of another coexisting disease. Different diagnostic findings do not cohere into a single object.

The first line of action in such "generally sick" cases is always antimalarials. These are usually given after a blood slide is taken but before the result is received from the laboratory. Clinical knowledge takes precedence over pathological or imaging knowledge.[4] Dr. Wali, the registrar in the pediatric ward, which faced similar challenges, explained the dilemmas that accompany the treatment of "generally sick" patients:

A patient came in. They had fever and they were crying a lot and had irritability. That was all. They weren't having convulsions or showing signs of the Central Nervous System. We are unable to do LPs here.[5] So we have to think of malaria. But the blood slide was negative. So then we put them on chloramphenicol. This is the first line drug. We also treated them for malaria. The blood slide was negative but it had a fever so we treated them anyway. That is the diagnosis dilemma. It could be malaria or meningitis. So we just cover for both. If the blood slide was positive we would have put them on antimalarials alone. If they got better then we would know it was malaria. These are the problems that we have. After forty-eight hours the child was doing a lot better. We are happy that we know we are dealing with it.

Often the bodies that are made visible at the intersection of bureaucratic and biomedical technologies in the hospital are not individuated biological bodies, distinguished and categorized by the diseases they suffer from, but what doctors call "generally sick." Action cannot simply follow on from diagnosis in such cases. Intervening in the "generally sick" patient is a much more murky affair.

Sometimes, moreover, the doctor is not the one doing the diagnostic work. In 2003, the ward was staffed by a single registrar, Dr. Bosa. Dr. Bosa was unable to complete his specialist training because there was no physician available to supervise him. Similarly residents could not be placed in the ward for lack of supervision. This meant that Dr. Bosa was essentially running a forty-bed ward single-handedly, with the assistance of a resident health extension officer, Eric, who was also completing his training before going to work in a rural health center. Health extension officers are trained to deal with simple medical problems in a rural context and to be able to clinically diagnose and refer complex cases to the hospital. Dr. Bosa worked hard but he was exhausted by his workload. He did the work of a consultant but felt this went unrecognized by the fully qualified consultants working in the neighboring wards, who looked down on him as a junior doctor. Sometimes he did not turn up after lunch. Sometimes he was away at conferences or training events in Port Moresby. At those times, Eric had to do the ward admission. Frequently, he admitted, he was stumped. If the HEO in the rural health clinic that referred the patient could not diagnose them, why would he be able to do a better job during his residential training?

BED TRAJECTORIES

Once the moment of admission has passed, the patient becomes absorbed into the daily routine of the ward, which is organized around the regular dispensing of medicine, nursing care, meal times, washing, and visits from family. The doctor is largely absent from much of this routine, attending consultation clinics elsewhere in the hospital or doing paperwork in his office. For most of the day the ward is the domain of the nursing staff, the patients, and their relatives.

For patients in beds 1–3 nurses must take hourly observations of vital signs, including pulse, temperature, and blood pressure. These are written onto graphs that sit in a small plastic slot at the end of the bed so as to be available for the doctor to look at when he returns to the ward. These observations also inform the nurses' perceptions of "how well the patient is doing" and whether, for example, they might be moved along the row of beds to a number a little further away from the nurses' office and, by implication, the possibility of death. At the end of each shift the officer in charge writes a report for each bed number and reads it out for the incoming shift:

Bed 2. Woke up early, gained consciousness but still confused, walked around. Condition stable. Hasn't eaten anything.

Bed 4. Had chest X-ray. No sign of TB. Fainted. Under observation. Had fever. She has been bedridden all morning.

Bed 5. New admission. Second grade malaria. Fully conscious but she looks pale. But she is still walking about. X-ray her tomorrow.

Bed 6. Remains much the same [the other nurse tuts] pale. Dehydrated. At first took offence if you went near her, but now less so. Not eating well.

Bed 7. She's up and about. No complaints this morning.

Bed 8. New admission.

Bed 9. Fully conscious, alert. But sleepy. Collect blood for hb test.

Bed 10. Sick looking. Complains of dizziness. Sleeps all day. Got a drip 4 percent extra.

Bed 11. Waiting for results of blood test. Continue treatment while awaiting blood. Hope relatives will donate.

Bed 12. Slept till 6 then got up and told story to me about his niece. I took him to the toilet. He ate and drank.

Bed 13. Snake bite. Quiet. Up and about. No complaints. But still pale so continue treatment.

Bed 14. He keeps bending over. They told his relatives he should straighten out but they just said this is how he is comfortable.

Bed 15. Waiting for drug transfusion. Sick looking, pale, wasted.

Bed 16. Our friend Rose. We thought her name was Anna because she kept writing Anna on her forms, but then she insisted her name was Rose. Turns out she was writing her sister-in-law's name on them. Need to collect forms back from pathology otherwise they will be looking for Anna, then we can do the blood transfusion. Think someone donated this morning. Quiet morning. Confined to bed, too dizzy to walk around.

Bed 17. Mobilizing. No complaint.

The observations in the report focus on practicalities; whether the patient has eaten anything, whether they have passed feces, whether they took or refused their medicine, whether they are mobile, whether they are talking to the relatives or to the staff. A patient's practical actions are combined with observations of their pallor and inform a judgment about whether the patient is "very sick" or is "getting better," which is written in the notes. The notes might also include information on a change in bed number according

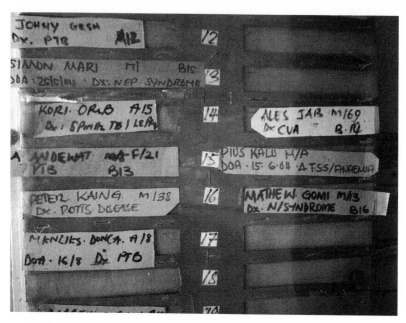

4.1. Medical ward map, used to identify patients with beds for purposes of care and treatment.

to whether the patient is considered to be getting worse and needs to move closer to the nurses' office for closer observation or is getting better and can be moved further down the ward.

This ordering of patient trajectories is facilitated by important but simple bureaucratic technologies such as the ward chart, a long piece of cardboard covered in plastic that provides a rudimentary map of the ward's beds. Next to each hand-scrawled bed number is a space where a slip of paper bearing a patient's name can be slotted in between the cardboard and plastic. When the patient moves to another bed, the slip of paper can be moved around accordingly (see figure 4.1). Such devices are crucial for ensuring the correct patient body is aligned with the correct bed number. With so much movement around the ward it is on this system that, for example, the correct allocation of treatment depends.

BROAD-SPECTRUM PHARMACEUTICALS

At 9:00 AM, two days after Daniel's admission to the ward, Dr. Bosa prepared to carry out his daily round of the ward's patients. The nurses shouted at the relatives to leave. With several relatives often sharing the bed with the patient it is crucial that at ward round a single bed number is aligned with a single body rather than, as in the rest of the day, a highly flexible family unit. Dr. Bosa piled the medical charts, X-rays, and the folder of treatment charts onto the ward round trolley, which he wheeled between each bed. The trolley also contains copies of laboratory request forms and sample bottles, which can be pulled out of their slots on the trolley at each patient's bedside.

At bed number 4, Dr. Bosa paused. Daniel was lying on his bed, barely moving. The antimalarials had not worked. After a brief examination and a short exchange with Daniel's wife, who told him that Daniel had not eaten or passed urine, Dr. Bosa decided to put Daniel on chloramphenicol, in case of meningitis.

One of the first broad-spectrum antibiotics to come onto global markets in 1949, chloramphenicol is no longer used in much of the Western world because of its potential adverse side effects and growing bacterial resistance. But in 2003 it was the first-line treatment for bacterial meningitis in Papua New Guinea.[6] In the medical ward Dr. Bosa explained that they used it all the time. While it was the first-line treatment for meningitis, chloramphenicol was also effective against other unspecified bacterial infections in "generally sick" patients: "This will cover a wide spectrum—meningitis, malaria, and typhoid. This is just a precaution because we don't really know what she has but we need to treat her quickly."[7] However, growing resistance to the drug also meant it was difficult for doctors to know whether the drug or diagnosis were at fault when the patient failed to recover.

Often Dr. Bosa explained, he didn't have much choice. Chloramphenicol is much more affordable than other more specific antibiotics and is ordered by the Department of Health in Papua New Guinea, as in many developing countries, in large supplies. Indeed, despite growing evidence of resistance to chloramphenicol in hemophilis influenza meningitis infections, it took a long time to change the standard guidelines (eventually changed in 2009), and even longer to change clinical practice, precisely because the alternative drug on the market, ceftriaxone is much more expensive and subject to delays in supply. The hospital is always more likely to have chloramphenicol than ceftriaxone in stock.

At ward round a few days later, Daniel was looking much better. He was sitting up in his bed and talking lucidly. His wife was smiling widely. Daniel grabbed Dr. Bosa's hand and shook it vigorously, thanking him for saving his life. Dr. Bosa removed his hand calmly and told Daniel to lie down. "Save your thanks until you are discharged," he said grimly.

"He looks like he is getting better," he told me later. "We don't know why. Is it because of the antimalarials or the antibiotics? I think it is the chloramphenicol. He had severe anemia, which made him susceptible to infection and the antibiotics killed it off. But we don't know what the infection was. We can't do the tests to find out so we just treated him." Dr. Bosa was very excited that Daniel was improving, "This is a day that makes me happy to be a doctor." But he didn't want to celebrate too soon. Daniel still had a low-grade fever and abdominal swelling. He was still very weak.

Sure enough, only two days later Daniel had begun to deteriorate again. He had difficulty passing water. His hemoglobin levels had dropped dangerously low. He had become increasingly confused. He still had swelling of the abdomen and legs and he was having difficulty eating. For several days Dr. Bosa persisted with the antibiotics and antimalarials. But after a further week of treatment Daniel failed to improve. Now Dr. Bosa decided to put Daniel on TB treatment.

If a patient neither recovers nor dies in the first few days in the medical ward, Dr. Bosa always considered tuberculosis. Tuberculosis, he explained, could take many forms and is very difficult to diagnose. Someone with tuberculosis of the brain could show the same symptoms as someone with bacterial meningitis, or someone with tuberculosis of the abdomen could show the same symptoms as someone with liver cirrhosis. Antibiotic treatment for tuberculosis became a default treatment for patients who did not recover on broad-spectrum antibiotics and antimalarials. Doctors are well aware of the side effects that accompany all of these drugs but argue that they cannot consider such issues when they are fighting against time to save lives. Bodies are deteriorating in front of their eyes, demanding intervention, and only certain options are available.

After two weeks on TB treatment Daniel was moved from bed 13, on the opposite side of the ward back to bed 4. This was a bad sign. These are the beds where nurses and doctors say they have to expect that the patient may die. Daniel wasn't getting better on TB treatment. At ward round Dr. Bosa looked at his hands and put them next to his own. They were very pale. He said he would check Daniel's blood and try to organize another transfusion. He wasn't sure where the blood would come from. Daniel's relatives had already come to donate and he didn't have any more *wantok* in the town to help out. Dr. Bosa said he would have to call around the wards and ask if any of the staff were willing to donate their blood.[8]

Sometimes the work that the doctor does on ward round is diagnostic work. He or she wonders whether a patient is suffering from fungal rather than bacterial meningitis and orders an Indian ink stain. A second X-ray has arrived, which is much clearer than the first, and clearly shows an enlarged heart. He or she might order further investigations; for example another malaria test for a young married man who presents with severe fever and is deteriorating despite a negative test on admission; or liver function tests for a patient who has not improved on antimalarials and antibiotics, which is later returned by the laboratory because they don't have the correct reagents. But the majority of ward round work is not diagnostic work. In the back of the medical chart the doctor writes the date and underneath scrawls a terse summary of how the patient is doing: "looking better"; "looking worse." Like the nurses, their concern is whether the patient is improving or getting worse; whether further intervention is necessary. As Doctor Bosa put it to his medical students: "What are the two outcomes for a patient? They live or they die. So you have to check them progressively. Every day make routine assessments. And then do action. Lots of action while the patient is in your care because as soon as they leave the hospital there is nothing you can do for them."

Examination of each patient at ward round might take no longer than a few minutes. Those who did not get diagnosis at admission are unlikely to be given one in this moment. The focus has already shifted away from diagnosis and onto what can be done. Dr. Bosa's priority, he explained, is to save lives. With limited manpower and resources there are only so many things he can do for the patients. Broad-spectrum antibiotics, antimalarials, and TB treatment are used simultaneously or sequentially in a process of trial and error. Drug dosages are adjusted. Blood transfusions are organized. The doctor notes that he will need to follow up an urgent blood cross-matching with the laboratory workers to make sure it is done. He spends time cajoling the nurses into taking the samples that should be done by an entourage of doctors and are really above their pay grade. There is an urgency to these interventions. The goal is not to locate disease within the interior space of the body but to move that body out of beds 1–4 and on to a trajectory out of the ward.

COLLABORATORS

The wide array of patients who were on TB treatment during my fieldwork in 2003–4 revealed another factor affecting the kinds of knowledge practices that are possible in the ward. Collaboration, of the kind Mol describes as enabling the enactment of disease, cannot be taken for granted. When a physician visited from Lae hospital to help establish a Directly Observed Treatment Short Course (DOTS) program at Madang, he explained that a key part of the program was for patients to be diagnosed with a sputum test prior to treatment. But after he left Dr. Bosa explained: "The sputum is good. But the thing about the sputum is you have to do a lot of work. You have to label the samples, instruct the patient how to collect the morning sputum. And who is going to take it to the lab? Sometimes they are taken and no one takes it [to the lab], not even the nurse. It is good to say take a sputum, but who is going to do it? It is important to do but who is going to do it? The physician would realize soon that he will have to do it himself." Instead Dr. Bosa put patients like Daniel on treatment for tuberculosis and watched for improvements.

It is not only laboratory and imaging technologies assistants that doctors find to be poor collaborators. The cooperation of other workers, such as nurses, cannot be assumed, and certainly cannot be guaranteed by the giving of verbal orders or the signing of pieces of paper. When a new registrar, who had previously worked as the director of medical services in the hospital administration, arrived on the ward to help out, for example, Dr. Bosa laughed at the abundance of laboratory request forms left on the ward round trolley after he completed ward round every morning. Dr. Bosa was not pleased about Dr. Masib's sudden arrival, nor the air of superiority he felt had no warrant considering Dr. Masib had been in a desk job for several years.

"The problem with Dr. Masib is that he comes and says a million tests should be done but he does not think about who is going to do them. If he hangs around for a couple of weeks he will realize that it is him who has to do them." What Dr. Masib needs to learn, Dr. Bosa explained, is that he cannot do things by the book. While Dr. Masib shouts at students to follow international protocols when writing up their cases, and to carry out every test possible when trying to diagnose a patient, he cannot assume that simply giving these orders will ensure they are carried out. "Dr. Masib thinks he is in control, but he isn't." The implication was that Dr. Masib had spent too much time in administration. He was overconcerned with protocols and rules and out of touch with the realities of the ward.

Sure enough, a few days after Dr. Masib's arrival, he arrived at a patient bed during ward round and requested the patient's medical record. A student handed it to him and Dr. Masib flicked through to the back where the laboratory results should be pasted or stapled to the cover. As he opened the cover, however, numerous white slips fluttered to the floor. Silently,

Dr. Masib picked up the next patient chart on the pile and opened it, again watching as all the laboratory result forms that he had ordered flew out in all directions. "What is this?" he shouted. "Someone is leaving the slips in the back here. Who is doing this?" The nursing officer standing a few feet away did not look up but continued to write notes in her large nursing tasks folder. Run off their feet with other tasks, the nurses complained that it would be impossible to carry out all the tests Dr. Masib requested before lunchtime, and it was unlikely the laboratory technicians would carry out the tests if the samples arrived in the afternoon. Nurses described laboratory test forms as "just talk" and argued that doctors, who do not enter into relationships with patients and so do not find out what social conflicts or sorcery could lie behind their ailments, are only able to see "skin deep." The tests were pointless, the nurses complained and just increased their workload when they were already understaffed.

"We aren't just dealing with disease here," Dr. Bosa told me. "You can't just give the nurses orders, they might start working back at you." Instead, he explained, you have to work with them, recognize they have different agendas from you, and avoid instituting a hierarchical relationship. The mistake that Dr. Masib made was thinking that writing a request on a form was enough to get things done. Instead, Dr. Bosa explained, he regularly found that he would have to do things himself.[9]

Berg points out that when doctors successfully align multiple actors in a collective goal, diagnosis appears retrospectively as the product of the individual doctor's agency, and he or she is established as an autonomous expert (1997, 134). It is the effective *distribution* of agency that simultaneously makes agency *appear* to be located in doctors as individual autonomous agents.[10] In Madang Hospital, nurses, patient bodies, and laboratory technologies frequently refuse to cooperate, techniques of delegation do not establish "centers of calculation," and doctors are forced to recognize their dependence on others. It is not disease that is rendered visible by such messy collaborations but the collaborations themselves.

GIVING UP CONTROL

Dr. Bosa and other doctors working in the hospital readily admitted to me that this way of operating was not what they had been taught in medical school, or during their training in Australia, and frequently invoked the gaze of the "white doctor" who they suspected would disapprove of their work.[11] As Wendland puts it in relation to medical students in Malawi, "encounters with medical tourists . . . could reinforce a sense that real medicine was what happened elsewhere" (Wendland 2010, 135). They argued, however, that being able to adapt to the particular conditions of work in Madang Hospital, negotiate relationships with other staff, work around the unreliability of medical technologies, and accept that patients did not subscribe to biomedical models of disease, was itself a form of expertise. "To be a good doctor here," Dr. Bosa told me, "you have to be able to give up control and do what you can."

Western textbooks are deemed largely irrelevant to this situation. "The thing is," Dr. Bosa explained, "the Australian doctors would never be able to function here." Other doctors agreed that Western doctors who were obsessed with diagnosis would not realize that there were only limited treatments to give patients. "It might look like bad practice," Dr. Wali explained in relation to the overprescription of broad spectrum antibiotics, "but we don't always have time to diagnose disease. We are trying to save lives." Meanwhile, white doctors' obsession with control and hierarchy it was suggested, would only be self-defeating in a context where attempts to control other people and technologies could provoke them to "work back at you."[12]

Asking "what can we do?" does not depend on asking "what does he have?" In fact, keeping multiple possibilities of diagnosis open is often preferable to closing them, and ancillary pathways for action, down. Here uncertainty is not a problem that leads to controversy, nor does it demand strategies of coordination or distribution between different answers. Uncertainty is an expert system that involves "giving up control," understanding Papua New Guinean medical "beliefs," resisting the impetus to assert "given" professional authority, and accepting the contingency of biomedical knowledge. This network of relationships is not concealed by the successful enactment of disease but is rendered explicit as the object of doctors' work. Dr. Bosa asserted that his ability to practice medicine in the particular circumstances of Papua New Guinea depended on his ability to give up control and certainty rather than to assert it.[13]

PURSUING CERTAINTY

Dr. Bosa's way of practicing biomedicine was shared by some other doctors in Madang Hospital, but it did not go uncontested. This was made explicit when Dr. Masib arrived on the medical ward. In his fifties, Dr. Masib was several years older than Dr. Bosa, but like him he had not yet completed his training to become a consultant. Instead he had for several years pursued a managerial career in the hospital and had most recently been acting as the director of medical services. Now this position had been filled, and he had been sent back to the medical ward to help out.

The two doctors had a difficult relationship from the beginning. Dr. Masib felt his greater experience gave him some authority over Dr. Bosa and he disapproved of the way Bosa was managing the ward. Dr. Bosa, meanwhile, was disgruntled by the suggestion that Dr. Masib might be able to tell him what to do; he was not a specialist after all, and he had not been running the medical ward single-handedly for several months. Dr. Bosa felt that, as an administrator, Dr. Masib was out of touch with the realities of clinical medicine in Papua New Guinea. Frequently when Dr. Masib turned up during ward round, Dr. Bosa would simply leave the room. Without any clear way of determining seniority between them, and without a consultant physician to assert hierarchical authority over them, the two men were incapable of working together.

Dr. Masib was keen to do everything by the book, to conform to international standards, and to follow national protocols. This, in his view, meant diagnosing patients before treating them. On ward round, trainee HEOs who could not find a patient's diagnosis in the medical chart would incense him. He would shout at the nurses to complete their tasks more quickly, complain that crucial tests had not been carried out, and scrawl all over the medical chart demanding further investigations or suggesting further diagnostic possibilities.

One day, several weeks after his arrival on the ward, Dr. Masib decided to do a round of the chronic side of the ward. When Dr. Bosa examined patients here the objective was usually to free up beds.[14] Many of the patients in the chronic side of the ward have never been given a clear diagnosis, but their condition has either stabilized or improved on treatment. Many of them are on treatment for tuberculosis. Although the DOTS program requires that patients are discharged on treatment, Dr. Bosa preferred to keep those patients from remote villages in the ward. He could not be sure they would be able to get medication at their nearest health center, or that they would be well enough to walk there. These were the issues at the forefront of his mind when he examined the patients on this side of the ward. Are they improving on treatment? Do they have transport to return to the village? Who will look after them? Will they be able to return for follow-ups and medications?

With Dr. Masib, however, the round of the ward was a very different affair:

We arrive at bed 16. This is a man in his forties from Bogia along the coast. He has come to the hospital without a guardian and is quiet and subdued. Dr. Masib asks Eric, the HEO, for a summary of his condition. "Swollen glands in neck and abdomen. He is on TB treatment," Eric says. "Right. Was a biopsy done?" demands Dr. Masib. Eric says he asked the surgeons to do one but they just said to continue treatment. "They would never just say that." Retorts Dr. Masib. "Right. What else could it be? How does it feel? Does it feel like one mass or multiple or matted?" Eric says it felt like it was single. "Right. If it's single it is usually something else, not TB. TB is multiple and feels rubbery. Or in a late stage formation some will be matted. But if it is single we need to be careful *not* to say it is TB." He looks at the man's abdomen. "His abdomen has swelled up. He has ascites. How did the liver feel? What sounds did if have? Was it nodular?" Eric mumbles incomprehensibly. "So we need to think about acute bacterial infections, viral infections, a tumor—lymphoma. We need to exclude it. TB treatment won't work on lymphoma. This is why we need a biopsy. Did you do a scan on the liver? No? If ascites is present in most cases it is liver cirrhosis." Eric says he thinks the liver felt enlarged. "Well, enlarged liver suggest other problems. If it is cirrhosis then you can't feel the liver at all. It shrinks in size." He feels the patient's abdomen. "This is not an enlarged liver."

He points to the blood vessels on the side of the abdomen. "What do you notice about these blood vessels? What do they tell you? If the blood vessels are retaining the blood like this then you need to think of cirrhosis. . . . We need a biopsy on this patient. It could be a swollen lymph node. Or what else could it be? Could it be the thyroid gland? Of course it could. Some people have their thyroid glands in strange places. It could be a thyroid gland. What else? It could be an abnormality in the blood vessel. If there is a weakness in a blood vessel then it tends to balloon out. But what will you see? You will see it pulsating. But this is not pulsating.

"He is on TB treatment already. This is taking a short cut. Continue treatment but best to get a biopsy first. Get a biopsy and get a scan." He states these orders out loud but he does not write them down. No one does. I ask him whether we are looking for one thing, whether these symptoms are related. He says, "We are probably seeing three different disease processes. Firstly swelling in neck. This may be connected to the cirrhosis, I don't know. Second TSS. Thirdly cirrhosis. We look at investigations, then try to tie them in. You have done a liver function test?" he barks at Eric. "No? Why not?"

We move onto bed 17 where a middle-aged woman who was admitted to the ward about two weeks ago lies quietly on the mattress. She is also on treatment for TB. Dr. Masib looks at her and notes that her skin is hot. "She has a fever." She tells him she has pain in her chest and legs. He presses below her shoulder. She whimpers and pulls away. "Oh sorry. Pen i stap [that is painful?]?" He looks at her chest. "Her respiratory rate has increased. There is throbbing between the ribs. What does this mean? So this tells you she has moderate to severe pneumonia." He points to the abdomen and the back of the neck. "Why are they tightened up? Is it related to the fast breathing? Of course it is. Of course it is."

He asks her to lift her arms. She can't lift her right arm. "This is because she has an enlarged thyroid gland. So the problem is the fever. Take a blood slide. She has signs of bronchial pneumonia. She has cross crepitation on right lower side. The left lower is alright. We can hear the breath in this side going in alright. Her pulse is 120. Can't hear murmurs. Treat for malaria and pneumonia now. Treat acute problems first. But do the investigations too. Give her aspirin. She should have an IV line. Give her antibiotics. She has arthritis in her shoulder. The fever could be part of pneumonia but we need to exclude malaria. Do a chest X-ray, and do a lymph node biopsy. She has enlargement of the neck vessels. This usually means obstruction. There are signs of septicaemia or another bacteria infection in her. You should do a blood culture. For example she could have typhoid fever. Blood culture is the only reliable test to know exactly what is causing the illness both for aerobic and anaerobic bacteria. And with that comes sensitivity of drugs. Try penicillin for forty-eight hours. See how she does and then change it if necessary."

He turns to Eric, who is looking baffled by the number of orders he has just received. "When she came did she have rashes or fever? Usually the fever reduces with treatment if she has TB. If it continues then we need to think about other infections, or else reactions to the TB drugs. To make things complete you should take blood pressure, pulse rate, respiratory rate, temperature etc. before you give IV or aspirin." He takes out the X-ray and holds it up to the light. "You can see patches on the right side. This is not a good picture. We should not interpret pictures like that. You will only make a wrong judgement. We will find out what is wrong with the X-ray and get a new one. Her thyroid is enlarged. It looks like thyroid toxicity. What test would you do? A thyroid function test."

Dr. Masib didn't accept that "generally sick" patients should be on TB treatment as a default option; he didn't accept the category "generally sick" at all. If he suspected cancer in a patient he pursued it, demanding biopsies that the surgeons would later refuse to carry out (they saw no point when treatment was not available) and liver functions tests that the laboratory often had no capacity to do. Dr. Masib often wrote his suspected diagnoses in the ward round notes at the back of the patient files. On other occasions he spoke out loud, stating the investigations and tests that would need to be done. What he didn't do was follow up on these orders, check with laboratory staff, take the samples to accompany his laboratory request slips. He didn't follow up on the blood he demanded for a patient, or check whether their relatives would be able to donate. This, he felt, was not the way the hospital should work. He should be able to state what needed to be done, and the next time he opened the patient chart the results should be there, in plain view. This, he told me, is how hospitals work everywhere else.

Each time Dr. Masib looked at a patient he started from the beginning. He wanted a full summary from the HEO, which Eric often failed to give him because the multiple diagnoses stated in the patient chart didn't conform to Dr. Masib's idea of a proper presentation. He refused to accept treatment as a solution to uncertainty, and continued to pursue diagnostic closure instead. He was less concerned at ward round with finding out whether a patient was improving or not improving and more concerned with whether a pathological cause of their sickness had been found.

When Dr. Masib arrived on the medical ward, Daniel had already been there for two months moving backward and forward between beds 4, 5, and 6. At ward round on that first morning, Dr. Masib set to work. He noted that Daniel had a collapsing pulse. "Aortic valve incompetence," he wrote in the ward round notes at the back of Daniel's chart. "Rheumatic heart disease. Do chest X-ray, ECG, increase Lasix." One week later, he did ward round again. "Do chest X-ray. Do ultrasound scan," he wrote. One week later, neither of these investigations had been carried out. Dr. Masib assumed that writing these directions would make sure they were done. Daniel's condition, meanwhile, continued to deteriorate. When he died, a few days later, no final diagnosis was written on his medical chart. Dr. Masib's notes about rheumatic heart disease were hidden away in the ward round notes at the back of the chart. On the death certificate the cause of death was filled in according to the treatment Daniel had been on: "tuberculosis." Just as treatment substitutes for diagnosis in life, so in death it retrospectively provides diagnosis in a single, complete form.

CONCLUSION

Doctors and patients alike experience the medical ward as a place where they wait. Here, precise "enactments" of disease (Mol 2002) are not prefigured by and make possible different actions. A pervasive opacity of the patient body, and the inability of the laboratory or of imaging technologies to effectively open it up to an expert gaze, creates a space of perpetual uncertainty where patients move slowly around the ward in a trajectory toward discharge or death.

Proceeding from an understanding of biomedicine that equates it with processes of diagnostic knowledge, we might expect that the nonenactment of disease would lead to a sense of helplessness and inadequacy among doctors. Certainly doctors are frustrated by the gap between the medical infrastructure taken for granted by their training and the medical infrastructure they must work with in practice. However, doctors do not only respond to these frustrations with feelings of failure. Instead, uncertainty sometimes provides the basis for alternative biomedical knowledge practices. It is another productive form that biomedical knowledge can take.

Here the patient body is not individualized as a site of disease (Foucault 2003).[15] The patients in the ward constitute variations on a single spectrum of sick rather than different "cases" of disease classification. Uncertainty revolves around the opposition between life and death and not the multiple underlying diseases that could be causing the patient's deterioration. Here biomedical work does not focus on the location of disease in the individual body but the movement of that body around the ward on a trajectory toward life.

In Madang Hospital, I argue, technologies of not knowing, which enact "generally sick" bodies, enable pragmatic collaborations and move those bodies toward discharge.[16] Action is not here dependent on specific enactments of disease. Action is instead correlated to what is feasible and then attenuated in relation to patients' responses to particular treatments. "We are acting blind" is a popular refrain for doctors working in Madang Hospital.[17] Within the medical ward, practices of not knowing enable networks of collaboration to expand through the production of uncertainty and the making of "modest" experts (De Laet and Mol 2000) who are visibly dependent on their relationships with other actors.

Dr. Bosa was fully aware that this way of doing medicine departed from the "international standard." He did not claim that this way of doing biomedicine was "better" than that described in the textbook written by the Western physician *in general*. Instead, he argued, it is "what we can do." In other words, that it is *locally* superior to the international standard. Like scientists in other postcolonial places of science, doctors in Madang Hospital "walk a tightrope between claims of difference from the global North and assertions of sameness (Crane 2010, 843; Johnson 2013). The comparability of Papua New Guinean medicine to medicine that is practiced elsewhere was of interest to Madang Hospital's doctors, as well as its anthropologists, as they "sought recognition but also desired a sphere of autonomy for their work" (Lowe 2006, 12). Unlike medics elsewhere, however, they do not walk this line by claiming universal legitimacy for "hybrid" forms of science. Rather they claim that their way of practicing medicine is *locally* superior to Western biomedicine, which does not adapt effectively to the contingencies of place. At the same time this requires that they acknowledge that their knowledge does not have legitimacy or authority beyond the confines of Madang Hospital. This was a compromise that Dr. Bosa, but not Dr. Masib, was willing to make.

CODA

Despite established links between HIV and tuberculosis, at the time of my first period of fieldwork in 2003–4 doctors in Madang Hospital did not regularly screen all patients on tuberculosis treatment for HIV. Indeed very few patients were tested for HIV at all. In addition to the diagnostic process being slow and unreliable, antiretroviral treatment was still only a faint possibility on the horizon. Doctors did not see any value to be gained in burdening patients with an increasingly stigmatized diagnosis that they could do little about. They also worried that a sickness that had a recognized "name" within "white people's medicine" but which doctors were nonetheless unable to cure could result in relatives implicating the doctor in the patient's death. Patients on TB treatment were "generally sick." They might recover on treatment or not, but they did not have a firm diagnosis—it was just "something we can do."

By 2009, this situation had dramatically changed. The rapid growth of the HIV epidemic in the country had attracted the attention of international philanthropic organizations already working in Africa and elsewhere. Funds and resources from institutions like AusAID and the Global Fund for HIV, Tuberculosis, and Malaria had been ploughed into the development of new HIV/AIDS related institutions such as the National Aids Council and had enabled the rollout of numerous new technical fixes, including free antiretroviral drugs, rural STI clinics, and the provision of laboratory equipment to rural laboratories and referral hospitals such as Madang, which would enable them to provide faster and more reliable tests for HIV.[18] With the global rise in multi–drug resistant tuberculosis the importance of diagnosing patients before treatment had also become a priority.

The medical response to HIV was now closely tied to that for tuberculosis, with a renewed emphasis on the DOTS regime and WHO protocols for monitoring and treating tuberculosis patients who were HIV positive. Compliance with these protocols was a basic requirement of Global Fund funding for the national TB program. In the medical ward this led to several transformations. An old empty ward at the back of the grounds had been renovated and converted into a TB ward with donor funds. All TB patients were now diagnosed with a sputum test and screened for HIV. Patients were regularly weighed and had their CD4 count measured. Everything was carefully written down on graphs, which the doctors had been specially trained by the WHO to draw and analyze. Here, specific diseases became visible and bodies were enacted in ways susceptible to micromanagement. A level of funding and governance that was out of all proportion to that associated with the routine running of the medical ward had created a diagnostic enclave within that institutional space.

Yet the new diagnostic infrastructure that surrounded these infectious diseases had little impact on the "generally sick" patients who were not tested or who tested negative for HIV or tuberculosis.[19] In 2010, for example, the hospital ran out of Giemsa stain, which is used to stain blood slides and color the different malaria parasites. The area medical store did not have any in stock. The national laboratory in Port Moresby was too low on supplies to send any to Madang. The microscopist in charge of malaria testing was able to appeal to contacts in the Institute of Medical Research and Divine Word University, but when even these supplies ran out, she closed the laboratory down. For a few days before Divine Word University gave a further donation, the referral hospital for the entire province was unable to test patients for malaria. Even the new TB ward is not immune from such systemic challenges. Doctors still question the reliability of laboratory tests for TB or HIV. The necessary reagents for these tests sometimes run out. A shortage of nursing staff means that sputum samples are not sent to the laboratory on time. In such circumstances doctors fall back on other ways of doing things that rely not on the exercise of an expert medical gaze, but the pragmatic engagement with people and technologies that might be able to assist them in "getting things done."

As new kinds of medical infrastructures emerge around specific diseases, so do spaces of exclusion from the diagnostic gaze continue to open up at the heart of the public health system. In Madang Hospital such blind spots emerge inside rather than outside the national health system. They might therefore be thought of as spaces of omission as much as exclusion. Spaces where persons are admitted as patients and yet where they fail to be individuated as a particular body suffering from a single disease.

Within such opaque spaces nonconventional biomedical knowledge practices, which inscribe medical technologies with new kinds of meanings and effects, are produced. The everyday and explicit contingency of diagnostic knowledge in the medical ward of Madang Hospital suggests that scientific and medical work is not always oriented to the production of fact. The activities of doctors are focused on the reorganization of relationships between persons, technologies, and bodies so as to direct a patient's trajectory away from death and toward discharge. It is these relationships and the kinds of persons (generally sick patients and distributed expert doctors) who make them up that are made visible in medical practices, not individual disease.

The next chapter examines biomedical uncertainty in Madang Hospital from another angle. What does it mean to be a "generally sick" person? The chapter explores the interferences between the production of knowledge and the making up of persons in relation to patients' attempts to transform their own bodies, and the frictions and power relationships entailed by alignments between biomedical and nonbiomedical relationships as hospital technologies become mediators in patients' relationships with both hospital workers and kin.

CHAPTER 5

The Waiting Place

■ The wailing had already begun. A nurse shuffled into the ward with a grubby white screen, which she pulled perfunctorily around the bed. It wasn't only for the family's privacy. If the body were there for some time patients would become scared that the dead man's angry and confused spirit might roam around the ward. The man, Daniel, had been in the ward for several weeks. The doctors didn't know what he had: "We can't do the tests to find out so we just put him on chloramphenicol."[1] It had looked like he was getting better. Only a few days earlier he had been laughing and talking with the neighboring patients. Now he was dead. Apart from the distressing sound of the family's grief, the ward was silent. The other patients and their guardians retreated to their beds or, if they could move, escaped the ward to the shady walkway outside.

The nurses retreated to their office to decide whose turn it was to deal with the body. After some discussion, Galang and Lorna emerged. They collected bundles of wide white bandages from the medicine room and walked back into the ward. The first job was to stop the flies getting to the body. Behind the screen, while Daniel's wife looked on, they set about rolling the bandage around the body, starting at the feet and moving their way up to the head. Grunting, they heaved the white mummy-like corpse onto a hospital trolley and rolled it down the central aisle, past the silent watching patients. The man's family followed behind wailing in grief as they walked.

They weren't on their way to the morgue. It had stopped working days ago and couldn't take any more bodies. The smell from the building was already starting to seep across the hospital grounds. Instead they took the body to a small side room off the walkway outside. Used for storage of old broken equipment and the occasional ward meeting, the room, which could not have been more than two meters square, also provided a substitute for the funeral tent (*haus krai*) that would traditionally be set up in a village when a person died. Here the family and friends could come to grieve, and to discuss arrangements for removal of the body.

Back in the ward, the patients were uneasy. This was the second death that week. Patients hadn't expected Daniel to die. His sudden death seemed arbitrary. Any of them could be next. Like Daniel, many of the patients had not been given a clear diagnosis by the doctors. They didn't know whether the doctor knew what was wrong with them, whether they would get better, or whether the hospital medicine was working. "Here," they say, "we just wait." There are only two ways to leave the hospital, patients say: discharge or death. They anticipate their own future departure in the daily occurrence of others. They watch as some patients pack up their sheets, plates, and clothes into brightly colored string bags and swing them over their head as they walk through the ward and out of the entrance toward the hospital gate. Meanwhile others, like Daniel, leave through the back door; their body destined for the morgue or the side room, while relatives deliberate over how they can afford to transport the body back to the village, no mean feat in a wet, mountainous country with few roads. Patients knew their own guardians must be thinking about those costs as they watched Daniel's body being wheeled by.

The first death that week had been less surprising, but equally disturbing for the patients. A few months previously Malu, a young boy of thirteen or fourteen, had taken to sleeping at the hospital. He claimed to have no family or village. Some of the staff took pity on him and gave him money or food. One of the nurses in the medical ward let him come to her home to wash and eat. But soon he began to refuse anything they gave him except for branded soft drinks. Eventually a group of nurses discovered him collapsed at the back of the hospital grounds and carried him to the medical ward, where he was admitted for severe malnutrition.

Malu was a curiosity to the other patients. How could he have no family? No support network? Some refused to believe it possible. He must be choosing to stay in the town rather than return to his family in the bush; his refusal to drink anything other than fanta or cola a sign of his rejection of village relationships. Others said they had heard of homeless people in countries like mine; now Malu's plight suggested they were appearing in towns in Papua New Guinea too. The patients watched as Malu became thinner and thinner. The doctors tried to put in a feeding tube but Malu thrashed around so violently they were unable to complete the procedure. The patients and guardians watching the procedure tutted their tongues and shook their heads. He still refused to drink anything other than store-bought fizzy drinks, but the doctors banned anyone from giving them to him.

For other patients, Malu's death resonated with fears that they too might be abandoned by family now they were in the hospital. His demise served as a sober reminder that one could cease to be socially significant to the extent that relatives might indeed leave one in the town hospital to die. People had heard rumors that families unable to afford the cost of transporting bodies back home were abandoning their dead relatives in the hospital morgue and that the hospital was burying them in mass graves outside the town. This was a terrifying thought. To not be buried on one's own land was bound to leave one's spirit restless and angry and to create problems for one's children whose claims to inherit one's land may be contested back home in the village.

Clearly, other patients remarked, Malu had decided to die. But even those who committed themselves to hospital medicine, who tried to forget the possibility that sorcery or social conflict in the village could be causing their sickness, and to focus instead on their relationships with hospital workers, were plagued by uncertainty. If their kinship relationships could not make them better, how could they navigate this institution defined by white people's knowledge and machines? How could they know that they had really been *seen* by the doctor, that he had recognized their condition and would treat them? Such anxieties were exacerbated by the fact that the doctors were often unable to give patients a clear diagnosis (*nem*) and were themselves often uncertain what patients were suffering from, whether they were improving, and how long they might be in the hospital for.

This chapter explores patients' experiences of confinement, kinship, and diagnostic technologies in the hospital and uses these experiences to reflect on the processes of person-making and bodily transformation that interactions with state institutions of biomedicine in contemporary Papua New Guinea afford. How are these experiences shaped by the biomedical limits that have come to characterize the state hospital, the changing relationships

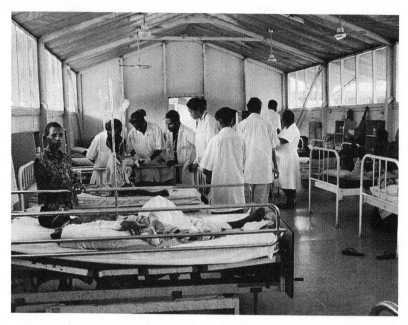

5.1. Medical ward round. Trainee health extension officers attend to Malu.

between rural and urban economies, and the pressures placed on kinship relationships in conditions of adversity? Here I focus on the story of one patient in particular, who I call Michael.[2] I follow Michael's exchanges with relatives in the village (mediated by garden grown foods), relatives in town (mediated by money, food, and commodities), and doctors in the hospital (mediated by biomedical technologies) as he experimented with new relational possibilities for recuperating his body. I argue that both food and X-rays might be understood as "relational technologies" that transform bodies through the social and symbolic processes that they engender. As technologies of knowledge production, both food and X-rays are the medium through which patients struggle to make themselves visible as socially viable and well persons.

Patients find that to put such relationships in motion constitutes a major challenge from the vantage point of a motionless hospital bed. The temporal and spatial organization of the ward inhibits patients' visibility as a social actor within either kinship or biomedical relational fields. They struggle to establish the network of relationships and exchanges through which they might be recognized as and materially transformed into a healthy person. Many patients, like Michael, ultimately experience failure in their attempts

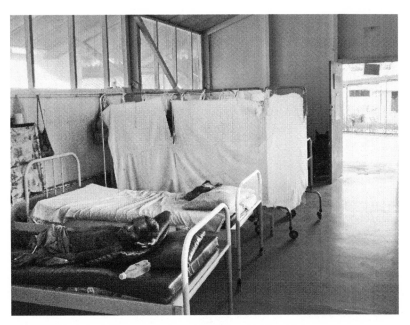

5.2. Medical ward screen. The screen is pulled around a dead body.

to activate hospital technologies and find themselves confined instead to a place of stationary inertia and death.

FORGOTTEN RELATIONS

After two months in the ward Michael was one of its longest standing patients. Michael was not sure whether the doctor had "found a name" (*painim nem*) for his sickness. He had been admitted and treated in the hospital for tuberculosis (*tibi*) a year previously, but he was not sure whether he was now suffering from the same sickness. The doctor rarely spoke to him and when he did, Michael found it difficult to ask questions. Michael's father had worked as the cook for the high school on the Rai Coast and he had learned some English, enabling him to overhear one of the doctors talking about an enlarged heart at ward round. But nothing had been followed up.

Michael was proud of being able to speak English and often bought one of the national newspapers from outside the hospital gates. He had managed to procure an old rusted classroom chair from somewhere, which he set up next to the ward entrance, where the light and air streamed in, and where he sat daily, carefully scrutinizing the national and world news or studying the Bible. After so long in the ward he and his mother, who was acting as his guardian (*wasman*), had established good relationships with their neighbors, with whom they regularly shared provisions such as salt, and for whom Michael's mother sometimes helped carry out tasks such as collecting food from the hospital kitchen. But Michael could also be aloof and irritable. His days were full of pain, discomfort, and boredom. He hated the hospital. Like other patients he complained that it was hot and airless, that the food was bad, the water unclean, and the wards full of mosquitoes at night. And like other patients, Michael spent his eventless days dreaming of returning to the village. "All the time I have been here," he told me,

> I have been thinking about the village. When we eat I think about the food in the village, the bananas, the taro and the yams. When I wash I think about the sea and the clear water on the Rai Coast. Look at my skin. The water here makes us itch all over. There is rust in the pipes here. I think about washing in the sea. And I think about money all the time. In the village there is no money. There is no need for money. But here you need money for everything and it makes me worry.

Mary, Michael's mother, was also tired of the institution. She compared the sense of movement, both physical and social, that characterized life in the village with the permanent stasis of the hospital ward.[3] "Here we don't do anything," she said. "We just stay in the same place. Look at the same place, sit doing nothing. In the village we move around, work in the garden, walk around to other places. Here I could go to town but I have no money so why would I go? In the town you need money to pay for food, but in the village the food just grows by itself! In the village you can wash whenever you want, but here it is difficult and the water is bad."

Through such active remembering the village and the relationships that animated it became a constant presence in Michael's daily life of the hospital. As his condition deteriorated, and hospital medicine seemed to do little to ameliorate it, he began to worry that social conflict in the village could still be causing the sickness. He had been ill in the village for a long time and many people had looked after him without receiving anything in return so it was possible that they were angry. Patients often worried that people may have committed sorcery against them in the village. But people's anger, conflict within one's household or one's own worries and anxieties about other people's thoughts and intentions were also considered to be capable of causing sickness. In the hospital people referred to sickness caused by such social conflicts as *sik bilong ples*.[4] In particular, Michael was worried that all the time he was in hospital he was not contributing to the shared garden he had with his brother who might now be having bad thoughts about him that could stop the hospital medicine from working. To worry (*wori*) about the thoughts and attitudes that relatives were cultivating in one's absence was common in the ward. Patients and nurses alike remarked that wori of this kind could stop the hospital medicine from working and could even lead to death.

One day I came into the medical ward to find Michael and his mother looking enthusiastic and happy. They were going home tomorrow. When they had told the doctor at ward round that morning that they wanted to return home to "straighten their relationships" (*stretim ol samting bilong ples*) he had agreed, giving them a special form to sign so they could go.[5]

As we were chatting the nurses began to distribute the 10:00 AM medicine. They reached the bed next to Michael where a new patient was lying. As they began talking Michael fell silent, listening to their conversation.

Nurse: Where are you from?
Patient: Rempi
Nurse: Where is your wasman (guardian)?
[The patient is silent and looks at the bed]
Nurse: You haven't got a wasman?
Patient: No
Nurse: Why? You must send talk to the village and get a wasman. All patients must come with a wasman. It is not good to come without a wasman [turns away and moves to the next bed].

When the nurse had moved on, Michael and his mother turned back to me to say that they had heard that in England there are homeless people who don't have family and to ask whether this was true. They thought this was also beginning to happen in Papua New Guinea. Their *wantok* (people from the same language group and exchange networks) in the town didn't visit them, give them money or food, and often got angry when they went to their house. Such concerns were shared by other patients. Those who came from the villages or settlements near the town frequently worried about why people did not visit them.[6] They claimed that their relatives must be angry or have hidden resentments against them causing them to stay away. Patients from *longwe* (far away, a term used to describe people from areas that were difficult to access by road) knew that people from their village would be unable to visit because of the costs and difficulties of transport, but they worried that people in the village had forgotten (*lus ting*

ting) them, had ceased to think of them, or that their gardens and houses were being stolen or taken over by others while they were in the hospital. Those relatives who did visit the hospital often brought news of houses being broken into and objects or food being stolen, adding to the fear that people may have jealousy or resentment toward them, and to patients' experience of their powerlessness to do anything about it from the vantage point of their bed in the hospital ward.

Such anxieties contributed to Michael's desire to return to the village. The failure of the hospital medicine to make him better convinced him that he needed to make himself present again in his village relationships. If he could ensure other people's good intentions toward him he would begin to get better.

A month after Michael left, he and his mother returned. He had a follow-up clinic appointment with the doctor, but they didn't have anywhere else to stay in town so they asked the nurses if they could stay in the ward for the night. They couldn't stay with their wantok, Mary explained, because they hadn't been able to bring any food from the village. Michael no longer worked in his garden, and she had developed a sore shoulder that had prevented her from being able to grow any food in hers either:

> We feel ashamed to go and stay with them if we haven't brought any food. Also sometimes our wantok are cross with us. They are angry because we ask for money when we are in town. Or we get cross with them because they don't give us any money. I know that our wantok find it hard in town because they don't have enough money sometimes. In the bush there is always food but in town if you don't have the money then you go hungry. Wages are not enough. So we were scared when we turned up in town with nothing to give our wantok.

Michael provided a more critical slant on their experience: "When you come to the hospital people don't help you. We have wantok but they don't help. They have new customs in the town and they don't care. They think only of themselves now. This is what happens in the town." Patients in the hospital found themselves caught between the overlapping social worlds and economies of village and town; neither fully immersed nor able to operate effectively in either. On the one hand, it was impossible to engage effectively from the hospital bed in kinship relationships organized around the growing and sharing of garden food in the village. On the other hand, patients often turned up at the hospital with no money with them. They were unable to pay for extra food for themselves or their guardian, for transport home or for other valuable commodities such as cold fizzy drinks or salted biscuits that could stave off hunger between the routinely pathetic hospital meals. On one occasion I saw a newly arrived mother being refused food for her sick child because they had not brought a bowl and spoon with them from the village. The mother's protest that they had no money with which to buy the bowl went unheeded. Patients feared that they had been forgotten by or were despised by kin back in the village, and that they were deemed socially insignificant by wantok in the town.

Life outside the hospital continued to permeate its walls. As van der Geest and Finkler argue, far from being a "tight little island" as it is depicted in early sociological studies, the hospital in fact "cannot divorce the patient from his or her family, or from other social institutions" (2004, 1996). This is perhaps even more pertinent in an institution where routine biomedical uncertainty makes it difficult for patients to forget the other possible causes of their sickness that they may need to address. And yet containment in the hospital simultaneously establishes physical and social distance from those relatives. It is both a place of permeability and exception (Street and Coleman, 2012). This sense of the hospital as a place of stasis and divided thoughts, caught between different social worlds, was expressed poignantly by Michael through the idiom of money: "I think about money in the hospital because I don't have any. And I think about the village because you don't need money in the village, everything is free. If I had money in the town then I would forget about the village. But I don't have anything so I have divided thoughts (*tupela tingting*)."[7]

SHAMEFUL BODIES

Michael was given a bed next to Den, who had been a patient in the ward when Michael and his mother had left a month earlier. Den was a convict from the provincial prison. He had been involved in a local gang and was caught stealing from a shop in the town. After some months in the prison he began to find it difficult to walk, and later his eyesight began to deteriorate. The doctor had told him it was because of the poor prison food and that his eyesight would never return to normal. At first Den had been given a personal guard in the ward to make sure he didn't escape, but as his mobility and eyesight deteriorated further he had been left to his own devices.

While I sat on Michael's bed, Den and he chatted about the changes that had taken place in the ward over the weeks that Michael had been away.

Den told Michael that Tutas, another long-term patient in the ward had died in his absence.

Tutas was from a village along the north coast road, near Madang Town. Even when he arrived at the hospital Tutas was thin and sickly looking, but during his time in the medical ward he had became skeletal. The doctors were not sure what was wrong with Tutas, but it was suggested that he may be suffering from the advanced effects of AIDS. The psychiatric nurse was brought in to counsel him and to explain what AIDS was before he was given the test for HIV. This discussion also took place in the open ward as by this time Tutas was unable to move from his bed. Tutas told the nurse that he was ashamed because he was losing weight and everyone could see it. He was scared of having AIDS because this had "its own shame" and he thought that his wife already wanted to leave him for a better man. He also thought his wife's first husband might have committed sorcery against him. He was scared that when his wife left the hospital she would find another man and not come back. He also knew that other patients would see this and ask questions.

Tutas had married a large, vivacious woman from Buka in North Solomons Province. While Tutas hardly spoke to the other patients, his wife was quick to make conversation with their neighbors. When relatives visited, in the first few weeks, he lay silent on the bed while she sat around on the floor with them noisily chatting and eating the garden food they had brought into the afternoon, often ignoring Tutas entirely.

Soon after the blood sample for the HIV test was taken Tutas began to refuse food. Tutas's wantok in the town had ceased to visit him and the only food he could have eaten was hospital food. This was a cold pile of thick wet rice twice a day, with a spoonful of donated tuna from the nearby Philippine factory slopped on top. Patients complained that hospital food could not make them better, only garden food could strengthen their bodies.[8] A lack of visitors bearing garden food fueled patients' worries about the reasons behind their neglect. Conversely, visits from relatives who brought gifts of garden food or fresh coconuts were seen as signs of good intentions and portended the possibility of recovery.

Patients examined their bodies for signs of improvement or deterioration and related those changes to the gifts of garden food that were or were not brought to the hospital by kin. Bodily transformations were read as a direct index of a person's social relationships. When gifts of food were given, patients said they knew their relatives were *wanbel* (that their intentions are aligned with their own) and that they would get better. The physical

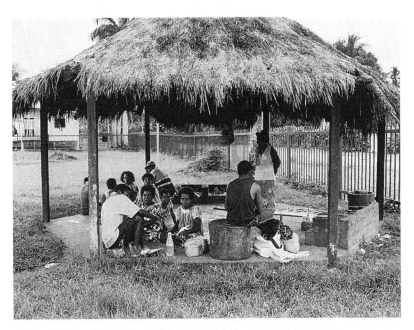

5.3. Patients cook in the hospital grounds.

sustenance such food provided was seen as inextricable from the social intentions that came with it.[9] Conversely, patients' unhealthy appearance, and in particular the loss of weight, *lusim skin* or *skin i go slak* (skin has become loose or lifeless), was a constant reminder to patients of their social failings as perceived publicly by others, and patients claimed to feel ashamed to be seen by the other patients.[10] According to this logic, rice was powerless to ameliorate the social conflict or failure that was depleting Tutas's body.[11]

When Tutas was barely conscious, the doctor attempted to force feed him through a tube, but it was too late. Tutas died the next day. A month later his blood test was returned from Moresby with a negative result for HIV, leading the doctor to assert that Tutas died "not from a disease but from shame." Tutas was described by staff and patients as someone who had become consumed by wori about his social relationships and had therefore had divided thoughts (tupela ting ting) about the hospital medicine. The other patients in the ward watched Tutas's slow decline and death with concern and a certain measure of fear. His neglect by his wife and his kin frequently fueled their own stories of having been forgotten or abandoned in the hospital.

When Den had finished telling Michael about Tutas's death, Michael shook his head. "The hospital is a bad place to die," he said quietly. Den agreed. He had heard that a person who was not buried in their village would not be able to leave the living world but would continue to roam the town trying to get home. He had also heard that the ghosts of those who die in town drive around at night offering people marijuana and enticing them into bad and violent ways of life.

The hospital was also a bad place to die because of the difficulty in transporting a dead body from the hospital to the village. The hospital had banned the use of its ambulances to transport dead bodies, and there was no car hire service in Madang for vehicles that could hold a coffin. It was sometimes possible to find individuals who would transport a coffin, but even then high fees were charged. Those who lived on the coast had an advantage in that they could transport the coffin by boat, but boat owners also charged high sums for this service. One young woman whose child died in the pediatric ward covered her dead child in blankets to transport her home on the PMV. If the bus drivers knew that the journey was in fact a funeral parade they would charge too much. When I met her in her home village some months later she told me that she had not been able to cry on the journey for fear the PMV driver would realize her baby was dead, and that the worst thing was knowing that she was not grieving in the proper way for her baby's soul.

The hospital made it harder for people to meet their obligations surrounding the treatment of the dead. But stories about abandoned bodies and roaming ghosts also took on a critical edge as people claimed that Papua New Guineans were no longer so eager to recognize those obligations.[12] Patients' fears that they might stop being recognized or remembered by relatives in the village or wantok in the town and that they might be cast out like homeless people in Britain were compounded by stories of abandoned bodies that lay unclaimed and discarded.

PERMEABLE BODIES

On his return home to the village, Michael had called a meeting for all his relatives. People had been invited to talk openly about any anger or resentment they might feel toward him. Several close family members had spoken out, saying they were angry because they had been looking after him for so long while Michael made no contribution to work in the garden or community: "I didn't work, but I ate their food. They didn't say anything but I could feel that they were cross, and I was getting sicker. It made me worry, it made my sickness get worse."

Following the meeting Michael provided a meal, including corned beef and tinned fish from the local trade store, for those who had spoken out about their anger toward him. After eating, they apologized for making him sick. The process, he said, had made everyone wanbel (in agreement) and he felt confident that the hospital medicine would begin to take effect.

Establishing wanbel relationships in the village enabled Michael to refocus on his relationships in the hospital. It was now important that the doctor looked at him properly and that he took all his medicine and followed the doctor's orders properly. But the hospital remained a stressful place to be. Like other patients, Michael said he did not know how hospital medicine worked, this was only known by white people and doctors, who had acquired white people's knowledge at university. He just had to "follow the doctor." But this did not mean that Michael was not anxious about exactly what the doctor was doing and what his intentions might be. In fact his anxiety was heightened by his self-conscious ignorance of the doctor's "white peoples" knowledge.

In the medical ward those anxieties often center on the circulation of bodily fluids. At ward round doctors regularly take specimens from patients for analysis.[13] But patients are not sure exactly why these samples are being taken, where they might be going, or what people might be doing with them. In Papua New Guinea the removal and circulation of body parts is a powerful idiom for sorcery. It is by magical work on bodily exuviae that sorcerers are able to take control over their victim's body through a kind of "contact sorcery" (Gell 1988, 103). People are therefore highly attentive to where nail filings, shorn hair, and bodily discharges go, and will usually burn or bury them if they can. Certainly, the association of the circulation of body parts with sorcery needs to be understood as a meaningful context for the circulation of samples and specimens within the hospital. And yet patients are adamant that doctors do not practice sorcery and that this is not where their anxieties about body parts are directed. Hospital medicine, they argue, is "white people's medicine," and white people do not have sorcery or sik bilong ples. Hospital medicine, in other words, occupies a parallel moral universe to that of sik bilong ples. It has, they assume, its own motivations and modes of transformation, but they do not profess to know what these might be.[14]

In fact, it is this sense of ignorance and exclusion from doctors' knowledge and exchanges that fuels patient fears about the circulation of bodily fluids in the hospital. These worries are all the more potent because patients have often been told they are "short of blood."[15] If they are short of blood, patients ask, why are doctors taking it from them? And who are they giving that blood to? If patients from urban settlements or villages near the town are also short of blood, patients from longwe wonder, might they have the resources to pay doctors or laboratory workers for the blood of other patients? In other words, the fear is not that their blood has become subject to acts of sorcery, but that it has entered a system of circulation based on access to money and knowledge that are concentrated in the town and from which longwe patients are excluded.

The hospital's Red Cross blood bank is always short of blood. People in Papua New Guinea rarely volunteer to give up their blood to anonymous strangers and the institution is instead dependent on a relative replacement system whereby the patient receiving a transfusion obtains a replacement donation from their kin. For patients coming from longwe, however, extracting blood from their relatives is difficult. How will they have the money and resources to come to town? Where will they stay? How will the patient even contact them from the hospital ward? The absence of relatives to give blood reinforces patients' sense of isolation from those kinship networks, and at the same time, the drawing away of their blood by doctors makes visible to them their exclusion from what they presume are urban and institutional networks of exchange based on money. This makes patients who profess to have forgotten about sik bilong ples all the more determined to learn how to engage with the hospital technologies in a productive way.

RELATIONAL TECHNOLOGIES

Within a few days of his readmission to the ward, Michael began to worry that the doctor seemed uninterested and that he had still not been given a "name" for his sickness. Michael saw the doctor walking in and out of the ward each day, but he would march past the patients in the chronic side of the ward, heading straight for the nurses' office and carry out a ward round on the acute side.

Michael took great care to ensure that he followed the doctor's orders, comparing himself to other patients who did not take their medicine properly. He also spoke often about the doctor's diagnosis, saying that he had seen the tibi because when he first came to the hospital the previous year, he had an X-ray taken. However, he now wondered what had happened to that X-ray. He explained that the first time he had been admitted with tibi the doctor had looked at the X-ray and shown it to Michael, but this time Michael had not seen it. Moreover they had done an ultrasound scan at admission, but he wasn't sure what, if anything, the doctor had seen. When the doctor did ward round for the other patients in the ward, many of whom were on treatment for tuberculosis, and took out the X-ray from its sleeve and held it up to the light, Michael was one of the few patients that did not have an X-ray for the doctor to look at.

Other patients similarly put emphasis on their X-rays. Most important, patients claimed that the X-ray led the doctor to "painim nem," to "find a name" for their sickness within Western medicine. The doctor's special powers, derived from white people, consisted precisely of his ability to see inside their bodies to find their sickness, much as traditional medical diviners, often described as having *ai X-ray* (X-ray eyes) are able to penetrate the patient's body to see what social relationships lie behind their illness. When telling stories about their referral through health centers and hospitals patients always pinned down the moment when the doctor painim nem. A small number of names were recognizable to patients as *sik bilong marasin*, including malaria, tuberculosis (tibi), and asthma (*sot win*). Patients would say that they knew they had tibi because the doctor had shown them on their X-ray. Doctors often followed up a diagnostic reading of an X-ray by telling the patient that there was medicine for this kind of sickness and that if they took it properly they would recover. For patients the act of painim nem was closely associated with the possibility of treatment.

When a patient was "given a name" by a doctor it instilled new confidence that the hospital medicine would work. Patients with a name often claimed that they had stopped thinking about sik bilong ples (village sickness) and worked hard to forget about relatives who might have forgotten them or who had abandoned them in the hospital. They no longer had divided thoughts, but focused on the fact they had sik bilong marasin and attempted to follow the hospital rules and conventions more strictly.

In a context of heightened uncertainty, X-rays operated for patients as objects of hope. They potentially facilitated the establishment of positive relationships with doctors who patients felt otherwise ignored them. Patients were very proud of their X-rays, and they played a central role in narratives of admission. As one female patient, Rose, described:

> TB began in my body. I got a bad cough. I had it for quite a long time, like a month. When I got it I was still working in the garden. But then it got worse, and I came to the hospital. I didn't know it was tibi but when I came to the hospital they showed me the picture and I saw the tibi. And in the ward the nurses told me it was tibi. When I came they

took an X-ray, and it is still there in the office [she points towards the nurses' office]. . . . They sent me to have an X-ray taken. I waited with many people. One by one they went inside. Then I went in. I stood up and they put something in front of me and something behind me. Took off my clothes. I put my arms like this. They took the picture. Ok, it was done and I went back outside, and another person went inside again. I took the picture back to outpatients. [The doctor] put it on a screen and we looked at the picture. Ok finished, he put it inside a long brown envelope and I carried it with me to the ward. Now at ward round they all look at this picture.

Other patients similarly narrated the story of the X-ray image's circulation; how the X-ray was taken, and how it subsequently moved around the hospital. At every moment patients with an X-ray knew where it was. In fact, patients placed so much value on their X-rays that doctors often gave the film to the patient on discharge, saying that the patients would reliably bring the film to the follow-up consultation while X-rays stored in the hospital frequently went missing.

Sometimes, however, even when patients have an X-ray taken they remain anxious that the doctor may fail to look at the image properly. Complaints that doctor "only looks skin deep" (*skanim skin tasol*) are common. At the time of Michael's readmission, the doctor had also arranged for his mother to have her shoulder X-rayed. Two weeks after their return, while the doctor was doing ward round in the chronic side of the ward, Michael summoned the courage to ask the doctor whether he had looked at the X-ray. Dr. Bosa apologized—he had completely forgotten he had agreed to look at the image. He told Michael's mother, Mary, that she should come to see him after ward round, and he would write a note in her clinic book so that she could take the X-ray to the surgeon to examine.

After ward round, however, I found Mary standing in the corridor waiting for the doctor. He was nowhere to be seen. While we were standing there, another doctor, Dr. Masib walked past. I called him over and explained the situation, asking if he would write the note for Mary so she could go to the surgical ward. Dr. Masib took the clinic book but passed it straight to the resident health extension officer, Eric, who was hovering behind him, before briskly walking on. Eric looked confused about who Mary was and what he should be writing in the book. I explained again and he scribbled a few words in the book before handing it back to Mary, who stood silently throughout the entire interaction. "We feel ashamed to ask," she said to me later. "It is up to them if they want to help us." While Michael felt he was being ignored, this sense of invisibility was equally profound for Mary as a guardian: "I don't have a name here. Michael is the patient. He has a name. They look at the file and know his name. But I am just a guardian (wasman)."

Patients' interest in X-rays suggests novel possibilities for the theorization of technological processes in the hospital. X-rays are conventionally understood as technologies of knowledge production that represent and provide insight into the hidden interior bodily space of disease (Cartwright 1995; Crary 1990). The importance of the X-ray lies in its ability to objectify the natural world in a comprehendible and ordered form. For patients in Madang Hospital also, the significance of the X-ray lay in its ability to help the doctor diagnose their sickness, or "painim nem." Yet the importance of "painim nem" was not that patients could now know and see what was inside them but that, in being rendered recognizable and knowable within the conventions of biomedicine, of which patients continued to profess ignorance, doctors would feel compelled to cure them.[16] The X-ray rendered the body in an appropriate, partible, and visible form.[17] Crucially, however, this did not mean that patients came to understand their bodies in biomedical terms, that they became biomedical subjects. Patients were not concerned with the meaning of the X-ray, which was deemed to be part of an exclusive realm of white people's knowledge; the issue was whether they could present themselves in the correct form.

Where biomedical knowledge practices construct representations through disease classifications or X-rays in order to attribute order to disorderly bodies, patients seem less inclined to construct explanation in their engagement with hospital technologies than to act experimentally in the hope of provoking a conducive response. Patients' engagements with X-rays were full of anticipation in the sense that they kept open the possibility of materially transformative relationships with hospital workers. Another way of putting this, following Miyazaki (2007), is that hope was patients' "method" for engagement with hospital technologies. As a technology of knowledge that would normalize patient bodies and render them comprehendible to the biomedical gaze the X-ray could simultaneously transform patients into the kind of person that doctors would recognize and treat. We might think of the X-ray as a bodily form with the affective power to elicit a medical response.[18]

Patients viewed the X-ray that enabled doctors to "find a name" as a personal achievement. An X-ray that showed their sickness revealed the

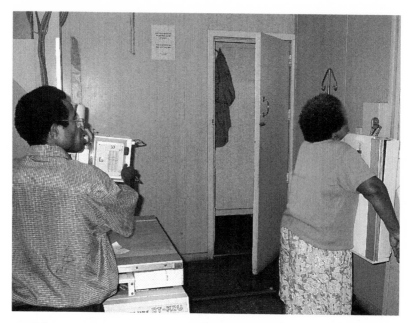

5.4. Taking an X-ray. The technician positions the patient and the machine.

patient retrospectively to have been successful in establishing the novel kinds of relationships required of them by the hospital. Rather than just producing knowledge, they also produced the kind of "person" that the doctor might want to engage with. They had appeared in the correct reified form. Such technologies are "relational technologies"; they do not only represent things, but simultaneously transform persons through social and symbolic processes (Dobbes and Hoffman 1999). Like garden food, X-rays were rendered effective by the relationships that they enacted.

Michael soon had his own occasion to hope that the doctor might "take a picture" and look inside his body. On ward round one day, the doctor told Michael that he would do another scan of his abdomen to check what was wrong with it. To do this he would have to borrow the portable ultrasound scanning machine from the obstetrics ward. Michael would have to wait until it was available. Michael became excited, telling me that the doctor was going to do a scan to "painim nem." But after a few days, the doctor seemed to have forgotten about his promise, and Michael began to lose hope that the scan would ever take place.

Michael began to worry that not only was he far from those relatives in the village who could be contributing to his sickness, but that he was not receiving any attention from the doctor in the hospital. Like other patients, Michael complained that the doctor did not listen to him, make eye contact when he walked through the ward, or show any sign that he intended to make him better. This sense that he was socially invisible to the hospital staff was bound up with broader perceptions of government corruption and failure:[19]

> I don't think the doctor here cares about sickness. He is not committed to his work. He does ward round too quickly. He doesn't sit down and listen to patient worries. In the beginning another doctor did a scan and told me I had TB but now the doctor says I have something else. Now I don't know which it is. Doctors like this are not doing their jobs. They just come and go but they don't actually look at the patients. They are stealing off the government, they take pay but don't do work. But then the government is also corrupt. They are like other corrupt people in government—the government doesn't care about village people. They get lots of money and women and buy cars and houses but they don't put any money into health and education or services. The hospital is a service but we are not getting a good service. Now the government is getting aid from foreign donors. I want to set up a cocoa drying business. I need a cocoa dryer. Can you help me get foreign aid when you go back to England. Will you think of me now you have taken my stories?

Such outbursts indicate the profound sense of marginality experienced by patients on the ward. The disdain with which they are treated by some hospital staff and the failure of doctors to "find a name" are collapsed with patients' experience of neglect by the state. Doctors and politicians appear to have access to white people's knowledge, technology, and money, which they keep secret from those Papua New Guineans who continue to live in the village subsistence economy. They refuse to enter into relationships based on reciprocal exchange and mutual recognition, which it is anticipated could lead to both economic development and the recuperation of the body.

Mattingly similarly describes the significance of small dramatic moments, such as the interpretation of an X-ray or MRI scan, for the production of hope in parents of children with cancer in American hospitals. The African American mother of a four-year-old girl with a brain tumor looks at the X-ray alongside the oncology consultant. The doctor, Mattingly argues, is like a detective who "can travel into the very recesses of [the] body and bring back secret messages that he then deciphers and delivers" (2010, 154). The mother follows the doctor's clinical gaze, becomes his detective assistant in their shared attempt to demystify their child's illness, but ultimately relies on him to tell her the meaning of the image. Her trust that he will do this and that he will give her daughter the best care possible, despite the fact that they are poor and black and she is a single mother, arises not only from his specialist status, but because while he discusses the X-ray he holds her daughter and strokes her hair, and because after discussing the X-ray he exchanges jokes about Thanksgiving. Mattingly describes such moments as "border crossings," moments in which people are able to exchange, communicate, and generate shared trust and hope in the future despite their social and economic differences. The kind of hope that X-ray technologies generate for patients in Madang Hospital might be quite different from those genres of hope specific to the popular American psyche.[20] But, as for the African American families who Mattingly works with, it is for their evidence that social recognition has taken place, the confirmation that they are indeed socially visible (and viable), as much as for the medical information they contain, that X-rays and the interactions they engender hold value for patients as objects of hope.[21] Patients in Madang Hospital do not appear to be concerned with doctors' "othering" of them so much as the fact this "otherness" is not construed as the basis for a relationship; their otherness is not specific and therefore visible (see also Stasch, *Society of Others*).

Often other patients who, like Michael, have not been given a name by the doctor or who share Michael's sense that the doctor is ignoring them turn to Christianity. Patients describe the ward as a place that has become like a church (*kamap lotu*). Although the majority of patients profess to be Christian, many also describe the intensification of their commitment to God (*bikpela*) in the hospital. The doctor may not be able to see what kind of sick they have, patients told me, but "God can see everything." Den, Michael's neighbor, who had been told by the doctor that he would never regain his eyesight, was able to maintain a hopeful disposition by focusing on his relationship with God. "I am not distracted by this," he told me. "He is only a doctor. He only has knowledge of this ground. Only God above can know whether my eyes will be ok or not."

Christian patients argue that the doctor cannot make them better, only God. As another patient explained to me: "The doctors talk about science and medicine, but God made all men and medicine comes underneath God, it is his work. If medicine will work or not is up to God. But it is not good to put medicine above God."

Michael tried to stop worrying about his kinship relationships in order to focus on following the doctor's orders and cultivating a relationship in which the latter might recognize and seek to cure him. Some Christian patients, meanwhile, sought to stop worrying about both kinship relationships and their relationship with the doctor in order to focus on God. Taking medicine and following the doctor's orders was still important, along with praying, giving up betel nut, and going to church. These were all actions that, it was hoped, would demonstrate their unified commitment to God and draw him into a harmonious (wanbel) relationship with them (Street 2010). While Michael also professed to be a Christian, he did not resort like other Christian patients to the popular refrain of "it is up to God. Only God can know." A stubbornly proud, educated Papua New Guinean, whose father had worked for the district high school, Michael was determined that he should not be excluded from the knowledge and powers that the hospital doctors had acquired from "white people." If only this knowledge were not concealed from him. If only the doctor would look more carefully at his body.

After two weeks back on the ward, Michael began to experience intense back pain. The trainee health extension officer gave him a prescription for Prednisone, a steroid used to control inflammation, but told him that the hospital didn't have any in stock. Michael would have to go to the pharmacy in town and buy it himself. Michael didn't have any money to buy the medicine: "Wantok will give you money if they feel sorry for you. Last week my father came to visit and he brought us drinks and some food. But he didn't bring any money. That is a problem for patients from longwe. We don't have any money." Michael felt increasingly isolated: from kin in the village, wantok in town, and from the hospital workers who he had hoped would "make a picture" of his sickness and treat it. The failure of the hospital to provide medicine and the failure of relatives to assist him in purchasing it from the pharmacy were made physically salient in the untreated pain that seared through his back. The social, governmental, and medical networks through which Michael's continued, undiagnosed, and untreated pain was made possible were as visible to him as they were to the anthropologist. Like other patients, he experienced the ongoing decline of his body as a direct reflection of his social failure, rejection, and neglect.

DEATH OUT OF PLACE

Confined to the hospital, Michael felt himself to be wholly abandoned and disconnected from multiple social worlds. He feared that relatives in the village could still be harboring bad sentiments, that wantok in town saw him only as a nuisance, that the doctor had no interest in treating or curing him, and ultimately, that the government in Port Moresby was stealing votes, money, and resources and leaving poor villagers like himself to die. It seemed there was no one to whom he remained visible as a significant person, whether in the guise of a relative, a citizen, or a biomedical body. To undergo social death in this way is for the hope with which patients orient themselves toward both hospital technologies and kinship relationships to come to an end.

One day I came in to the ward to find Michael sitting up tensely, gripping the sides of the bed. A nurse was fiddling with an IV line while one of Michael's brothers, who had come to stay in the hospital while looking for work in the town, was stroking his back. Mary sat on the floor by the bed looking very worried. It turned out the IV line, which they had put in the night before had become blocked. Michael's face was screwed up in pain and every now and then he let out a groan, calling to the nurse for pain medicine. Mary explained that they hadn't slept all night because he was throwing up and in so much pain. The doctor came at noon and gave medicine and the drip (*wara*) and Michael had felt better for a while. But now the pain was beginning again in his abdomen and back. Mary began to cradle Michael's head while his brother stroked his back. Michael took a tiny bottle of clear liquid out of his shirt pocket and gave it to his brother who started rubbing it hard into his back. It smelt like tiger balm.

At this moment Dr. Bosa walked past and down the aisle as if to leave the ward. "Doctor!" Michael called out. The strangled sound was somewhere inbetween a greeting and a desperate plea for help. The spontaneous outburst cut across the ward, leaving silence in its wake. I had never heard a patient ask for help or even address the doctor publicly before. The doctor seemed equally shaken. He hesitated, quickly nodded his head in Michael's direction, but kept walking.

Later that afternoon I was talking to another patient in the acute side of the ward. As we were chatting, Michael's brother came running from the chronic ward to the nurses' office between the two sides of the ward and shouted out for the nurse to call the doctor. The nurse went into the ward to take a look at Michael, and then went back into the office. By this time many other patients and relatives were gathering around. The commotion was even felt in the acute side where people started moving toward the chronic ward, standing in the connecting corridor trying to get a look at what was happening. I felt very uncomfortable. I was worried about Michael but did not want to add to the spectacle. Wails now sounded from where Michael lay in the ward. The patient I had been sitting with, Margaret, turned to me and said, "Death is like a thief. You can't know when it will come to take you."

The nurse had called the doctor and was waiting for him to arrive, but suspected it was already too late. Michael's brother came out of the ward and collected a mop. Several patients were now standing up in the chronic ward looking at Michael as his mother rubbed his chest. His brother started mopping the floor. Then he went to get the cloth screen that was stored outside the nurses' office. He placed the screen around the bed and he and Mary went inside it. There was now total silence in the ward. As people walked past outside it seemed as though they could feel the heavy silence and many peered inside. When they saw the screen they muttered "a person must have died" (the tok pisin has a finality to it: "wanpela mas i dai pinis") and walked on.

I went into the office. Two of the nurses were sitting down looking visibly upset, waiting for the doctor to arrive. They explained that patients should not die in the chronic side of the ward. They were sad because Michael had been staying there for so long that they had got to know him. The patient file with the death certificate waiting to be filled in was lying between them on the desk. They began to discuss logistics. One asked if they should put the body in the side room. The nursing officer in charge told her that they should let the family stay a while first. The nurse explained that they would let the mother and brother stay in the hospital for the night, and maybe the next day if they couldn't arrange transport.

I went and stood outside the ward. Den was standing alone in the shade. He had gone for a short walk and when he returned found that Michael had died. He didn't want to go back into the ward:

I worry about this. That you can die at any time. I did not expect Michael to die. He did not look like he was going to die. [Other patients also standing outside nod their heads.] It makes me worry because the other day I was cross with Michael. I was walking over there and I saw someone come out of the washroom and because of my eyes I couldn't see who it was. I called out "Who are you?" but they didn't answer. Then I saw that it was Michael and this made me very angry that he didn't respond. I came back to the ward and was thinking about it and I couldn't sleep because I was so angry. In the morning I shouted at him and then I left the ward and went and sat in the operating theater waiting area. Then in the afternoon Michael found me there and he apologized and said he should have responded when I called out and I said sorry too and then it was ok. But when he died I remembered this. I shouted at him and then he died so now I am worrying and thinking a lot.

This is not the way that death should be. In the village people should not be standing around talking like this doing nothing. We should be crying and we should go inside and cry. But in town people have other things to think about. They look at other things. They are not too busy with thinking about the dead. But in the village you think about him and that is all you think about, you don't look at anything else. In town you go around the stores and then you look at other things and don't help your dead wantok.

Den's account of his argument with Michael and his fears of his own culpability in Michael's death illustrate the emotional and physical stakes that patients have in their relationships with each other in the hospital. When one has already been forgotten and rendered invisible by everyone else, the refusal of a fellow patient to acknowledge one can provoke intense fear and anger. Michael's subsequent death and its aftermath only confirmed to Den that the hospital was a place where people ceased to be properly embedded and remembered in social relationships, where social and physical death collide.

The next morning I came into the ward to find Michael's brother packing up their belongings on the hospital bed. Mary was in the side room with Michael's body, which lay wrapped tightly in white bandages on a trolley in the center of the room. There was barely enough space for Mary and two other relatives to squeeze around it to stand in the corners of the room. They asked me to join them, holding hands and crying over the body. The nurse came to the door and asked Mary what her plans were. They wanted to know whether to move the body to the morgue or whether they would be taking it today. Mary explained that they needed to get in contact with Rai Coast High School where her husband used to work and ask the headmaster if he would send the school's dinghy to come and collect them. If they couldn't find a dinghy they would have to take the body to the settlement outside town where some of their wantok were living. She didn't know if they would help them to transport the body home or whether they would have to bury him in town.

By the afternoon they had heard through the hospital radio that the high school would send a dinghy, but the doctor had still not signed the death certificate. They needed the death certificate to access the money that Michael had kept in his bank account in order to pay for the food to take back to the village for the funeral. For Michael's relatives, the doctor's delay in signing the death certificate only reinforced the connection between the doctor's dismissive attitude toward Michael and the failure of the hospital technologies to make him better.

THE INVISIBLE BODY

Adam Reed describes how, for men in Bomana Prison in Papua New Guinea, separation from kin enables them to engage in alternative forms of relationship within the prison (Reed 2003). It is the substitution of one set of relationships for another, he argues, that enables them to apprehend their own transformation within the institution. Bomana is characterized as a "place of men" and likened by the inmates to the seclusion of boys during initiation. Extending the terms that Marilyn Strathern devised in her description of Melanesian sociality (1988), Reed claims that their separation from women (their mothers, wives, girlfriends) and what Strathern refers to as "particular" and "cross-sex" relationships, reveals the inmates as a unitary body in a "collective" and "same-sex" relationship with one another. In such a state their cross-sex relationships with women are eclipsed, but also anticipated insofar as it is these women who will meet them upon their release and judge their progress. Like initiates secluded in the Highlands long house or Sepik spirit house, it is their seclusion that effects their transformation insofar as it enables bodily change to register in the regard of others (women). In this respect, the prison and spirit house operate as transformative technologies that work through closely controlled modes of spatiotemporal containment.

Unlike prisoners, patients did not make analogies between their containment in the hospital and initiation. But the extension of this metaphor to the hospital is revealing of patients' concerns with concealment as a predicate to social efficacy. Patients often talked about their admission to the hospital with a degree of pride or relief. They said that when they were ill in the village and unable to engage in productive work or exchanges people lost respect for them or became angry with them, thus making their illness worse. In being referred to Madang they felt that their sickness had been identified as treatable by both the health center workers near their village and by the doctors who admitted them, thus opening up new opportunities for realizing their social and physical capacities. Like prison and initiation, the hospital initially appears to offer the simultaneous possibility of seclusion from kin and the substitution of new kinds of relationships through which to work on the body, in this case with doctors. Like those other versions of institutional containment, patients anticipate that when they return to the village their kin will look at them and admire their visibly healthy bodies, their shiny eyes, and plump glowing skin.[22]

In his ethnography of Reite, a Madang Province village, James Leach also employs the idiom of visibility to describe the temporal process of recognition. Recognition is "the emergence of a socially effective, temporally sequenced, whole person who is visible, as such, to others" (Leach 2003, 151). Visibility is described as the "power to make themselves apparent as a particular thing (a desirable person/place, a man)" (Leach 2003). While the mother and father in Reite provide growth through the sharing of food within the hamlet, exchanges with the mother's brother differentiate the mother's brother and the sister's child. Such exchanges, Leach argues, also produce the mother's brother as a "perspective" on the child, from which he can be released from his "containment" in relationships with his parents and siblings, and recognized as a man.

The hospital does not appear to function as an effective container in this sense. No one takes a perspective from which a patient can be recognized as a particular kind of person. Patients describe themselves as trying and failing to forget neglectful relatives. Kin seem to be both too distant (patients are unable to activate these relationships and their obligations) and too present (those relationships still dominate patients' thoughts and demand action). At the same time, patients are often unable to elicit a positive response from the doctor, and there is intense uncertainty over whether the doctor has looked beyond the surface of their skin to find the sickness. They are neither able to make themselves visible as a socially effective person in the regard of kin nor hospital workers. Their thoughts about and orientation to these multiple relationships at once condemn them to a kind of social stasis. To escape this static state of worry (wori), Christian patients profess to reduce multiple thoughts to one by focusing solely on their relationship with God.

Patients are perhaps more similar to prisoners on remand who spend all their time "thinking about court" (ting ting long kot) (Reed 2011b, 529) and who are described by fellow inmates as "half freedom" and "half-kalabus [prison]" (Reed 2011b, 534). The contrast between inmates who have already been sentenced and those on remand who are waiting for the court judgment "is between a subject who has still to find out what he will become and one who knows what has happened to him" (Reed 2011b, 530). Convicts, like patients who are on the verge of discharge or death "are, quite literally, the endpoint of a process" (Reed 2011b, 530). Like prison for those on remand, the hospital is a place where patients wait to find out who they will become and what kind of body they will be found to have. It is a place "where we just wait." Some forms of waiting, Reed suggests, following others in hope studies (Crapanzano 2011; Hage 2003), can be intrinsically connected to hope and the cultivation of a prospective, future-oriented disposition (Hage 2003; Reed 2011b). Patients constantly look to their own body, the garden food they receive from kin, and the attentions they receive from hospital staff for signs of how they will leave the hospital—whether they will walk out the ward entrance carrying their belongings and accompanied by their relatives, or whether their bandaged body will be wheeled out of the back of the ward on a metal hospital trolley. The doctor's failure to respond to Michael's cry for help seemed like a final refusal to engage, confirming Michael's fears that the doctor had never "seen" him at all. The time of waiting, hope, and experimentation had come to an end.

CONCLUSION

The story about the mass graves, it turned out, was true. The hospital does indeed periodically resort to mass burials of abandoned bodies on the outskirts of the town. These are the bodies of persons that had ceased to be recognized by kin and that in many cases also remained biomedically unknown. They are invisible to family, medicine, and the state. That neither one's family nor the hospital would be able, or perhaps want to, help them, is a real possibility patients countenance on an everyday basis as they monitor their relationships (with their guardians, with their relatives in town, and with hospital workers), and as they examine their bodies for minute signs of improvement.

Critiques of biomedicine have often rested on the ways in which biomedical knowledge practices reduce personhood to the biological body. In Madang Hospital, however, the problem as experienced by patients is how to make themselves knowable as a biomedical entity and therefore compel the doctor to cure them. Here the biomedical gaze is disrupted by weak state infrastructure and unstable technologies. Amidst bed shortages, drug shortages, and staff shortages, patients easily fall through the "gaps in the gaze" (Gibson 2004), making new, indistinct pathologies and forms of abandonment possible.

The extended process of waiting and uncertainty on the ward spurs patients to action. They travel backward and forward to the village, engage proactively with biomedical technologies, and resolutely follow the doctor's orders. Uncertainty is not an epistemic problem so much as a relational one. Like Whyte's account of the Nyole in Uganda, patients in Madang Hospital are "engaged in a quest for security rather than a quest for certainty" (Whyte 1997, 3). In this sense, when patients such as Michael invoke notions of sik bilong marasin and sik bilong ples, they do not apply contrastive "explanatory models" (e.g., biomedical and social) to their condition (Kleinman 1986) within a pluralistic medical framework (Frankel and Lewis 1989). Patients' knowledge practices in the hospital consist less of reflective attempts to provide comprehensive explanations for their condition than pragmatic experimentation with relational technologies in the hospital and in the village, which they hope will materially transform their bodies.[23] To presume that explanatory meaning is the goal of patients' improvisatory ventures is to negate the intrinsically future oriented, anticipatory mode of being that makes the hospital "a waiting place" (Miyazaki 2010).[24] Uncertainty is an integral characteristic of social relationships in the hospital and demands an experimental response. Patients do not seek to *know* their body as a reified form, but to *turn it into* a form that might be seen by others.

The hospital is not a place, like zones of abandonment that Joao Biehl documents in urban Brazil, where "living beings go when they are no longer considered people" (2005b, 2). But it is a place where people can undergo a slow process of social disappearance at the hands of family, medicine, and the state. Here patients become aware of their profound marginality to urban political and economic life. Doctors' biomedical failure to effectively know and heal patients as biological bodies (described in chapter 4) is recalibrated by patients as a personal failure to make oneself seen.

CHAPTER 6

Technologies of Detachment

■ "If I could change one thing, it would be access to information. We don't have the Internet here. There is nothing to back us up." I was reminded of the comment, made by a surgical registrar during an interview in 2003, several years later in 2011, while searching for the doctors that I had worked with in Madang on Biomed Experts, a professional networking site for medical researchers. By 2011, the Internet's value for medical professionals lay not only in the ability to access information about disease, but the capacity to access information about one another. The site profiles include information about the individual's research projects, previous and currently held posts, publications, and collaborations. For each individual profile, the site creates a digital map of professional links and associations around the world, based on their coauthorship of journal articles. This is depicted on a world map as a series of black lines, like flight paths, emanating from the medic's location. By clicking on one profile it is possible to trace an entire network of medical professionals working in a thematic area across international space.

Madang Hospital's connection to the Internet is still fragile: a single, old, virus-ridden, desktop computer sits in the office of the institution's public relations officer. The only Papua New Guinean doctor whose completed profile I could find on Biomed Experts was that of the director of the Institute of Medical Research, who had been appointed to the position in 2006. Through his international collaborations (described in more detail in chapter 8) a series of crisscrossing lines take the viewer to Australia, Europe, Africa, North and South America. The networked person created and displayed to others through this digital medium is extended in time and space. Their names have traveled, along with grants from international bodies, data from the field, and journal articles, to other places. The circulation of names and knowledge in digital form constitute international "space-time" (Munn 1986) and scale relationships between persons, and therefore those persons themselves between the "local" and the "global." The scientist apprehended on the website is a global scientist. As journal articles move around the world it is not only scientific facts that become consolidated and stabilized (Latour and Woolgar 1986) and accrue scientific value, but particular versions of personhood.

Warwick Anderson has commented on similarities between Melanesian and scientific prestige economies: "In the drive for credit, whether among Melanesians or scientists, it is necessary to keep extending and confirming networks through strategic exchange" (2008, 155). Thus Anderson describes how the kuru scientist, Carleton Gadjusek, who spent several years conducting research among the Fore in the Papua New Guinean Highlands, gifted Fore brains to pathologists at the NIH laboratories in Bethesda and scientists in Australia in order to compel them to recognize his scientific prowess and assist him in his work. He "anticipated the extractive perspective of his fellow scientists and set about manipulating the emerging economy of his kuru blood and brains" (Anderson 2009, 154). Through the circulation of scientific goods and manipulation of social relationships Gadjusek made himself into a "big man" within the mid-twentieth-century scientific economy. "As these novel things circulated, they acquired the power to create social relations, to move other persons, to make persons visible in surprising ways. For recipients, these objects were personified around the figure of Gadjusek. That is, these things, once Fore, were now Gadjusek's kuru valuables" (2009, 155).

In the twenty-first-century knowledge economy, meanwhile, with its new exchange networks and practices of institution building (Fischer 2011), scientists seek to amplify their public presence through the research grants, journal articles, and "hits" that are registered and made visible on their Biomed Experts profile. Across these different scientific economies, scientific personhood has continued to entail a peculiar version of individual creativity: the individual, heroic scientist is only made visible through the exchanges and collaborations that they establish with others. Scientists are regarded as individuals, but their individuality is enhanced by their public capacity to enroll other scientists and scientific objects into their scientific network. From the perspective of any one scientific profile on Biomed Experts the scientist's collaborators are visible only as subsidiary elements of their person, the means through which the scientist's creative capacity gains expression in the world. The agency of other persons is thus encompassed within the figure of the "global" or "great" scientist, but as the container for and assembler of these relationships credit accrues to his person as a unitary rather than composite person.[1] Collaborators thus have both an internal and an external function in the constitution of scientific personhood; internally their actions contribute to the scientist's creative capacity, externally they provide social recognition of that capacity.[2]

Anthropologists have similarly described Melanesian gift exchange as a mode of objectifying persons. Nonetheless there are significant differences between scientific and Melanesian personhood and exchange as they have been reified in ethnographic literature. By contrast with the international scientists described by Anderson, Strathern argues that gift exchange in Melanesia is not oriented toward the *construction* of social ties, where otherwise there would only be individuals, but rather to the *differentiation* of persons and the *revelation* of particular relationships that make those persons up.[3] Each exchange reveals certain relationships and eclipses others. Social action is undertaken in order to draw out of persons the relationships they are capable of establishing and in making them visible, mobilize their effects. The "global scientist" is a figure of encompassment in which other persons' actions contribute to and make visible one individual's creative agency. They are the author of both their own *and* other's actions. The "Melanesian person" is, by contrast, a composite of their relationships with others. The act of giving is always apprehended as compelled or elicited by the actions or gifts of someone else. Their actions are not self-authored so much as they are elicited or caused by others (Strathern 1988, 268–306).

In both prestige economies, however, personhood is dependent on external recognition. International scientists rely on the actions of others to make their own capacities visible. As in Melanesian ceremonial exchange, scientific recognition also depends on the flow and exchange of things. Anderson's study drew attention to a moment when the generation of scientific prestige through exchanges of body parts, paper, and technologies was, perhaps, more explicit but, as this chapter shows, such exchanges are no less significant today. The digitally mapped global scientist depends on, as well as enables, the flow and exchange of material resources through his/her relationships and across space and time. For doctors in Madang Hospital controlling (or eliciting) these flows and exchanges across the borderlands of professional and kinship, national, and global identities is particularly challenging. Indeed, it is doctors' inability to keep the entanglements of kinship and biomedicine separate, and the persistent flow of objects and persons across this contact zone (Pratt 1991) that is experienced as the greatest constraint in becoming a scientific (as opposed to Melanesian) "big man."

A NATIONAL PROFESSION

All the doctors in the hospital except one were Papua New Guinean and had been trained at the School of Medical and Health Sciences at the University of Papua New Guinea in Port Moresby. The school was established in 1970 when the Papuan Medical College, which had opened a decade earlier, was incorporated into the new university.[4] This was a period of intense social and political change in Papua New Guinea. By 1960 the UN had established a Decolonization Committee and the Australian government was under pressure to move the territory toward self-governance. Local councils were established in 1960, replacing *luluais* and *tultuls* (see chapter 2), the number of native members in the Legislative Council grew to seven in 1961, and a House of Representatives with elected native members was established in 1964. By 1973 the territory had achieved self-governance, and by 1975 gained independence. It was during this same period that national doctors began to graduate from the Papua New Guinean medical school.[5]

Many of the senior doctors in Madang Hospital were trained in the immediate postindependence era, when hopes for national development were running high, and when doctors were expected to play a central role in bringing that development about. They were educated in the newly established national high schools and at the University of Papua New Guinea, where they met other students from all over the country.[6] Indeed this centralized system of education was designed in the preindependence period precisely in order to inculcate a sense of national identity and belonging in the educated elite. The anticipated importance of doctors to the development of a national consciousness in Papua New Guinea was based on the notion that the rational and objective universal principles of science would shield them from the partiality of ethnic or kinship ties and would inculcate a commitment to the social good. As elsewhere in the colonial world, science was associated with both modernity and the birth of national consciousness (Prakash 1999). In Papua New Guinea, however, the colonial administration was keen to encourage rather than clamp down on the blooming of this national consciousness, partly because it was considered far too nascent to represent a threat to the colonial order.

Indeed many early health professionals and medical graduates did play an important role in public and political life in the 1960s and 1970s, but they often represented a conservative as opposed to revolutionary position on independence. The newly elected native member of the House of Representatives, Tei Abel, who had been trained as a medical orderly in Wabag in the 1950s, for example, argued strongly that Papua New Guinea needed more time for education and more time for preparation before full independence could take place.[7] Many of the new educated elite felt the rest of the country was still too backward to be able to operate without Australian supervision. In this people like Tei Abal echoed the sentiments of Australian politicians such as Paul Hasluck, the minister of territories, who sought to resist the pressure from the UN to move rapidly toward independence on the basis that Papua New Guinea was still far too primitive to cope without the paternalistic overview of their Australian neighbor.[8] The country could not depend, he argued, on a tiny educated minority, but needed slow and "even development," including education for all, before a self-sufficient national economy and political system would become possible.

Doctors in Madang refer to this pioneering generation of medical graduates as "the first national professionals" who had been lifted out of "traditional" village life. Senior doctors describe their time at university and in the national high schools as moments of radical transformation when they fostered ties to people beyond their kin networks and when they learned from their expatriate teachers that the work of medicine could contribute to development and the improvement of people's lives on a national scale. Like indigenous doctors trained in colonial and postcolonial contexts elsewhere, Papua New Guinean doctors "came to view themselves as modern and cosmopolitan intellectuals, not mere colonial subjects," people to whom science had bequeathed "a sense of anticipation, of limitless potential, of national futures" (Anderson and Pols 2012, 111). This was a time that the senior doctors describe as full of optimism and hope in the contribution a national medical profession could make to their young country's future. Doctors talked, for example, of the desire to "help Papua New Guineans" and contribute to development as important in their decision to study medicine in a way that scaled up their own agency and personhood to a "national" level, in contrast to their village counterparts.[9]

Today, however, many doctors told me that they had come to realize that they couldn't really have any impact on *national* development at all. As Doctor Bosa explained: "Most patients arrive too sick for us to do anything for them. The real impact is made through prevention work in the rural areas. That is where the health of the population can be improved, not in the hospital. We don't save lives here." In Madang Hospital doctors are stuck at the far end of decline in a population's health, where all they can do is struggle to save an individual life with inadequate resources. Their medical effects are not registered on an epidemiological scale. Much of this frustration is directed at the Papua New Guinean government. The state, doctors argue, is failing in its duty to provide basic services and lift its people out of ill health and poverty. Until this political situation is changed, they argue, individual doctors working in urban hospitals will be unable to improve lives. The truth and rational principles of science, doctors in Madang Hospital have come to realize, is not enough; national development also requires political change. In contrast to Adams's account of doctors in Nepal, who also saw political change as central to the achievement of medical goals (Adams 1998, 23), the doctors in Madang Hospital do not aspire to use their positions in urban public life as political leverage. Rather they grieve the loss of national capacity that they had once associated with medical work.[10] Doctors thus find themselves in an awkward symbiosis with the state (Iliffe 1998). They are both dependent on it for their training, employment, and wages, and increasingly see themselves as a victim and external arbiter of its failures.

Doctors have also learnt that the world of science is itself riven by inequalities. In the 1970s and 1980s becoming a doctor had been a way of becoming equal with the European doctors who taught and worked alongside national doctors. But doctors also remember their frustration at the time that expatriate doctors had continued to live segregated lives, to earn more than nationals for the same job, and to treat them as if their medical practice was substandard.[11] If they were to lead the development of a nation, the doctors felt, they should also have international recognition of their professional status. Doctors might not have been instigators of revolutionary anticolonial struggle, but many remember taking part in strikes in the 1970s against unequal pay and poor treatment by their expatriate colleagues.

Today concerns about the way they are perceived by an international community of medics and scientists continues to shape doctors' professional identity. Their medical training plays a crucial role in this. At the time of the new medical school's opening, there had been vigorous debate about the extent to which the curriculum should mirror that in Australian hospitals or should be made "appropriate" to Papua New Guinea. On one hand there were concerns that Papua New Guinean doctors would not be recognized and would be treated as "second-rate" by an international scientific community. On the other hand, it was deemed inappropriate for Papua New Guinean doctors to be trained in a corpus of medical knowledge that they would have no occasion to use in Papua New Guinea itself (Denoon 1989, 97). The compromise reached was that the degree program would include a greater focus on community health, but Papua New Guinean doctors undergoing specialist training would also spend a period of residency at an Australian hospital in order to learn procedures and the use of technologies unavailable in the hospitals in Papua New Guinea. Fully qualified specialists therefore return from Australia with experience and knowledge of complex procedures that they have no foreseeable opportunity to use in their everyday practice in Papua New Guinea. Many specialists are consequently resistant to moving back to a provincial hospital, where the resources available to deal with complex cases are limited and where the large medical community and social network established at Port Moresby Hospital is missing. Doctors who are undergoing training as residents or registrars, meanwhile, would prefer to work in Port Moresby where there is a greater concentration of equipment and specialists to learn from. Doctors complain about the crime, cost of living, and ugliness of Port Moresby by comparison with Madang, but many admit they would still prefer to have a government position in the capital city.

PROVINCIAL MEDICINE

In describing their reasons for wanting to become a doctor, many of those working in Madang Hospital recalled their desire to work in rural areas. One surgical registrar, Dr. Kalim, had grown up on Karkar Island off the mainland of Madang Province where, during the Second World War, a German Missionary, Edwin Tscharke, had established a rural hospital. Dr. Kalim saw Tscharke as a role model: "He was on Karkar for many years and he has done a lot for the people and they absolutely loved him. He was well loved and respected right up until his death." Doctors describe the ideal of being loved and respected by people in a small community as one of their main inspirations for wanting to study medicine.

Dr. Nabik, who had grown up in a village near Mount Hagen in the Highlands, recalled becoming very sick as a child and the health extension officer who treated him in the village. Many years later, when at National High School in Port Moresby, he sat on a flight to Madang and read about another health extension officer in the on-flight magazine: "I was reading this flight magazine and there was a particular story about one HEO [health extension officer] in one of these AID posts in the bush who was treating people and there were some pictures of kids with these very big bellies and so on. And I was thinking about these things in the past like when I was in Grade Two. And then the thing is on the plane I made up my mind. As soon as I go back I would do my foundation science." He later went to work on Karkar:

> Working wise I really enjoyed it because you are working in the rural setting. You are situated right in the village. And then there are times when you really see the people in the village [and] they really appreciate a real doctor working with them. They really appreciate it, you know. That was the thing about [the hospital] I really enjoyed. I could have been there longer if I had been looked after in a way that I could have settled. In Moresby people had choices. . . . But in the village they had no choices, and when you were there they were very appreciative.

The medical authority and prestige that doctors can ostensibly cultivate in a rural community is impossible to realize amid the complex teamwork and internal hierarchy of a large urban hospital. Doctors who had worked in rural areas described their enjoyment at being the only doctor, of treating all medical problems not just those in their specialty and not having to negotiate treatment or management plans with anyone else. As Dr. Nabik explained, working with the theater staff in Madang was very difficult after having worked at two rural church hospitals in Madang Province: "It is mostly to do with the theater staff. Because when I was working [on Karkar] I was on my own, I would do most things . . . I will do this operation now and I could get the patient ready. So because I was the boss I could make decisions about how to do things. But here I could not do it." In particular, surgeons who had worked in rural areas found it difficult to work with the senior anesthetist in the operating theater, who saw the theater as her domain of authority. One of the frustrations and perks of working in rural hospitals, surgical doctors told me, was that they did not have to work alongside anesthetists.

For Dr. Bosa the difficulties of working with other colleagues in the hospital was heightened by his ambivalent position as both the only doctor on the medical ward and being perceived as less qualified than the specialists who presided over the other wards. Consultants have a whole team of people underneath them who recognize their authority and contribute to their creative agency in precisely the same mode of individual encompassment as is visualized at a global scale by the Biomed Experts website. Dr. Bosa did not have any trainees. The other consultants in the hospital did not treat him as an equal or ask him for advice in the way they might a physician. And yet it was precisely the work and the responsibilities of a consultant-level physician that Dr. Bosa felt had been imposed on him as the sole doctor in the ward. Over the year I spent at the hospital in 2003, he became increasingly resistant to asking for assistance or advice, for fear he would be treated as junior by the other consultants, and avoided spaces in the hospital, such as ICU or the private ward, where he was forced to collaborate with the other doctors in managing the care of patients. Like the rural doctor he was "the boss" of his own ward, but outside that ward he had to negotiate professional relationships with other more senior doctors.[12]

Despite the role that fantasies of rural medicine play in the educational biographies of many of Madang's doctors, none of those I spoke to wanted to return to work in a rural hospital. In fact, the shortage of medical doctors willing to work in rural areas presents a significant human resources problem in Papua New Guinea (Hongoro and McPake, 2004). The Lutheran mission hospital on Karkar today depends on foreign doctors recruited through the mission to staff the hospital rather than national doctors. The isolation of the rural village is attractive because it enhances the doctor's standing within that community, but ultimately it exacerbates their isolation from a global medical community and specialist professional network.

And yet, in other ways, the provincial hospital in Papua New Guinea too closely resembles the rural hospital. The number of medical specialists employed by a hospital and the size of the population served determine its "level" within a national referral system. From rural aid posts, staffed by a basically trained community health worker, patients are referred to a health center, which should have nursing staff and where the officer in charge is usually a health extension officer.[13] From the health center patients are referred to the provincial, Level 1 hospital (such as Madang), which should have at least one specialist in each department. Regional, Level 2 hospitals (such as Goroka or Lae), should have specialist units able to deal with particular conditions, such as cancer or psychiatric care. The last resort would be the national Level 3 referral hospital in Port Moresby. Despite its status as a Level 1 hospital, consultant positions in Madang Hospital are often unfilled. Meanwhile, the doctors who work there find that the resources that are meant to flow from the capital to the province rarely do so.

Drugs and equipment are sourced from overseas by one of six medical supplies companies operating out of Port Moresby. Medical doctors complain that the suppliers starve the health system of drugs in order to bypass the official tender process and that Department of Health officials who then buy the drugs through "emergency procedures" at raised prices, get substantial kickbacks.[14] There is also widespread concern about corruption in the tendering process and the effective regulation of the drugs procured.[15]

Even when the supplies reach Port Moresby it isn't given that they will get to Madang. Drugs and medical equipment are stored in the Central Medical Store in Badili, Port Moresby. From here they are shipped to Lae and then transported by road to the Area Medical Store, which is located on the hospital site in Madang. The Area Medical Store is responsible for making frequent orders for drugs and equipment. However, the administrators often only make their requests when stock is already running low. Meanwhile, the stores in Port Moresby regularly take longer than expected to respond to such requests. In addition the black market in drugs has also become a major source of supplementary income for many of those involved in this supply chain and large quantities of drugs and medical goods frequently go missing. The interlocked public and private circulation of basic pharmaceuticals in Papua New Guinea reveals the "morass of economic and moral paradoxes" that characterizes pharmaceutical markets worldwide (Petryna 2005, 2). The hindered flow of medical supplies to the hospital, coupled with the free flow of drugs toward Port Moresby and out into the black market, means the hospital is frequently short of the most basic drugs, equipment or laboratory reagents.

Doctors' frustrations often center on these shortages. "The most difficult part of my job," one doctor explained, "is trying to secure materials." Doctors often have to locate drugs or pieces of equipment around the country and persuade their colleagues in other hospitals to send them on. In 2010, the Area Medical Store in Madang was closed down altogether after the building was condemned by the Department of Public Works. The province went without a medical store for several months before an alternative location was found. When the hospital ran out of vital supplies during this time, doctors and technicians resorted to calling their equivalents in Port Moresby. However, the capacity to compel staff in Port Moresby to send those supplies often depends on the ability of the Madang staff to invoke an established connection, for example of shared schooling or employment in the past. When relationships cannot be mobilized to move resources, doctors frequently end up writing private prescriptions for basic medicines, which they tell patients' families to purchase at the pharmacy in town. All too often they know that the families will not be able to afford the medications or that by the time they had found the money it will be too late for the patient. "Most deaths are preventable," I was told, "if we had the resources." People living a cosmopolitan lifestyle in Port Moresby, doctors suggest, have a lack of concern for what happens in the provincial institutions they are meant to support.

As described in chapter 4 doctors often find they have to locate resources themselves or seek pragmatic alternatives to standard testing and treatment protocols. This would often make Dr. Bosa furious:

Well the question is if I see that there is something we can do but we have constraints. I suppose I feel angry. I feel angry and what I do is I go and look for that thing. And if there is something we should be doing I try to do it as it should be done. And quickly . . . intervention. I try to put in interventions quickly so that we actively manage the cases or if I am not able to do that I must go and get other officers who are able to do that. Well I feel angry and it's not a good feeling to have. Frustration, like if there is an urgent lab test that they are not able to do and the outcome of that test might have determined the management of the patient. If we had a person, say, with chest trauma or a patient with *sotwin* [asthma] we want an urgent X-ray. If they had a chest injury the lung might be collapsed. So the X-ray will help to see that and do something about it. Then if they are not able to do an X-ray—then it is that kind of example that makes the doctors frustrated. Then sometimes it makes you angry.

Doctors' sense that they cannot rely on a system but have to 'do everything by ourselves' is articulated through comparisons with Port Moresby General Hospital. As Dr. Nabik, who completed his residency in Port Moresby, explained:

The thing is [in Port Moresby] in the lab if you just ask for the blood then it is done. Then you've got the blood the next day. If you want the blood in the night then it is done. And the medicines are there. Good quality X-rays. If you wanted good quality advice there was good teaching there. But [regarding] the support service certain things were there [and] you didn't have to go and look for them. But here, you know how reliable the lab and you don't know how reliable the results are. . . . The thing is if they are not there, then you have to go around looking for them. That was not like in Moresby. Especially a big hospital like . . . Moresby and Madang. . . . Moresby is a better place to work in as a doctor because the support services are up to date, the laboratory is up to date. And they wouldn't complain.

People as well as medical goods and test results refuse to flow to the provinces. Senior staff in Port Moresby, it is claimed, never visit Madang. Indeed, in the fifteen months I spent in Madang between 2003 and 2004, the physician at the regional hospital in Lae made only a single trip to supervise the registrar in Madang Hospital's medical ward. This reinforced Dr. Bosa's sense of marginalization from a national professional community and his growing resentment about the lack of recognition he received for his work in the hospital.

Madang does not offer the individual autonomy and authority imagined to exist for doctors in rural hospitals. It is not far enough away from the medical establishment for doctors to achieve the status of heroic lone doctor akin to the rural missionary doctors of an earlier era. Nor, by contrast with Port Moresby or the Australian hospitals where many have trained, does the provincial hospital enable doctors to practice the up-to-date interventions from their specialty. Obstructed flows of persons and things make Madang feel a very long way from both the capital and the well-funded research hospitals in the West where new progress in their field was being made. Disconnected from the Internet and with limited equipment, doctors complain they have to resign themselves to the routine treatment of preventable infectious diseases, to a version of medicine that works for Madang Hospital but which has no legitimacy beyond it (see chapter 4).[16]

THE WHITE LIFE

Doctors' lifestyles in Madang also fall short of the expectations that were instilled at medical school, especially through the example of their European teachers. The doctors' houses in the compound behind the hospital were once built for the expatriate doctors at the hospital and were more spacious and airy than the cramped concrete blocks that were built for the "native" hospital workers and that are now the homes of the hospital's nursing staff. Nonetheless the doctors' houses have received no maintenance since independence, and are today dilapidated. There is no alternative affordable accommodation available in the town, especially since a growing number of NGOs and the development of a nickel mine along the coast have pushed up the cost of rent. One senior doctor at the hospital described how he had been forced to move out of a hospital-owned house into rented accommodation because the hospital had allowed their home to become derelict. Now the hospital was failing to pay his landlord the rent and so the landlord was refusing to do any maintenance on the house, which he complained had broken furniture, a leaking roof and no washing machine. The inability of the hospital to provide a large freestanding family house with the kinds of white goods that doctors considered necessary to urban living was widely described as central to the lack of interest that newly qualified physicians showed in applying to a position at the hospital. As Iliffe noted of living conditions for East African doctors in the 1940s and 1950s, "To be a paragon of modernity in these circumstances was hard indeed" (1998, 83).

Partly because of the shortage of doctors, those who are employed in Madang work exceptionally long hours and are often on call. But where they see doctors in the rest of the world, and especially Australia, compensated for this hard work with large pay packets, plush houses, and new cars, doctors in Madang Hospital complain that they do not enjoy any of these perks. Doctor Nabik described his envy when he saw peers from his university days who had taken different employment trajectories: "When you are really over worked and you see other people you were at college with and they all have cars and nice houses like this materialist kind of thing and then you are really like, you are working your guts out and you don't seem to have anything in the world." The demands on their salaries from extended kin means there is little money left over for consumption of the kinds of household goods that white people have. "Working for government" means living amidst the colonial detritus of institutions that might once have fulfilled ideals of modern living, but which are now long past their heyday. This was one reason why Dr. Nabik saw life in Port Moresby to be so attractive: "To work effectively, to work really effectively and keep your full concentration on your work you have to have all these things, like your house and things. The only thing about Moresby I really enjoyed was that they take care of your outside life. Like housing was taken care of. It meets your daily needs, [and when these] were taken care of . . . you didn't need to think about those. You just needed to think about your work."

For doctors from Madang itself or its neighboring provinces living in Port Moresby also means your house is less likely to be full of *wantok* visiting from the village. Dr. Bosa from neighboring Morobe Province lived in the compound with his wife and children, his mother, father, brother, and several other relatives from the village who slept on the floor in his living room. This was why their home life was so different from that they imagined for European doctors, and why they said it distracted them from their work.

Doctors in Madang Hospital are highly aware of the links between colonialism and science. They often see the world of global science as a space of gross inequality where some kinds of medicine are more closely aligned with truth and rationality than others, and where those superior truths always belong to European doctors. Today those inequalities are made visible in the very different opportunities and values accorded the work of national doctors and the work of foreign medical scientists in the hospital (see chapter 8). Doctors in Madang Hospital find they are unable to participate in the kinds of medical practices, have the kinds of development effects, or create the kinds of consumerist lifestyle that make one either a national or global doctor.

UNCERTAIN EXPERTS

A key means by which doctors know themselves as different from Papua New Guineans in "the village," and understand their biographical transformation into individual medical experts, is in terms of their movement away from "belief" in witchcraft and sorcery. Doctors often talked about their time in medical school as a time of personal transformation. When they arrived at medical school, they told me, they still believed in witchcraft and sorcery. All sickness could, they thought, ultimately be traced back to social relationships. But their teachers in medical school taught them to cut the body open and "see the disease." Through their years in medical school they gradually learned that disease was caused by microbes and germs: "We have these beliefs in Papua New Guinea. But when I came here I saw that all the sicknesses that they say are caused by sorcery in the village, White people have these sicknesses too. So then I knew that these are the same sicknesses. It is just microbes and bacteria—they cause all sickness." Dr. Wani described the terror entailed by this process of medical conversion:

I went to [university] late, I arrived a couple of weeks late because of fighting in Enga province. When I arrived, my friend who was also at college told me that they were cutting dead bodies. I had just arrived and I didn't have a lab coat but he said they were going to cut the bodies, so he lent me his lab coat and I started cutting the cadavers. At the beginning I was very scared. I couldn't sleep at night, I was having nightmares. But this went after a few weeks. Then I carried bones and things and kept them in my room, studied the bones. I realized they were just bones. This really motivated me, that I could do it. I started to develop an interest in medicine. We were also watching films on how to cut bodies and this motivated me. This was my first contact that was why I was scared. I hadn't touched dead people before.

Many of the doctors in Madang Hospital profess to no longer believe in "village sickness" (sik bilong ples) or spirits. "It is my job to believe in modern medicine," Dr. Bosa told me, "I can't go believing in something that contradicts it." Their distinction between such "traditional beliefs" and their own "medical knowledge" is the basis for knowing themselves as a different kind of person from "village people."

Where Christian patients tend to view belief (belip) as a relational orientation and commitment to God (see chapter 5), doctors see belief as a representational stance, which implies the possibility of alternative stances.[17] For doctors "belief" is a mental image of reality that, by comparison with scientific and biomedical knowledge, is not based on empirical evidence. Their modernist distinction between "knowledge" and "belief" is fundamental to their understanding of their own transformation into modern experts and is perceived as the basis for their medical authority.

It is tempting, in hospitals that are located in Papua New Guinea, to search for a "Melanesianization" of biomedical knowledge practices.[18] But doctors' stories of absolute conversion to a biomedical way of seeing disease demand to be taken seriously.[19] A distinction between biomedical knowing and Papua New Guinean "culture" or "belief" is central to their experience of being a doctor. Through their medical education and experience, they feel that they have become modern rationals and cosmopolitans. Here science is yoked to modernity and "culture" to tradition. By comparison with doctors elsewhere, however, Papua New Guinean doctors do not seek to accommodate medicine to what they understood to be Papua New Guinean culture; they do not seek to make a kind of hybrid medicine or seek to recontextualize it within familiar cultural terms.[20] Instead they seek to make a complete break with Papua New Guinean "beliefs." As I described in chapter 4, if doctors make claims to a peculiarly Papua New Guinean way of doing medicine, this is based on the ability to work with and adapt to technologies and persons who do not share their medical agenda rather than the hybridization of medical knowledge.

Certain bureaucratic instruments are used by doctors to maintain this separation within everyday medical practice. One day, the resident HEO who worked in the medical ward, Eric, brought a chart into the nurses' office with a note fixed to the front, signed by the patient and the doctor, stating that the patient was "leaving hospital at their own risk." The patient had been diagnosed with Pott's disease (TB of the spine), explained Eric. "She was getting better on treatment. She was in C ward doing physiotherapy and some of the feeling was coming back. But they didn't think that she was getting better. They thought it was sik bilong ples. We tried to tell them to stay. But the family was very strong. They say they will go to the village and straighten everything and then come back. But they don't come back. They go to the village and then they get worse and then they know it is sik bilong ples. If they die, then for them that proves it was sik bilong ples."

Doctors use the "Leaving hospital at own risk" form to manage the otherwise unruly movement of patients in and out of the hospital. This bureaucratic form concentrates their authority, and therefore responsibility, within the hospital walls; establishing a legal boundary between the social relationships of "traditional" medicine and those of modern biomedicine. In fact one doctor explained that it is "useful that patients believe in black magic because it takes the pressure off me a bit." Indeed a major fear for doctors is that patients might see them as responsible should their treatment fail and that the doctor might be pulled into a world of social recrimination, compensation claims and potential violence. When a patient has a clear terminal diagnosis, or the hospital does not have the facilities to treat the patient, the doctor will often tell the patient and their family "we don't have medicine for this kind of sickness. There isn't medicine for this sickness anywhere, not in hospitals in England or America. You should go back to the village and look at things there," or simply, "this is not sickness for hospital medicine [sik bilong marasin]," the clear implication being that it must therefore be "village sickness." Such comments encourage patients to distinguish between "village sickness" and "hospital sickness," even as doctors refuted the very existence of sik bilong ples and insisted that "all sickness is biological." For doctors enforcing a spatial and bureaucratic distinction between sik bilong ples and sik bilong marasin enables them to control and even refuse social relationships with patients and the obligations and modes of accountability that those relationships potentially carry with them.

One afternoon Dr. Bosa came back from the town market pale faced and subdued. He had met an old patient who he had diagnosed with HIV and he explained that he had found the encounter deeply upsetting because he knew that this man associated him with the fact he was going to die. He had felt shaken by the way the man had looked at him, Dr. Bosa explained, and had tried to hide his face and quickly walk away. Stories were circulating at this time about a Madagascan doctor who had been posted to the Lutheran hospital at Yagaum, outside Madang town, but had been forced to leave the previous year because of death threats and personal attacks. There had been a cluster of recent deaths at the hospital and the locals had accused the doctor of sorcery. In 2003–4 doctors acknowledged that their fears about being blamed for deaths by patients' relatives was one reason they often let unsigned death certificates build up into huge piles in the medical ward office. Death certificates also often circulated between wards as doctors tried to claim these patients had been seen by another doctor or that they should have been in that doctor's ward, thereby passing on responsibility.

Doctors fear that patients seek to draw them into particular relationships that might implicate them in bodily transformations in much the way that other relatives are implicated in *sik bilong ples*. Even as they strive to keep the medical and the social separate, patients who refuse to acknowledge this separation in their relationships with doctors emerge as a persistent point of resistance. This creates a dilemma for doctors in how they negotiate their personal interactions with patients. In formal interviews doctors frequently explained to me that the most important factor in good medical practice was talking to and building a relationship with the patient, understanding their cultural context and "going down to their level." Indeed doctors regularly expressed their exasperation with lab workers, who they say take far too long to carry out important tests because they "don't care about the patients." In this regard doctors echo a broader normative discourse about biomedicine that portrays it as exercising a cool, rational gaze on patients that inhibits the creation of social relationships. Imparting the importance of a comforting "bedside manner" and relating to the patient as a "whole" person rather than objectified body have become a central tenet of medical education internationally.

And yet in their everyday practices doctors do not struggle to overcome the distance created by medical knowledge in order to establish relationships with patients. The challenge that they encounter is how to avoid an abundance of relationships and prevent them from proliferating out of control. Distance and detachment have to be actively cultivated (Candea 2010). In fact doctors often talk about the lengths they had to go to in order to avoid relationships with patients. They told me that they avoided eye contact or talking too much with patients because they were concerned that once they had engaged with them patients would start demanding things of them. The slightest gesture, they complain, could be taken as evidence of a relationship, and attendant obligations, having been recognized. Doctors say that they fear any intimacy with patients will result in them asking for money or food, that patients might then have unrealistic expectations of how much attention the doctor should give them, or expect that they will receive special attention. They might also worry, if they don't begin to improve, that their relationship with the doctor has soured. In these circumstances detachment has to be cultivated, it does not follow automatically from doctors' location in a hospital and their exercise of biomedical knowledge.

Doctors' attempts to establish a separation between hospital and village, sik bilong ples and sik bilong marasin, are further complicated by the presence of traditional healers within the hospital walls. Patients who are too sick to travel home to the village often consult traditional diviners or healers within the hospital grounds. The consultations are usually done secretively; the patient or their *wasman* (carer) would meet the glasman on the grassy area behind the ward. The doctors are aware that such consultations take place. "If we tell them not to see the glasman they will just leave. They have these beliefs. So we try not to interfere." As the director of nursing services, Sister Mairu, explained to me on my arrival at the hospital: "We can't control the patients here or tell their families what to do. We have to let them make decisions. Otherwise they will disappear. There is nothing we can do to stop them. So we let the patient families use their own healing methods in the wards, or if they don't think the hospital medicine is working we let them take the patient out to pursue other causes or remedies. This is how we do medicine in Papua New Guinea." But the presence of the glasman also makes doctors uneasy. Dr. Bosa explained: "The family came and asked me first and I said yes they could ask a glasman in but that no food or drink should be given to the patient and there should be no piercing of the skin with needles. What is important is that they do not interfere with the medicine. Whatever else they want to do, wave a leaf around, that is fine. But if they don't obey me then I tell the family to take the patient away, I will no longer treat them in the hospital."

Doctors respond to the infringement of the glasman into the hospital and a space marked by their own expertise by remapping the boundaries of their authority onto the patient body. It is only by penetrating the skin or giving the patient something to ingest, according to the doctors, that the glasman will have a material effect and therefore that their medical work will interfere with that of the doctor. Interestingly, medical materialism also leads doctors to accept the use of herbal remedies, for example for snake bites, within the hospital. Because they involve ingestible substances doctors are willing to countenance their efficacy and are generally enthusiastic about the possibility of further medical research and clinical trials to examine the usefulness of Papua New Guinean traditional remedies. By contrast, "talking," gift exchanges, or "waving a leaf around" neither challenge their medical capacities nor offer opportunities for future biomedical practice because they are intangible interventions.[21]

Doctors are also often uncomfortable about the local pastors who regularly visit the hospital wards uninvited. Pastors will often wander into the wards and preach to the patients using excerpts from the Bible or giving ad lib sermons, usually extolling the healing virtues of prayer. Some of the doctors, such as Dr. Lima, the hospital's consultant pediatrician, who are religious themselves, are happy for the pastors to talk to patients, but others are less sure. As Doctor Bosa told me after one pastor passed him on his way out the door:

> I have a problem with the church people who come in. I don't mind church visitors to the ward. I am also a church man, but I don't like the way they come. They just come and preach aggressively in the middle of everyone. It is badly organized and they don't come and ask first, they just come and do it. The preacher just goes and sits down and talks to them, and if it is obvious the patient doesn't like it but he just talks to them anyway. I have thrown two preachers out of the ward since I have been here. I don't like people just coming and preaching because sometimes they tell them the wrong things, like medicine won't help them, they just have to pray. The preachers also avoid me as the doctor. This makes me angry because the thing is they should recognise me as boss. That is the way this place should run. They should respect that I am in charge and then they should organize visits through me. I should be in charge of what happens in this ward. But here anyone just comes in.

There is more underpinning these frustrations than anxiety about patient safety. Doctors also fear that patients will attribute medical agency to the glasman or God rather than to themselves. The different actors in the hospital, whether nurses, patients, glasman, or pastors, refrain from acknowledging the doctors' creative energies and medical authority and instead pursue creative avenues and relationships of their own. The hospital's status as a hospital must be constantly negotiated in relation to the nonbiomedical knowledge practices that take place within it.[22] Nonbiomedical knowledge practices cannot be excluded from the hospital, but doctors must nonetheless differentiate it as a place of biomedicine from other social spaces, such as the church or the village, in order to maintain their own unique authority. In other words, they must constantly work to *make* it a different, modern, kind of place, a place where individual experts have hierarchical authority. As I described in chapter 4, the fragile balance that doctors seek to establish between the hospital's permeability and its separation from everyday social space has important implications for the kinds of knowledge practices that take place within it.[23]

Despite their claims to medical conversion and assertion of difference from their rural kin, Madang Hospital's doctors continue to be entangled in kinship and exchange networks in the villages where they had grown up.[24] Many doctors return to the village for several weeks' leave every year and make substantial contributions to important events such as the payment of bride wealth or contributions to funerals. Far from freeing them from kinship relationships, familial investments in their education made doctors even more obligated to their family. As the eldest or most successful sibling in their family, many doctors pay for their younger siblings' school fees, which constitutes a major drain on their wages. Dr. Wani described some of these financial pressures:

> It was very hard to find the school fees. My parents found them by selling vegetables in the market, mostly sweet potato they sold in the market. Other people in the family couldn't help because they had their own children to try to find the school fees for. I was the oldest in the family. The second, a girl got married but she died. The third is at university and the fourth is at National High School. The two others are at secondary high schools. I support them now. My parents just stay in the village so I look after everything now. It is a big drain on my salary, I have to look after my parents, and I pay all the university and school fees for my brothers and sisters.

Many also send frequent gifts of money to family who look after their land, in the hope that they will retain the right to return to the village once they retired. However, some doctors also express skepticism that they will actually be able to return, saying that they do not know how to live in the village anymore. They instead invest hope in the education of their children who, it is anticipated, will be able to gain employment and house their retired parents in the town.

And yet at the same time doctors in Madang Hospital continue to assert their difference from rurally based Papua New Guineans. Doctors often talk about "feeling sorry for" the "village people" they see when they return home, because of their "poor clothes," their "simple thinking" or "ignorance." Sometimes they describe the gifts of food, money, and consumer goods that they make when they return home as motivated by a sense of charity. As Dr. Wani explained: "I go back to the village when my Mum is sick or when I am on leave. The people there regard me as someone who is higher.

There is much respect, I have many people coming to me. Not because they want money but they just want to see me. When I go someone in Wabag town passes on the information so when I turn up there are many people there waiting for me. I contribute a lot to the village, to bride price. When I see them too I feel sorry for them. The way they dress, they look sick and dirty. I give some money to them. But I also give money to bride price and to doing moka and compensation payments. To solving problems with the family or clans."

At other times, doctors describe the gifting of money and consumer goods to village relatives as a major expense and drain on their salary, which is compelled by kin who insist on continued obligations. Dr. Gawale, the hospital dentist, had not returned to his home village for more than ten years because of the expense it would incur. "I am seen as a big man and many people ask me for things. Last time I went it cost me 10,000 kina for two weeks. I came back totally broke. This was too big an expense so I am reluctant to do it again. Even when I am in town the wantok system is a problem. People phone me every day asking for money. Mostly I give excuses, I lie to them to tell them I cannot help them. But every fortnight I still send money back to the village."

Whether it is given as charity or out of obligation, the gift of money is used by doctors to distance themselves from their village-based kin and assert their own modernity and individualism in contrast to the "tradition," "poverty," and "backwardness" of the village. As in other contexts of development the generic notion of "the village" crystallizes a whole set of ideas about Papua New Guinean culture and its opposition to development. Widely circulating representations of "village life" help to construct a "social map" of contemporary Papua New Guinean society and have become the symbolic basis for people's attempts to mark social difference (Pigg 1992). If gift exchange has always been employed as a technology of detachment in Melanesian societies, a means by which productive differences and therefore future exchanges can be set in motion, then doctors' gifts to their rural kin are intended to establish social distance of a different order. Giving money is a way of temporarily holding off the demands that their kin can make of them, a means of temporarily eclipsing the relationship, and of objectifying the different status of the two parties to the exchange: these are gifts that will not be reciprocated and do not therefore entail an exchange of perspectives. Detachment is not here imagined as the basis for productive engagement but as the basis for the cultivation of professional relationships elsewhere.

Like other middle-class professionals in Papua New Guinea, doctors draw on a broad set of symbolic distinctions (between village and town, uneducated and educated, "grassroots" and "national") to mark themselves off as different from their rural kin (Gewertz and Errington 1999). Gewertz and Errington have described how participation in urban networks such as the Rotary Club (which several of Madang Hospital's doctors were members of) help to sediment and naturalize hierarchical distinctions based on kind rather than degree (Gewertz and Errington 1999, 57). Through these social distinctions, "relatively affluent 'nationals'" are able to "present themselves in an apparently diverse array of contexts . . . as fundamentally superior" (Gewertz and Errington 1999, 1).

The pressure on doctors to realize this distance from village relatives through participation in a global professional community is intensified by their training and employment in a government hospital. As websites such as Biomed Experts demonstrate, participation in an international network of professional links, collaborations, and exchanges has become central to the idea of what a medical professional does. But despite this pressure, doctors in Madang Hospital find they are unable to effectively mediate the circulation of money, medical goods, and infrastructure in such a way that these social attachments and detachments are made possible. Doctors have not become so embedded in an everyday middle-class habitus that they are able to take "differences of fixed kind" rather than "fluctuating degree" (Gewertz and Errington 1999, 2) for granted. Their professional training has led them to aspire to a version of modern personhood in which such differences, and their social visibility as doctors, might be given, and yet their conditions of work and living prevail against it.

CONCLUSION

Doctors in Madang Hospital aspire to a certain kind of professional personhood, often modeled on Western images of the heroic doctor, that is premised on the hierarchical encompassment of others' creative agency. But in this institution it is difficult to become that person. Madang doctors find they are neither the heroic pioneer in an appreciative rural community, nor do they have the equipment and resources to become top of their game in the global medical community. Everyday interactions between the country's medical institutions, the flow and movement of medical goods and drugs, and the medical specialization system all contribute to the perception among doctors in Madang Hospital that it sits on the periphery of a global network of biomedicine and excludes them from a global community of biomedical professionals. The latter do not afford recognition of their scientific status.

It is perhaps because of uncertainty as regards their participation and visibility within a national and international medical community that doctors in Madang are ambivalent about reinforcing their separation from rural kin. Doctors depend on the external regard of others to make their status as doctors visible. If they do not know themselves as important medical experts through their relationships with other medical experts, then they are dependent on their kin in the town or the village for this self-knowledge.

Doctors complain about the drain of kinship obligations on their salaries, but they do not want to completely cut those ties. They often talk with enthusiasm about the number of pigs or amount of money they have contributed to a bride wealth ceremony, or boast about the respect and admiration with which they are treated when they return home. The way they are viewed by people in their home village continues to be important to them. For doctors to realize themselves as modern experts is not as simple as cutting themselves off and establishing an absolute difference with "grassroots" Papua New Guineans and rural kin. Doctors also need their rural relatives to recognize this difference, and to know them as modern, urban individuals. Paradoxically, this recognition can only be achieved within the very kinship networks and rituals that, on other occasions, doctors eschew. Doctors seek to differentiate themselves from their rural kin through participation in the very exchange practices that reinforce their connection to rural centers.

Doctors' closest relationships continue to be with those very people who, from their perspective, "believe" in witchcraft and sorcery and from whom they seek to differentiate themselves. Very often those persons are their wives, husbands, parents, and other relatives who they live with. If doctors' claims to be rational moderns and their attempts to purify the "modern" and the "traditional" in their everyday work suggest that they have become colonized subjects who now themselves extend Western hegemony by asserting the superiority of Western science (Nandy 1983), this chapter has sought to illustrate the sheer impossibility of such a total transformation (colonization) of personhood given the relationships, exchanges, and material worlds in which Papua New Guinean doctors are emotionally embedded. These relationships, it turns out, cannot be detached like so many individual possessions.

Within scientific economies of exchange, gifts work as technologies of attachment; they create relationships across international borders where they would not otherwise exist. Within Melanesian economies, by contrast, gifts work as technologies of detachment; by differentiating persons who would otherwise be diffusely related to one another, they establish the conditions for particular relationships and productive exchange. Attachment and detachment might be regarded as two different techniques for making the person visible. In Madang Hospital, doctors must navigate between these different exchange systems. As Anderson describes, Gadjusek's Fore samples continued to bear the traces of his relationships with their original owners even as they became laboratory specimens (2008, 157). The network of associations between laboratory and field could not be cut. Similarly, doctors' attempts to establish the hospital as a place marked by their biomedical authority, where they are divorced from relationships to other Papua New Guineans and where they join instead an international community of medical experts are never complete. In fact they often find that it is their kin who most effectively provide external recognition of their scientific prestige.

If Gewertz and Errington describe a class of Papua New Guinean "nationals" who have come to view themselves as intrinsically different from the majority of the country's citizens, then the problem for Madang Hospital's doctors is that they are not different enough, or that they are dependent on external recognition for this self-knowledge. It is through their exchanges of money, medical resources, and domestic goods that doctors seek to sediment such differences and make themselves visible to others as doctors and global professionals.

In the final two chapters I continue to explore relationships between biomedical knowledge practices and hospital infrastructures through the story of public-private partnerships and internationally funded medical research in the hospital. Sites of research investment and donor intervention, which have increasingly revolved around the global focus on particular infectious diseases, generate landscapes of inequality where nurses and doctors become increasingly aware of the kinds of expertise they are not able to practice and the kind of expert person they are not able to become. The experience of invisibility that is integral to being a medical professional in Papua New Guinea, I argue, has become inextricable from one's relationship to both a state and statelike actors elsewhere.

PART III ■ INFRASTRUCTURE

CHAPTER 7

The Partnership Hospital

▓ In July 2003, when I first arrived at Madang Hospital, feelings of disappointment, frustration, and resignation to failure pervaded the clinical spaces of the hospital. Those frustrations centered on the deteriorating infrastructure of the hospital, its broken technologies, decrepit buildings, and crowded facilities. The material environment of the hospital clearly fell short of expectations about the aesthetics of development and compounded the sense among staff that this was a place where they could not effectively care for and treat patients. Instead, they portrayed themselves as invisible workers, toiling away in the hidden wards of the public hospital, while the government and, by extension, the hospital's management, turned a blind eye.

"The government doesn't help us here," I was told as staff pointed to the crowded rows of beds, the lack of bed sheets, of privacy, of space for the guardians who cared for the patients in the absence of an adequate workforce. Perceptions of the hospital's rundown medical services were, it seemed, inextricable from people's disappointments with government. Those disappointments were articulated through an ocular idiom. "Em i no lukim mipela" was the common complaint made against hospital management and politicians alike, with the tok pisin term *lukim* suggesting both the English verbs "to see" and "to recognize." To "see" someone is registered in the actions you take in their regard. Thus for the staff, their invisibility was evident from the hospital's physical neglect. The decrepit ward building, with its rusted gauze walls, broken fans, and torn linoleum, was presented as evidence of the state's failure to see or act in regard of either the hospital's workers or poor publics. "When we try to talk to the CEO he tells us he is busy and doesn't want to see us"; "He just hides away in his office, he doesn't come around the wards and see what we are doing." "He sends memos to the wards. He doesn't talk to us directly." The refusal of the hospital management to *lukim mipela* was shared, argued the nurses, with the country's bureaucrats and politicians. The state, they suggested, had turned away from the lives being lived within its own public institutions. People's affective experience of the hospital as a space of modernity and technoscience was fundamentally shaped by the institution's association with the workings of political power.

Hospital workers' experiences of the hospital as a site of failure and state neglect need to be understood in relation to the heightened circulation of narratives of state failure, both within the country and internationally, over the first decade of this century. The twinned discourses of state fragility and state building, which have emerged out of tight political and academic circles in the United States, Europe, and Australia (see chapter 3), reverberate through the Papua New Guinea media. In 2003 and 2004 a series of public comments by high-profile right-wing Australian academics and politicians, which suggested that Papua New Guinea was a "failing state" and that demanded more Australian control over the aid budget, strained diplomatic relationships between the two countries and generated media controversy. Headlines such as "On the Road to Failure" and "PNG Bashers Told: Leave" were equally commonplace contributions to the furor.[1]

Inside the country, Madang Hospital emerged as one of Papua New Guinea's own "problem spaces"; a site where ideas about public institutions, the state, and good governance were problematized by everyday events and where stories about these events fed directly into national debates about state failure. Madang-based reporters seeking local stories of controversy and intrigue found a bountiful supply at the hospital. Over the first year of my fieldwork in Papua New Guinea, for example, stories reported in the *Post Courier* newspaper included donated ambulances at Madang Hospital that lay idle for two years; the attempted rape of a hospital nurse by unnamed youths; the misappropriation of K10,000 (US$4,000) intended for the hospital's rural outreach services by the Provincial Health Office; the threatened closure of the hospital due to a budgetary shortfall of K560,000 (US$200,000), possibly attributable to payments the previous board made to themselves,[2] but also exacerbated by the suspension of Madang from donor health funding following the failure of the Provincial Health Office to acquit its accounts. Finally, the failure of Madang Hospital was encapsulated in frequent stories about nurses' strikes at the hospital, which often forced the institution to reduce services or close completely.[3] In both foreign and national debates about state failure in PNG, the decline of the public hospital had become an allegory for the development of the nation-state.

Yet it would be a mistake to take those reports at face value and understand Madang Hospital simply as a reflection of wider processes of postcolonial ruination. The prominence of Madang Hospital in media debates about state failure was made possible by repeated leaks to local journalists by disgruntled staff, who used the publicity as a discursive weapon in their own battles with the hospital management over the future of the institution. The public hospital does not only operate as an allegorical space where public perceptions of the state are formed. It has also become a place of state building in a much wider sense, where government employees, politicians, and international donors seek to reshape the Papua New Guinean state into a desirable form. Where chapters 2 and 3 focused on the kinds of racially distinct bodies and publics that were made visible and knowable to the state in the different spaces of the hospital, this chapter focuses on people's attempts to make themselves visible to a state otherwise perceived as blind to the problems and internal dynamics of hospital life. Hospital workers are just as involved in intensive state-building work as foreign aid agencies. But the kind of state being envisaged and built through these practices is, I suggest, quite different from that underpinning imported models of state building and good governance. A desirable state, according to hospital workers, is a state that sees. In this chapter I explore just what kinds of relationships such visibility entails. I do so through an ethnographic analysis of hospital workers' engagements with one of the key emblems of contemporary international state-building efforts in Papua New Guinea's public institutions: the "partnership."

POLITICAL LANDSCAPES

By 2003, the health sector in Papua New Guinea had became a prime site for experimentation in public sector reform, with good governance in health imagined as a means of shoring up state legitimacy at the same time as improving health indicators. Discourses of "good governance" and "capacity building" were translated into interventions focused on health management (Mosse and Lewis, 2005; Mitchell 2002). To this end, AusAID invested substantial funds in technical assistance, which was largely composed of Australian "management experts" who were placed in the National

Department of Health and Provincial Hospitals to advise on areas such as financial management, procurement and distribution, the development of hospital standards, and the improvement of health information systems. Between 2005 and 2010, AusAID invested a further A$70 million to finance a "health services capacity building centre" run by an international health consultancy firm and intended to transfer planning, management, and financing expertise to government administrators and health managers.

Madang Hospital received its first "Hospital Advisor" in 2002. At the same time AusAID funded the establishment of a Health Management Department at the Divine Word University in Madang Town and provided expertise to assist in the development and teaching of courses. A key message the management consultants sought to communicate to Madang Hospital's executive management was a new model of what a public institution might be. A crucial aspect of good hospital management, the hospital's managers were told, is the capacity to build relationships with nonstate organizations that improve the institution's economic independence from the state. The importance of extrastate financing and "public-private partnership" was championed in the 2001–10 National Health Plan, which had also been written with the assistance of AusAID funded "advisors" (NDOH 2001). While the state was still held responsible for governing a wide array of state and nonstate health service providers, this plan envisaged Public Hospitals as corporate-style entities run by trained managers as commercial ventures. Where the old model of the welfare state was construed to have failed, a new kind of state, which was based on "stewardship," "outsourcing," and "partnership" with nonstate bodies, would be built. Madang Hospital management was encouraged to seek resources from beyond the state through partnership with overseas hospitals, NGOs, church institutions such as the Divine Word University, and local businesses. This was the new world of state building. As Madang Hospital's PR officer explained to me, "We can't just rely on government now."

A key actor in mediating these new partnerships at Madang Hospital was Divine Word University, the rapidly expanding ecumenical Christian university located near the hospital, whose president was also the chairman of the Hospital Board between 2003 until 2012. The university was originally established as a secondary school by two Divine Word missionaries, who secured a lease on an old rubber plantation in 1964. The institution was turned into an institute and then a university by an act of parliament in 1996. The university continued to be privately governed by the Catholic Church, but as a university was also eligible to receive government funds.

Since then the university has enjoyed substantial success in attracting international publicity and donor funding, partly because it conforms to exactly the model of public-private partnership that has become popularized in international development circles over this same period. These funds have enabled it to rapidly expand by creating a new campus in the Sepik region, developing new departments and courses, and becoming increasingly involved in development activities (an example of which is the establishment of a development consultancy arm, Diwai Pacific, in 2007).

During the 2000s the president of Divine Word University saw particular opportunity for expansion in the field of health. By 2011, the university had taken over the allied health college next to the hospital, was providing degree certification for the nearby Lutheran Nursing College, and was in the process of lobbying the government to establish a second national medical school at the university to compete with the original national medical school housed at the University of Papua New Guinea in Port Moresby. If dilapidated hospital infrastructure has become the prime symbol of state failure in Papua New Guinea, infrastructure was also the focus of the university president's vision for Madang Hospital. The university had built a new research and teaching pathology laboratory on the paramedical college grounds, with space to house a new pathology laboratory for the hospital. The president had mediated the arrival of the Fred Hollows Foundation, which had renovated and extended the eye ward and had obtained a grant from the health sector improvement program (HSIP) fund, funded by AusAID, to renovate the maternity ward. Through a twinning arrangement with a Catholic Australian hospital the latter had funded the design of a new operating theater. The hospital also had a new agreement with the Institute of Medical Research, who had built a research laboratory on the hospital site and renovated part of an old unused ward to house a hospital library.

Increasingly tight links forged between the hospital's management, Divine Word University, and local politicians had provided the local foundations for these multiple infrastructural projects. The university president's declared vision for Madang Hospital saw it transformed into a major teaching and research hospital, with Divine Word University at its helm. As the president put it: "The message is always about partnership. A hospital cannot be alone. Partnership is the key to success." When asked to list his achievements since becoming chairman of the hospital board in 2003, he simply provided me with a list of donor-funded building projects over which he had presided.

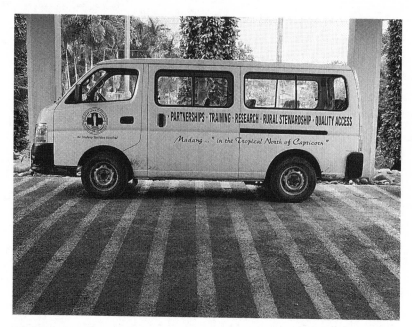

7.1. The hospital's new minibus in 2009, which advertises the hospital's new motto of partnership.

Knowing that the ongoing renewal of his chairmanship required the support of politicians in Port Moresby, the chairman had developed close relationships with government ministers and made frequent visits to the capital. In Madang he had developed links with local politicians and with an ex-health minister, who had helped raise funds for the construction of the new hospital block in 1995 and who was the owner of the town's oldest luxury hotel. In an interview in 2011, the latter told me that they hoped to "solve the problem of Madang Hospital," including the recalcitrance of the hospital staff, by eventually "contracting out the entire management of the hospital to Divine Word University. They will get people over from Australia to sort it out."

GROUND BREAKING

Accompanying the new partnership-funded infrastructure projects at Madang Hospital were a flurry of public ceremonies at which the products of partnerships were put on display. One project could involve three such ceremonies: a groundbreaking ceremony, at which politicians, hospital managers, and donor partners placed their footprints in a concrete slab located where the new building would be built; an official opening of the building; and a ceremony for the donation of technical equipment to that building. These ceremonies took a strictly conventional form, bequeathed by the Australian colonial era. A stage was set up in the hospital grounds for politicians, managers, and senior civil servants from the provincial government and donor partners. The hospital staff lined up in their uniforms in front of the stage. Members of the public were invited to watch from the sidelines or, if deemed important, from a series of plastic chairs laid out on the ground in front of the stage. A local village dance troop was rolled out and garlands of flowers were placed around the neck of the PNG and donor representatives. Politicians gave speeches in which they dwelt on the challenges faced by the hospital and the importance of donors for helping the staff do their jobs. Following the speeches a lunch, usually consisting of white sliced bread spread with margarine and fried processed sausages, was served for the politicians, donors, and hospital staff in the traditional bush material meeting house that had been built at the entrance to the hospital grounds. This was usually followed by an exclusive reception for the politicians, hospital managers, and donors, held at the town's five-star hotel, owned by the ex–health minister.

At these events infrastructure projects were presented as objectifications of the state's good intentions and capacity as well as counter-evidence for the narratives of state neglect that circulated through the institution. Local politicians played an important mediating role in these proceedings. In some cases they were themselves donors to the projects put on display, using their annual slush funds to help fund them. At other times they highlighted their role in pulling in the donations from overseas agencies and organizations. The hospital staff were addressed as project recipients. They were lined up in front of the stage and were fed following the ceremony. If the deterioration of hospital infrastructure is widely used to illustrate the failure of the state to fulfill its most basic obligations then the highly personalized donation of infrastructure to the hospital has also become a prime opportunity for elite bureaucrats and politicians to perform the state in a guise that hospital workers and wider publics were expected to recognize as legitimate. If hospital staff complained that they were invisible to the state's politicians and bureaucrats, it was these moments of gift giving that we might expect would fulfill their expectations for recognition.

Yet hospital staff in Madang were ambivalent about these infrastructural developments. On the one hand, as archetypal symbols of modernity, which embody the very concept of national development and progress, cars, buildings, and machines were taken to be appropriate gifts for politicians to give. Doctors and nurses often judged politicians by the infrastructure projects they had presided over. Whether a politician "has done anything for us" was routinely measured in numbers of ambulances and buildings. These ceremonies might thus be said, following Miyazaki, to operate as intensive moments of hope in the extensibility of indigenous Melanesian modes of exchange into state-citizen relationships (Miyazaki 2005). They were moments in which hospital staff hoped the gifts displayed would provide evidence that they had been "seen." "Em i lukim mi" or "em i tingim mi" are common ways to describe the presentation of a gift.

On the other hand when, over the ensuing months and years, staff scrutinized the material transformations that the donated infrastructure underwent, they frequently found retrospective signs that the relationship with the state they had anticipated in the moment of ceremonial display had not been successfully enacted after all. The funds for the Japanese donated hospital built in 1995, for example, had been secured by the minister for health at that time, a naturalized Papua New Guinean citizen originally from Australia, who also owned the town's prime tourist hotel and conference center. By 2003, the building had already become grubby and there was an increasing problem of mold growing on internal walls. The internal rooms were hot and needed to be cooled with air-conditioning, but the hospital could not afford the electricity bills. Nurses and doctors pointed out that the funds had been used to rebuild the more prominent main hospital building, when the preexisting building had been perfectly adequate, and left the crowded, hot, and stuffy public wards that were concealed behind the new construction unimproved. There were suggestions that it was the government's desire for closer trade links with Japan that had been at the center of this infrastructure project, not the hospital itself.

In 2009, a new pathology laboratory built on the Divine Word campus was still standing empty several months after its completion because of difficulty in acquiring the funds to equip it and because of some ambiguity over whether the hospital had ever agreed to move the laboratory's location. Among hospital workers, meanwhile, there was intense resistance to the removal of the hospital's laboratory to the university site. "It is the hospital laboratory, it should be on hospital land." The new building was a ten-minute walk from the main public wards and staff questioned how the samples were going to travel backward and forth from lab to hospital. Nurses suspected that they would simply have more work carrying the samples to the laboratory. The laboratory workers felt that they had not been consulted in the decision, and said they would prefer to see their current building renovated. By 2011 the hospital's malaria microscopy unit was based at the new building but the other laboratory technicians had refused to move. By the summer of 2013 Divine Word University had taken back the laboratory and were running a private laboratory service for international medical researchers and private clinics in the town. There were suggestions that the laboratory might also begin to provide private services to the hospital when its own pathology laboratory failed and that, ultimately, laboratory services could be outsourced to Divine Word University altogether. Meanwhile, as I describe in chapter 8, there was antipathy to the new building projects by the Institute of Medical Research on the hospital compound, which it was suggested were beneficial to foreign research scientists but did little to help build the hospital's capacity as a public health provider.

Donated technologies fared equally badly. Behind newly constructed buildings and alongside painted walkways lie scrap heaps of rusting wreckage from donated technologies. A digital sterilizer donated by AusAID in 2003 broke down every time there was a black out. The hospital's engineer was unable to fix it because the Brisbane based company from whom it had been purchased refused to provide the code to access the CPU, or to train the hospital staff to reset it. The hospital could not afford to fly the company's own engineers out to Papua New Guinea. In 2009 the hospital appealed to AusAID to buy them a replacement, but by 2010 this new sterilizer was also not working.

At the heart of people's ambivalent attitudes toward infrastructural developments is the disjuncture between the temporality of exchange and the biographies of the things exchanged. In Papua New Guinea, gifts that are donated in moments of ceremonial display are often secreted away afterward; the oscillation between concealment and revelation contributing to their affective power in moments of display (Dalton 1996; Leach 2002). But in a public hospital, gifted infrastructure is not hidden away unused; the places where it is stored are wards, operating theaters, and laboratories. Here those objects continue to be crucial to the capacity of nurses and doctors to do their jobs and their ability to save lives. All too often the things that are given quickly deteriorate and break down. Ambulances are crashed by drunk drivers, or break down and the hospital is unable to pay for repairs. Machines turn out to be poorly designed for the climate and fragile power infrastructure of Papua New Guinea. New glamorous infrastructures start to segue into the dysfunctional and old.

In the long term, nurses usually judged political gifts to the hospital as failures. New buildings and technologies became a part of the hospital's everyday neglect. In some ways this is a familiar tale of inappropriate technology transfer and top-down development. But for hospital staff what is significant about the material deterioration of hospital is what it retrospectively reveals about the moment of exchange itself. While the structure of the ceremonial displays that accompany new infrastructures foreground relationships between the state and the hospital workers, the deterioration of the infrastructure leads the latter to suspect that other relationships, from which they are excluded, were in fact taking center stage all along. In other words, it was suspected that hospital workers may not be the origin of the politicians' donations at all; they were not given with the hospital's inhabitants in mind. Rather, hospital workers told me, the managers and politicians used the hospital as a platform to establish other relationships elsewhere. Infrastructural projects and their attendant ceremonies objectified and strengthened ties between hospital managers, politicians, and overseas donors, corporate partners, and NGOs.

Gift giving in Melanesia has conventionally been analyzed by anthropologists as a kind of technology of visibility. In the moment of prestation what is made visible is both the capacity of the donor to mobilize the relationships necessary to produce the gift, and the capacity of the recipient to compel the donor to make that effort, to act in their regard. In other words, if relationships of reciprocal exchange are distributed across time and space, the moment of gift exchange condenses those relationships in a multitemporal image. But this is an image intended to generate knowledge in the form of effect rather than representation. Whether those relationships have been effectively mobilized is evidenced not by the gift itself but by the recipient's response to it. Gift giving is thus a moment of hope and uncertainty.

Who is being judged in ceremonial displays of infrastructure at Papua New Guinea's public hospitals? The ceremonies appear to make hospital staff visible as an object of regard for the state. Indeed when hospital staff deem politicians' gifts of ambulances, buildings, or technologies to be appropriate, the judgment is both that the politicians have successfully mobilized their relationships with foreign others to serve their relationship with the hospital, and that to do so at all the politician must have wanted to make an impression on the hospital workers. The understanding is that he saw them as significant persons with whom a relationship must be maintained. The fact that, over time, those gifts are usually deemed inappropriate does not only tell the hospital staff that politicians are corrupt, but also that they may not be acting in their regard at all. It is the capacities of hospital staff as well as the state that are brought into question by the later judgment of such events as failures.

Rather than politicians and managers harnessing relationships with foreign donors in support of their exchanges with hospital staff, the latter apprehend in the ruination of hospital infrastructure an inversion of this relationship. It is the state's benevolence to hospital workers that is being put on display for the judgment of foreign donors, NGOs, and corporate partners. The use of one relationship as a support for another is common-place in Papua New Guinean exchange systems; relationships propagate relationships. Exchanges of pigs between men eclipse the relationships with women by which those pigs have been reared (Strathern 1988). But here relationships between politicians, managers, and hospital workers seemed to appear *only* as an artifact of exchanges occurring elsewhere; there was no moment prior or subsequent to their value transformation when they took center stage. In other words, politicians and managers did not temporarily "eclipse" their relationships with hospital workers, but wholly encompassed them. The state thus appeared to be seeking to make itself visible to external others rather than "see" those it was meant to be governing. Political gifts of hospital infrastructure operated as technologies of visibility for politicians and managers (in their relationships with foreign donors) rather than the hospital staff.

Hospital workers used the idiom of consumption rather than exchange to describe the practices of politicians and hospital managers. They likened the hospital's managers to "white people" who are able to shrug off the social obligations of a Christian Papua New Guinean culture and accrue personal gain at the expense of others. An increase in hospital fees, for example, was taken to be indicative of the CEO's general greed and tendency to extract money from patients rather than extend services to them. The work of CEOs, nurses told me, was "surface work." They had high-up positions and friends in government but they did not make any actual contribution to patient care. As one nurse put it to me:

> We have no democracy here. No rights. We are the backbone of the hospital. The CEO doesn't come to the ward, give injections, look after the welfare of the patients. The CEO depends on us. Without us who are you? We are the simple ones clearing up the mess from the garden you have been eating from. Twenty-four hours a day we stand by the bedside of the patients, give them emotional support. The CEO doesn't do this. We

will do this work and he will be promoted because of us simple nurses. The doctor does the ward round. Will he stop and give medicine and injections? No, he comes and goes, just gives orders and the nurses will do the work. He just leaves and the work-load is on us.

There are resonances here with an opposition between "consumption" and "transmission" that runs through Papua New Guinea ethnography. If gift exchange is "the prototypical act of value-creation, the privileged means for defining and making visible social relations and identities" (Foster 1999, 167), then consumption without subsequent exchange exhibits a form of negative value creation (Munn 1986). It is through transactions that the symbolic value of the persons who exchange things is realized. Excessive or uncontrolled consumption, of the kind associated with managers and white people, is consumption that does not set up new "preconditions for future action" (Munn 1986, 179), that does not create possibilities for further exchange and therefore the extension of a person's relational qualities. It is in this sense that exchange exists as a form of "value transformation" (Munn 1986). In Gawan society, a selfish person is "one who eats" rather than gives: "Food that is caught inside the body . . . epitomizes what is not only consumed, but also cannot be released" (Munn 1986, 49). By contrast, food that is given away to overseas visitors "is perceived as initiating a spatiotemporally extending process—an expansion beyond the donors' persons and the immediate moment, and beyond Gawa Island—as visitors take away the favorable news of Gawan hospitality (Munn 1986, 50). The ultimate form of negative value transformation is encapsulated in the figure of the witch, who is perceived as the cause of illness, the depletion of gardens, theft, and death (in order to feast on the decomposing body) (Munn 1986, 216).

Considering the emphasis placed on food in these accounts, it is telling that the nurses likened managers (and aloof doctors) to pigs that guzzle from people's gardens and that are contrasted to "normal" humans, who might eat gifted pig meat on one occasion but know that they must return it on another. Pig meat here works as an implicit analogy for power. Managers, nurses often argued, forget that they are dependent on other people and instead act as though their authority is preordained by a fixed hierarchy. The comparison of pigs, that eat continuously until the garden is finished, to humans, who alternate between eating and giving, implies that the nurses' objection to this hierarchy was not that it involved an unequal distribution of power but rather that it involved a continuous as opposed to alternating temporality. Managers, like pigs and white people who eat without giving, seize all the power to themselves rather than recognizing its basis in relations of exchange and codependency.

The public hospital is clearly an important site of political theater as well as health infrastructure. At the heart of staff skepticism about the new "partnership" model of hospital management, therefore, lie concerns about the kind of state power that is generated alongside hospital reform. The interest of overseas agencies such as AusAID in partnership models of health-care delivery is driven by the perception that the highly politicized public service has failed as a service provider. By shifting the role of the state from provider to contract manager, it is envisaged that new, more efficient, neutral and professional organizations, like Divine Word University, will be able to substitute for failed state infrastructure and provide more cost-effective and efficient services. The concerns of hospital staff meanwhile imply that this new managership can in fact *contribute* to the personalization of state power, the creation of new local empires that empower political elites, and the development of new inequalities. Infrastructure is the material form through which such relationships become entrenched.

Such fears were realized in the most farcical way in February 2010 when the minister for health announced his plans to build a new "superhospital" in Port Moresby under a public-private partnership agreement. The superhospital, called the Pacific Medical Center, would, it was claimed, provide state of the art medical facilities, funded through a combination of government, NGO, philanthropic and donor support, and private investment. On April 2, during a visit to PNG as patron of the Clinton Foundation, Bill Clinton met with Michael Somare and the national planning minister. The government later claimed that the development of the Pacific Medical Center had been discussed at this meeting and emails from the ambassador to the United States, which were leaked to the press claimed that Clinton had indicated a willingness to support the project through the Clinton Foundation and that he would further use his connections to reach out to "the leaders of other nations that provide PNG bilateral development assistance, founders/CEOs of major foundations in the U.S. and CEOs of major corporations that have various business interests in PNG and other major prospective partners . . . to support the PMC as a major healthcare initiative for our entire nation and other Pacific Islands nations." Clinton's support for the project, it was stated, would be declared in a "major announcement" in September 2010 in New York City during the annual meeting of the Clinton Global Initiative.[4]

As the year progressed, however, and details of the project began to emerge in the Papua New Guinean media, the project and Clinton's involvement in it came to seem increasingly illusory. Clinton himself appeared to have been unaware of the support he had pledged, and the Clinton Global Initiative event in New York came and went without any announcement of support for a new superhospital in Papua New Guinea. A senior doctor working in Port Moresby told me that claims for support from philanthropic and church-based organizations had been entirely fabricated. "Yes, there was a meeting with Bill Clinton. Yes, maybe they raised the Pacific Medical Center and Bill Clinton said, "Yes, that's a great idea, you go ahead and do that," but that was it. These politicians don't even know how it works. They don't even realize that Clinton is only the patron, he can't pledge the foundation's money; he is just a figurehead." In fact, this doctor suggested, the only person interested in becoming a partner on the project was a U.S.-based property developer who had pitched to project manage the hospital on behalf of the government at a substantial cost to the state. The press subsequently revealed that enquiries with donor agencies had confirmed none of those countries stated in the superhospital proposal documents to support the plan in fact intended to provide any funding or support. The U.S. embassy, for example, remarked that they had no development presence in PNG and that they furthermore no longer invested in individual infrastructure projects, instead focusing on "technical support."[5]

The details surrounding the project, meanwhile, were exceedingly murky. Reporters and government ministers appeared to be confused over whether the hospital would be "not for profit," or whether it would be an investment opportunity for the government and private business, with the potential to "earn about K50 million [US$20 million] annually from medical, operational and other fees."[6] The government was pledged to provide $US500 million in start-up costs, but it was unclear where this money would come from. In October 2010, it was revealed that the minister for health had submitted a proposal to the National Executive Council for the redeployment of funds intended for medical equipment, static infrastructure, and housing from provincial hospitals to the superhospital. Rumors began to circulate that those pushing the project could in fact have a personal interest in closing deals with private consortia. The president for the Port Moresby Chamber of Commerce and Industry, for example, criticized the PMC and other large infrastructure projects as "shrouded in secrecy, created outside normal departmental channels, ignoring sound professional advice from many quarters, including the wide donor community who do not support this proposal, [so] that they inevitably end up with the scent of corruption on them."[7]

The project was also the object of increasing vitriol from the medical establishment. This was "a politician's project" remarked a senior pediatrician (quoted in Mola 2010, 3). In a widely circulated opinion piece written for the National Research Institute, another doctor stated that "diverting scarce health funds to this project could lead to the complete collapse of the struggling PNG hospital sector and a massive deterioration in health care capacity for ordinary Papua New Guineans" (Mola 2010, 1). The hospital would not be able to attract enough fee-paying patients to cover its costs, the piece argued, and would require ongoing government subsidies. Meanwhile, the hospital would only be able to provide the same level of services as Port Moresby General Hospital, and its main purpose would therefore only be to provide more "salubrious surroundings" for rich mine company employees awaiting medical evacuation out of the country. Even the health secretary, who was largely silent on the subject, asked when pushed, "Who is going to benefit? Is it for the urban population? Is it the right time for us to do it while we have the existing problems in the rural areas?"[8]

In November 2010, Prime Minister Michael Somare relented to public pressure and wrote to the health minister Sasa Zibe stating that the existing health budget should not be used to fund the superhospital. As there were no "development partners" interested in the project this essentially led to it being shelved. The prime minister pointed out that "many of the local and US global partners mentioned in the accompanying documentation as supporting the project have since disclaimed any interest to be a partner in or as having said they support the PMC. . . . It is also disingenuous to suggest that the PMC project will not take anything away—existing or future government—funded healthcare projects or programs. It is obvious that any money provided to the PMC project would come at the cost of existing and future government health projects and programs."[9] In September 2011, the new minister for health and HIV finally laid the project to rest, removing it from the government's priority agenda for health.

The nonappearance of the Papua New Guinean superhospital demonstrates the new dream zones that accompany the emergence of development models based on "partnership."[10] It is unclear whether the superhospital was the poorly imagined fantasy of a group of elite politicians, or a cleverly constructed "economy of appearances" (Tsing 2005) that started with the leaking of Clinton's (nonexistent) interest in the hospital and enabled those politicians to use the ensuing speculation to cultivate personal connections with international corporate firms and philanthropic bodies, potentially for private gain. Yet the story of the superhospital that never came to be demonstrates the propensity of new development models, apparently designed to constrain opportunities for political interference and corruption, to shore up existing forms of political power. Such stories swell already existing suspicions among those who inhabit the country's hospitals that corrupt deals and exclusionary power relations continue to lie behind the new modes of "good governance" and "health management" being pushed by the country's donors.

THE UNSEEING STATE

If politicians' ceremonial displays and political gifts fail as technologies of visibility (at least for hospital workers), then nurses have found other, more effective technologies for visualizing their capacities and compelling the state to act in their regard.

Nurses in PNG have become notorious for their strong unionization and repeated strike action. Nurses in Madang, for example, took strike action against either the hospital management or the national government in 2003, 2004, 2005, 2009, 2010, and 2013. Strikes in 2005 and 2010 were coordinated by the National Nurses Association in response to the government's failure to put the agreed 2001 pay deal into practice and their failure to carry out an agreed review of all salary grades. Independently organized strike action in Madang Hospital likewise made reference to dissatisfaction over pay but also focused repeatedly on the hospital's CEOs and their relationship to national politicians. In 2003, for example, the confident and outspoken leader of the Madang Nurses Association, who I call Deirdre, claimed that the acting CEO had failed to sign the forms necessary for the payment of their shift-loading allowances (shifts outside the public service hours) by the national payroll system and used this as the basis for mobilization. She also claimed that he had been illegally appointed to the position by the minister for health rather than through the Department of Personnel Management. The CEO's failure to sign their pay slips, she argued, encapsulated his "management style"—the fact he was more interested in his relationships with politicians than the hospital workers.

On February 21, 2004, following Deirdre's lead, the nurses declared that they would no longer work outside the public service hours of 8:00 AM to

4:00 PM. Every morning for the next two weeks the Nurses Association organized a public meeting in the meetinghouse outside the CEO's office where Deirdre and her executive committee vocalized their disenchantment with the hospital management, demanded in loud speeches and chanting that the CEO must go, and challenged him to come out and "speak to his staff directly."

The acting CEO remained locked in his office but continued to release numerous memos. On day three he left the office to attend a meeting and Dierdre tried to grab his briefcase off him as he fled to his car. The scuffle that followed resulted in the CEO falling to the ground and accusing Deirdre of assault. On day four, he circulated a memo declaring that the board had given him disciplinary powers to suspend the nurses involved. The memo was posted up on the wall in the medical ward and the nurses crowded around to read it: "We have no medicine, no gloves, no soap. He should put patient care first. When he has patient care he can have disciplinary powers. What has the CEO done for the hospital?" shouted the nursing officer in charge. The others agreed: "We should send a letter signed by us all in Ward 2 saying that we will recognize those powers when he gives us the resources we need to give patient care."

After several days of industrial action the Nurses Association began to clandestinely collect letters, testimonials, and memos from different offices and filing cabinets in the hospital, which they collated into a carefully indexed two-hundred-page document attesting to the CEO's bad leadership. The booklet accused the CEO of keeping hospital-bought items such as computers and cameras for himself, using hospital funds to buy himself clothes for a conference trip to Australia, and spending six thousand kina of hospital funds at the middle-class department store, Brian Bell, on the refurbishment of his house. The recent increase in hospital fees was presented as illegal because it had not gone through the proper protocols. The CEO's attempt to discipline striking nurses was illegal because he did not have the authority as "acting" CEO to take disciplinary action. The CEO's appointment of his own administrative support staff was illegal because he had not followed the correct procedures. Correspondence between the CEO and Deirdre, including his own threats of legal action for defamation, were presented as evidence of his poor communication with hospital staff. In sum, the booklet argued that the CEO displayed "undemocratic leadership," "poor governance," and "a lack of transparency" and used precisely these terms, imported from the same management schools in which the CEO had been trained, to argue the point.

In the following letter, for example, Deirdre accused the acting CEO of appointing staff to nonexistent positions and paying them overtime for work that should be done in office hours: "We condemn this action because there is no transparency, honesty and fairness in your action, which we can only regard as malpractice and a blatant disregard for set procedures regarding claims for, and payment, of overtime, and calls into question your integrity and conflict of interest. . . . Where is the transparency and Christian principle you are supposed to up-hold?"

Another letter demanded to know why the CEO had not made the hospital car available for the hospital outreach program: "No doubt the color of your character is now being shown. This is the type of leadership we call "AUTHORITATIVE or VERTICAL, or even DICTATORSHIP leadership style. Let me assure you it is not a healthy leadership style."

In public speeches and formal correspondence, Deirdre made repeated references to Christian ethics, often quoting from the Bible. "Finally as a Christian who fear the Lord, let me quote Proverbs 12:2 as food for thought for you:—"A good man obtains favor from the Lord, but a man of wicked intention, He (God) will condemn"; "Your leadership style demonstrates that you are a very vindictive person despite your public pretenses. I will quote Proverbs 29:2 because it sums up your leadership: "When the righteous are in authority, the people rejoice, but when a wicked man rules, the people groan." Sadly, your double standards and witch hunting is eroding the '[Madang Hospital] Culture' we once enjoyed."

In this correspondence, bureaucratic notions of transparency, accountability, and democratic leadership were realigned with a Papua New Guinean Christian culture. The very managers who had been put in place and trained through foreign development interventions focused on good governance and health management were now framed as corrupt within that same "good governance" discourse.

This booklet became the centerpiece of the nurses' protest. Nurses Association leaders held it in their hands and gesticulated with it during their speeches. It was ceremonially presented to the few members of the board who agreed to come to the meetinghouse and listen to the nurses' complaints. "When they read the booklet they will *have* to dismiss him, he has not followed protocol," Deirdre told me triumphantly.

The booklet was laid out as a quasilegal document. A table of contents gave sections for the different claims being made against the CEO. The documents and letters were carefully classified, as though they were pieces of evidence presented for exhibition at a trial. In the introduction the booklet made reference to Papua New Guinea public service orders, and the letters and documents it contained were dotted with references to illegalities and threatened legal action. In fact the booklet was strangely recursive. The items presented as evidence of illegal behavior were often themselves earlier letters to the CEO making the same allegations and threatening legal action.

The board members never directly addressed the accusations made in this booklet. Those who read it confessed it held some worrying documents but that they found it rather strange, strewn as it was with personal letters full of vitriol sent between Deirdre and the CEO. Eventually, however, the hospital board realized that the acting CEO had no legitimacy with the hospital staff and decided not to appoint him to the permanent position. For the nurses this was taken as a victory that they presumed had followed directly from their booklet of evidence. They had, in effect, established their own trial, with the board as judges, and the CEO, as they read the verdict, had been found guilty.

PLAYING THE LAW

In fact, this was not the first or last CEO to be ousted by the Madang nurses. They had also forced a previous CEO out of office in 2001 by barricading her office door. Again complaints had been made of misconduct, this time that she had favored people from her own church, the Seventh Day Adventists, in the allocation of hospital building contracts. In 2005, meanwhile, they initiated complaints against the newly appointed CEO following a visit by an American Navy Mercy ship to the hospital when he spent several thousand kina on food and wine for a reception. Again, the complaint was that he had by-passed hospital regulations and neglected patient care by wasting resources. In 2005, when the nurses joined the national nurses strike, Deirdre presented these complaints against the CEO alongside the national pay dispute as reasons for their strike and called for his dismissal. On this occasion the CEO took the strikers to court and requested a court order to get the nurses back to work. The order was granted, but the judge presiding over the case also gave a court order that prevented the CEO from disciplining the nurses involved in the strike while the pay dispute was outstanding.

Several months later Deirdre left the hospital for some days to attend a Nurses Association meeting without asking the CEO for leave of absence. Seeing her as a long-term troublemaker, the CEO immediately took the opportunity to dismiss her. The Nurses Association subsequently took him to court as the original court action preventing disciplinary action was still in force. By the time the case came to court, the CEO had left the hospital and was running the health services for a large corporate gold mine off the Papua New Guinean coast. The judge, an old colonial officer and now natural-ized Papua New Guinean citizen, found the CEO to have acted in contempt of court and sentenced him to six months in prison. The nurses were jubilant: "Now they can see what we can do," Deirdre told me. "He thought he didn't have to listen to the law, he thought he was a big man, but we brought him down."

How can we understand this turn to the law? Can the actions of the nurses' union in Papua New Guinea be understood, as the Comaroffs have argued, as a response to the disorder and division of interests that prevails in the shadow of the neoliberal state, with its dispersed systems of gov-ernance and overlapping sovereignties? The Comaroffs have argued that, amidst the corporate and state violence that has thrived alongside neoliberal reforms, law has become both a tool of the powerful (a kind of "lawfare") and a weapon of the weak.

The trouble with this reading of unionization in Papua New Guinea is that it suggests such engagements with the law are about the enforcement of social norms, that the law is turned to as a means of imposing order on a state seen to have become disordered and out of control. But the nurses in Madang Hospital did not care that the CEO had been imprisoned because of contempt of court proceedings rather than the original claims of mis-conduct they had brought against him. What mattered was that they had demonstrated their ability to use the legal bureaucracy to put him in prison, that they had won. The nurses he had disciplined were reinstated while he went to jail. Their adoption of a new language of governance, leadership, and transparency does not appear to entail the nurses' internalization of a new set of neoliberal rationalities, against which they measure others and govern themselves (Rose 1999; Mosse 2005). They did not turn to the law as a moral force that would bring a corrupt government back into line. Rather, by doing things properly, by producing the right kinds of bureaucratic docu-ments, by using the correct combination of development buzzwords and Christian proverbs, and by closely following legal protocol, they hoped that they would provoke a response. The hospital board or judge would be forced to recognize their capacities and act in their regard. Their goal was less about forcing hospital managers to conform to norms of international manage-ment than to provoke a response by which the nurses knew they had been recognized by those managers as persons of equivalent value. The dramatic staging of industrial strikes and presentation of official documents of complaint to the hospital board can be understood as attempts by the hospital nurses to make themselves visible in the form of the law. In other words they used this bureaucracy as a technology for instantiating a relationship between themselves and the state that was based on personal mutuality and equivalence.[11]

If politicians' gifts of infrastructure eclipse the work of hospital staff, the "gift" of law forces managers and politicians to recognize their powers. By presenting themselves in the forms required by the new discourses of good governance and state building, the nurses are able to tap into the legal powers those forms contain. They are able to harness the power of the state for themselves. In a sense, the nurses can be understood as using the law to produce an image of their own power. It is by no means incidental that this incident was widely reported in the national press, much to the glee of the nurses involved.

Literature on ceremonial exchange and initiation in Papua New Guinea has described the significance of public display as a moment in which the products of transactions and exchanges that have occurred offstage are presented for the judgment of onlookers (Strathern 1988, 2000; Biersack 1982; Leach 2002; Reed 2003). According to Strathern, the hope in such moments is that the audience will be sufficiently impressed that future exchanges, relationships, and marriages will result. In other words, that the person or group put on display will be recognized as persons worth engaging with for the future. The uncertainty entailed by these events follows from the fact that the response of the audience is not immediate. Those on display cannot know what their observers are thinking or what subsequent intentions toward them might be. This temporal dynamic produces an "exchange of perspectives" (Strathern 1988; Foster 1995b) whereby donors and recipients alternate positions and see in one another their own past and future forms. Agency is decentered; people always appear as the cause or effect of another person's actions.

As Eric Hirsch (2001) has suggested, power in Melanesia is better characterized by the attempt to "compel" or "oblige" others to act through display, rather than the discursive work of controlling meanings and norms. Power consists in the ability to *conform* to norms and thereby elicit a response rather than the ability to control others' behavior through the establishment of those norms. The exercise of such power rests on the capacity to make oneself visible in the correct form, often objectified in an exchange object.

In Madang Hospital, I suggest, a ledger of complaints might operate as just such an object, hence nurses' emphasis, in the construction of that document, on "the aesthetics of logic and language" (Riles 1998, 386). "We must follow the procedures" or "do things properly" were popular refrains of the leaders of industrial action. Letters and correspondence with the CEO and hospital board conformed to formal legal conventions of language and presentation, including the use of headers, references to sections of the law, and the inclusion of the author's formal title beneath the name and signature. This is despite the fact most of the correspondence was only ever moving a few meters between people's offices.

Nurses were not only interested in the style of the documents and letters themselves. A lot of discussion and consideration went into the composition of the ledger as a whole. Ultimately it was decided that the ledger should be prefaced with a petition from all the nursing staff declaring a lack of confidence in the management of the acting CEO. This would be followed by the assemblage of documents, which could only have been acquired from the hospital's filing cabinets and offices with the support of multiple administrators within the institution. Thus composed, the ledger not only provided evidence of the CEO's corruption and mismanagement (detailed within the content of documents themselves) but, in its physical formation, also served as evidence for the nurses' relationships and support across the hospital.

Likewise, the nurses took great care over the image they presented to the CEO when camped outside his office. The bush material meetinghouse was edged with benches, and Deirdre worked hard every morning to make sure that every bench was filled in order to create an unbroken line around the perimeter of the building. She likened this to the fence that is built around gardens in the village to keep out pigs. Nurses who didn't turn up to the demonstration were chastised "you must not break the fence!" The fence, Deirdre told me, was important to show the management that the nurses were a single body (*wanbel*) with a single agenda (*wanpela ting ting*). While the ledger provided an image of the heterogeneous support the nurses enjoyed across the institution, the demonstration in the meetinghouse provided an image of the nurses as a single unified force.

Gender symbolization plays an important, if implicit role in these actions. Across Papua New Guinea women's work often operates as a support for male value creation; relationships between men and women provide the offstage foundations for highly visible exchanges (Strathern 1988). Women are also more closely, though not exclusively, associated with witchcraft than men. Inversely, nurses in Madang Hospital, the majority of whom are female, accuse male managers and politicians of consuming their relationships with hospital staff, an image that is symbolically resonant with witchcraft. Managers and politicians "encompass" rather than "eclipse" their relationship with hospital staff; they do not acknowledge their dependence on that relationship (and its role in generating value for their identity). By presenting themselves in the form of the law, nurses respond to their consumption by the state by exercising the right to forms of power, exchange, and visibility that have conventionally been the province of men.

CONCLUSION

The aesthetics of hospital dilapidation in countries with poor state infrastructures like Papua New Guinea has become something of a development cliché. It is easy for the foreign visitor, such as development workers, consultants, or anthropologists, to take such conditions for granted. But for Papua New Guineans working in the country's hospitals, the dream of the modern hospital has never receded. Comparisons with the ideal hospitals supposedly existing in countries in the West continue to reinforce health workers' experience of their institutional environment as a place of disappointment and failure, where they are unable to save lives or effectively perform professional and expert identities.

This chapter has described the experience of these medical spaces as places of government by those who work within them. In the Papua New Guinean hospital the inherent challenges and uncertainties of patient care are intensified by a sense of abandonment by the state. Hopes in the possibility of a "proper hospital" are continually played up through the political donation of glossy new infrastructure, machines, and vehicles. But such projects and gifts are tinged with the suspicion that they are superficial gestures, which only pretend to incorporate the inhabitants of the public hospital into the sphere of international development to which politicians and elite bureaucrats already appear to have access. People's relationships to hospital infrastructure are therefore inherently ambivalent. Feelings of hope and of resignation to failure are coproduced through people's interactions with hospital space (Street 2012).

On the one hand, the public hospital is a place of intense visibility that is the object of media attention and the site of frequent public ceremonies and events. On the other hand, staff experience the public hospital as a place of invisibility, where the state refuses to acknowledge or engage with its publics.

The changing hospital landscape, increasingly transformed through partnerships with overseas development agencies, NGOs, and international organizations, raised questions for the hospital workers about what kinds of publics were being served by those buildings and who was expected to benefit from them. While new high-tech donor funded infrastructures are put on display in ceremonial events, the real "public" places of the hospital, which continue to depend on state investment, remain neglected. As the hospital is reconfigured into a "partnership" between state and nonstate actors, the fear is that the distance between these two hospital infrastructures will grow. The transformation of the hospital landscape is apprehended through the prism of increasing social inequalities and growing political elites.

Nurses responded to state neglect by adopting the very language of good governance that was being employed by hospital managers and promoted by the country's development donors. But the kind of government and, by extension, hospital management, that the nurses envisaged as "good" differed substantially from that portrayed in the reforms of international aid agencies such as AusAID. Indeed when they adopted the managerial language of good governance nurses did not appear to have internalized the meanings associated with such concepts, but rather deployed it in order to compel managers to "see" their workers and act in their regard.

Donors such as AusAID, meanwhile, tend to see the nurses as self-interested public servants who lack a sense of the public good, possibly because of their continuing ties to their villages and ethnic groups. These views are shared by people in the hospital management team. In response to the nurses' claims that the CEO's spending on fancy receptions for foreign visitors amounted to corruption, for example, the hospital's public relations officer stated that nurses had failed to understand the nature of modern management and the need to attract money from donors: "This is how you have to operate. You spend a little money when they come and then they send all the money afterwards. You get it all back. But people here are not operating in today's world. They are trying to run the hospital like thirty years ago and it doesn't work that way anymore."

The industrial action that has frequently erupted at Madang Hospital over the past decade cannot only be understood as a straightforward battle over workers' rights and wages. If nurses appear to harbor nostalgia for a postindependence, welfare state, then this is partly because it was a model that took relationships between the people who make up the state and the citizens they serve to be paramount. New managerial strategies, which incorporate notions of efficiency, partnership, and competition, meanwhile, appear to focus on the relationships that state actors form with one other and with "partnering" organizations. Elite bureaucrats and politicians are perceived to have tight personal links to each other and, increasingly, to foreign organizations and businesses, cultivated through conferences and expensive hotel receptions, which enable them to accrue and distribute money and resources as they wish and to live a Western consumer lifestyle. Frontline health workers and patients, meanwhile, are both excluded from those social networks. Nurses imagine that from the perspective of those elite state actors they have become socially invisible.

It is these relationships that nurses seek to transform when they reject managerial authority in the hospital. Indeed, the current CEO of Madang Hospital is a woman and a nurse, and yet in 2013 the nurses went on strike again. It seems that it is the office of the CEO and the kind of power invested in it that nurses refuse to accept.

The dramatic staging of industrial strikes by nurses and their presentation of official documents of complaint to the hospital board can thus be interpreted as attempts to force government managers to recognize them as persons of equivalent value. But their adoption of a new language of governance, leadership, and transparency does not appear to entail the nurses' internalization of those managerial rationalities. It is the bureaucratic form of good governance that they seek to assume. This, they identify, is how their capacities might be made visible and the state forced to see.

The following chapter continues to focus on the emergence of the partnership hospital, in this case through the increasingly dominant presence of medical research in the institution. Relationships between foreign medical researchers and Papua New Guinea's public health institutions are increasingly mediated through the governance of research ethics. The chapter examines how research ethics is shaping the ways in which medical research is carried out and the ways in which capacity in public health is defined, with important implications for public employees in the hospital.

CHAPTER 8

Research in the Clinic

■ From the entrance to the ward, I could see the Australian doctor leaning over the bed of a small child, a stethoscope hanging loosely around his neck. Next to him a Papua New Guinean health extension officer was busy taking a blood slide from the child for malaria testing. Nurses bustled to and fro, making observations, administering medications, and taking fluid samples for laboratory analysis. Here, in the pediatric ward of Madang Hospital, the institution's limited resources were very much on display. Closely spaced beds ran in lines along the edge of the room. The air was thick with heat, sweat, and chemicals, and the fans above the beds were encrusted with so much dust that they were unable to turn. In the absence of hospital issued sheets, the beds were swathed in multicolored and patterned lap laps, which did not reach around the plastic coated mattress and lay in crumpled piles around the patients. The beds were occupied by whole families: usually the child's mother and several siblings who might sleep in the bed with the patient or underneath it on the floor. From the doorway where I stood, this dimly lit tableau seemed an archetypal image of everyday life in a "third world" hospital.

But this was not a normal ward, or at least it was not *only* a normal ward. The Australian physician I was observing was not employed by the government hospital, he was a Ph.D. student at a prestigious university in Australia. And the blood slide was not only intended for diagnostic purposes. It would also be translated into data for a clinical trial comparing two different ways of administering artesunate antimalarials to children.[1] The crowded and busy clinical space of the pediatric ward was in fact a complex experimental system that had been designed to yield uncompromised facts about drug-disease interfaces in tropical countries. It was also the site of a global collaboration between an Australian university, a private Australian research laboratory and the PNG Institute of Medical Research, with funding from the WHO, the Royal Australasian College of Physicians, and the Australian National Health and Medicine Research Council.

Once inside the ward, subtle material-spatial differentiations between this global collaborative research project and the everyday functions of the hospital ward became apparent. Dr. Halland, the principal investigator, and his assistant, Paul, showed me the laminated signs on some of the patient beds that indicated they were part of the clinical trial and would be treated only by the researchers. They took me to their "office," a small, shabby side room opposite the nurses' office within the ward building. The space had originally been intended as an examination room, but doctors rarely used it, opting instead to place a temporary standing screen around a patient's bed when conducting an intimate examination. The room had since become a place for dumping unused or broken medical equipment and supplies, or for nurses to take quick naps during their breaks on night shift. Now it had been cleared out except for the bed and a couple of chairs, and a large freezer had been placed in the corner for the storage of samples before they were sent to the laboratory for analysis. As Dr. Halland and Paul showed me around, a hospital pediatrician entered the nurses' office opposite and sat talking to a couple of nurses. He did not acknowledge our presence.

INSTITUTIONAL ASSEMBLAGES

This chapter explores the interactions between the different but overlapping infrastructural assemblages that constitute the public hospital as a place of biomedicine and as a place of bioscience in Papua New Guinea. According to the doctors and nurses who work there, Madang Hospital today struggles to operate as an effective public health institution. For medical researchers, meanwhile, the hospital's deteriorating infrastructure and ample supply of patients suffering from common infectious diseases have epistemic value: the failing hospital is an important place for the production of bioscientific knowledge deemed relevant for the "developing tropics" in general. As this chapter shows, where weak public health infrastructures become a scientific resource, the alignment of medicine and research in the production of public goods becomes increasingly problematic.

In this chapter, I examine the ways in which science relates to the place where it is done, what I call emplacement, when that place is a public health institution where the everyday production of biomedical knowledge frequently fails. Social studies of science have conventionally focused on the epistemological value that particular places hold for science. A focus on the situated material networks of persons, technologies, and buildings that produce universal scientific facts has been crucial, for example, in illustrating the historical significance of particular kinds of places, such as hospitals or laboratories, to act as privileged "truth spots" (Gieryn 2008) that lend special credibility to scientists' claims (Knorr-Cetina 1999; Rheinberger 1997).[2] I refer to this process by which the specificity of place offers verification for scientific knowledge and enables its movement into the public arena (i.e., establishes a connection between the *specificity* of place and the *general* significance of the knowledge produced) as epistemological emplacement.

When the site of scientific research is not a research laboratory in the Global North, but a postcolonial hospital in Papua New Guinea, and when the epistemic value that science derives from that place depends on its poverty and apparent deficiency as a public institution, the relationship between place and knowledge often becomes governed by issues other than veracity and credibility. Many of the hospitals where today's medical scientists carry out their clinical trials are postcolonial institutions located in places with long histories of colonial governance, resource extraction, and poor population health indicators.[3] In such medical institutions, I argue, the question of how place contributes value to science becomes entangled with the question of what science *does* to place.[4] Indeed prior consideration of "local benefits" is today a prerequisite to accessing international research funding and to obtaining permission from government and institutions in developing countries. The relevance of research findings for the places where it is carried out and the investment in local human resources and the infrastructural improvements that an experimental apparatus makes to a site are now widely considered to be defining qualities of "good science." Insofar as those "commitments to place" (Kelly 2011) are increasingly assessed and evaluated by research ethics committees I call this mode of emplacement "ethical."

What kind of public hospital does the governance of scientific emplacement create? "Ethical emplacement" in Madang Hospital often entails investment in "capacity building," but what kinds of capacities are generated by encounters between public hospitals and research assemblages and how are those capacities distributed across research and medicine, scientists and doctors?

The value of science and the prestige of scientists are generated through the circulation of ideas, persons, technologies, and scientific objects. As I describe below, the infrastructural assemblage of Madang Hospital allows foreign scientists and their research findings to be simultaneously emplaced in Madang Hospital and recognized beyond its confines. Research is performed as simultaneously local and global. Hospital doctors and their idiosyncratic knowledge practices, by contrast, remain firmly entrenched in the particularities of the institution, while "development" is perpetually deferred into the future. As Peter Redfield puts it: "All knowledges, practices and objects may indeed be local, but are they *equally* local? Or are not some, as it were, more local than others?" (2002, 792). Following the anthropologist Nancy Munn's account of kula exchange in Papua New Guinea, I suggest that we consider the capacities of place in spatiotemporal terms as the ability to generate value through the movement and exchange of persons and things. It is only through the appropriate distribution of expertise, infrastructure, and scientific facts in time and space that one is able to appear to others in a global guise.

From the perspective of hospital doctors, as opposed to research scientists, the important relationships entailed by scientific research are not the collaborations between humans and material spaces and artifacts that enable the production of universal scientific facts, but the ways in which postcolonial scientific projects partake in the production of differences and inequalities between persons. Their interest in medical research is less in the potential appropriateness of research findings for the "development tropics" than in the potential of research projects as development projects that might transform the hospital, its relations and capacities in the present. As the locus for fragile intersections between scientific, public health, and development interventions, hospitals like Madang Hospital can, I suggest, provide anthropology and science and technology studies with important insights into the importance of place and infrastructure in the ongoing coproduction of historically situated postcolonial socialities and universally valid scientific knowledges.[5] What happens when development claims are made for medical research in a place like PNG?

MAKING THE "DEVELOPING TROPICS"

In chapter 2 I described the intense interest that PNG held for biomedical scientists under successive colonial administrations. A nascent scientific infrastructure emerged with Koch's makeshift hospital laboratory on the

Northeast Coast in the early 1900s and was reinforced and entwined with Australian white nationalist imaginaries with the emergence of Australian tropical medicine research in the 1920s. Koch's research had been confined to the hospital and the immediate communities surrounding the government station, but as the borders and boundaries of European contact expanded, so too—after a time—did the geographical locations for biomedical research. In the postwar period, the Australian-administered territory of New Guinea continued to be perceived by Australia's scientists and administrators as a valuable research site. The geographical extension of political influence and the opening up of the Highlands posed new public health challenges and new opportunities for research on an as yet unknown demographic.

Biomedical research followed the contours of political influence and power. By the 1950s the Australian virologist Macfarlane Burnet of the Walter and Eliza Hall Institute in Melbourne was in discussion with John Gunther, the director of public health in Papua New Guinea about the potential establishment of an Australian field station in New Guinea. Scientific interest had shifted by this time away from a concern with the native threat to white Australia and, in line with the postwar international development framework, medical research was increasingly focused on the island's distinct disease ecology and burden of morbidity. The agenda was no less nationalistic however. From the perspective of Australian scientists and administrators, New Guinea was an outpost of the Australian tropics and a valuable national resource that would enable them to make a distinctive Australian contribution to medicine and biology at an international level. New Guinea was to be Australia's own offshore laboratory for disease ecology.

The agenda to establish New Guinea as Australian research territory was nowhere more evident than in the case of research on kuru (Anderson 2009). The discovery of this degenerative neural disease in the New Guinean Highlands in the 1950s provided the opportunity for Australia to compete with the American research institutions that were dominating the growing international field of scientific research. As Anderson describes, the arrival of the charismatic American scientist, Carleton Gadjusek, in New Guinea in 1957 to study kuru represented a major setback for the Australian administrators and provoked a hostile response from John Gunther, who hoped to preserve New Guinea for Australian scientists (Anderson 2009, 57). The amicable solution that was reached when Gadjusek agreed to send his specimens to the Eliza and Walter Research Institute quickly deteriorated when it was discovered that he was in fact sending his best samples to the National Institute of Health in Bethesda, Maryland, in the United States (ibid., 83). So followed a series of ultimately futile political maneuvers by Gunther intended to remove Gadjusek and his collaborators from the field and to establish a parallel, Australian led, kuru research project.

Gadjusek's entry into the field and growing international profile located Papua New Guinea in the scientific imaginary of a generation of international biologists. At the same time he set a precedent for an "open door" policy to foreign scientists that was to continue to have implications for public health into the twenty-first century (Denoon 1989, 103). Gadjusek worked out of a makeshift clinic in Okapa in the Eastern Highlands and, as Anderson describes, struggled to hold the network of bodies, identities, and tissue samples together in this ramshackle space. Many patients were reluctant to attend the clinic, and Gadjusek had to hunt his subjects down and take valuable samples in rural villages. This research assemblage was dependent on Gadjusek's affiliation with the National Institute of Health in Bethesda, where he sent the majority of his samples for testing. He also sent samples to other scientists, both in order to utilize their technical resources and knowledge and to extend his relationships and scientific alliances (see Anderson 2009, chapter 4). The kuru laboratory began in rural Okapa, but ended in Maryland and Melbourne.

In 1968, Macfarlane Burnet helped established the Institute of Human Biology in Papua New Guinea, with Richard Hornabrook, a New Zealand neurologist who had worked at Okapa on kuru research in the early 1960s as the institute's director. The institute was initially located in the old European Hospital building on the site of the Madang Hospital. However, the hospital was not at this point a major site for the institute's medical research. Instead "community-based research" and access to remote populations now dominated the research agenda in Papua New Guinea. While in Okapa, Hornabrook had not spent a lot of time in the surrounding villages himself, but had disapproved of international scientists, who he felt swooped in for their blood samples before disappearing to their wealthy laboratories elsewhere and had an entirely extractive relationship to Papua New Guineans (Anderson 2009, 182).

For Macfarlane Burnet a strong rationale for establishing the institute in Papua New Guinea was to enable Australia to contribute to the U.S.-dominated International Biology Program, and therefore to mark out Australia's contribution to the growing field of international science. The International Human Biology Program (IHB) was established by the International Council of Scientific Unions in 1964 following discussions that had been initiated in the International Geophysical Year activities of

1959 (NAS 1975). In the postwar cold war era large-scale centralized research efforts such as the U.S. national space program, dubbed "Big Science," were gaining political currency. International collaboration (organized along cold war fault lines) was seen to hold new opportunities for scientific progress. The core theme of the IHB was broadly defined as "biological productivity and the welfare of man" with an emphasis on holistic, ecological, and systems-based approaches to synoptic data collection.[6] What distinguished the IHB from other Big Science of the day was that large-scale field-based data collection formed its primary goal and the basis for international collaboration, as opposed to the conceptual frameworks that drove the physics-based Big Science of the day (Aranova et al. 2010).[7]

As a site of rapid Western acculturation imposed on pristine biological variation, Papua New Guinea was considered an ideal location for generating scientific contributions to the human adaptability component of the IHB. The incorporation of the newly established Papua New Guinean Institute for Human Biology into the IHB meant the institute's funding and infrastructural organizations were tied into interdisciplinary and international research collaborations from the start. Under the directorship of Hornabrook, the institute established two interdisciplinary field studies, one on Karkar Island off the coast of Madang where a new field laboratory was established, the other at Lufa, a village near Goroka, with its established kuru research infrastructure, in the Highlands. The research program focused on climatic, genetic, and socioeconomic variations between the two sites and in line with the IBP systems-based approach involved physical anthropologists, geneticists, demographers, parasitologists, nutritionists, social scientists, and medical doctors (Hornabrook et al. 1977). The investment in these two field sites would result in outputs extending well beyond the lifetime of the IHB program itself, which ended in 1974. Resulting publications focused on the differences between genetic and environmental influences on disease incidence (Anderson et al. 1978), the implications of nutrition for subsistence economies (Harrison et al. 1975), the effects of social change on fertility patterns (Stanhope and Hornabrook 1974), and comparison of highland/coastal body composition (Norgan et al. 1982).

From its beginning tensions between international science and public health cut through the research agenda of the institute. When the PNG Institute for Human Biology was established in 1968 Richard Hornabrook published an open invitation in the international journal, *Science*, for interested scientists to apply to conduct research in PNG. While Hornabrook was interested in the welfare benefits that research could provide for the Papua

New Guinean population, he was aware that such concerns might not attract the international scientists he needed to carry out the research. Emphasis was given to Papua New Guinea's potential as a site for the exploration of the more fundamental questions of human biology: "The institute will initiate research into a wide range of problems relating to the biology of man in a country well placed for such investigations" (1970, 147). "Some problems do not occur more frequently in New Guinea than in other underdeveloped parts of the world" Hornabrook conceded "but they are possibly more easily studied in New Guinea" (1970, 147). Kuru was given as a perfect example of a study that initially appeared to be of only local significance but in fact presents "a new horizon in the study of so-called degenerative or system diseases of the nervous system" (1970, 147).

The IBP was ultimately branded a failure on account of its top-down, centralized institutional framework and the weakness of its ecological framework for mobilizing biologists' "pure science" interests (NAS 1975). However, the international, interdisciplinary research model it established in Papua New Guinea would continue to shape the institute in its future incarnations. In 1970 the institute was moved to Goroka, near to the Lufa research site and ongoing kuru research. Hornabrook returned to New Zealand in 1975, the year of Papua New Guinea's independence, creating uncertainty over the future of the institute. Hornabrook predicted its demise in the face of nationalist suspicion about biological research (Anderson 2009, 182). But in 1977 Michael Alpers, an Australian doctor who had already spent many years in the country studying kuru, took over the position of director.

At independence the institute was renamed the Papua New Guinea Institute of Medical Research, and under Alpers, the applied nature of the institute became more explicit. Alpers made it clear that, while a key part of what scientists do, scientific papers are not an end in themselves. "The IMR's [Institute of Medical Research] work has always been applied, problem-driven research, not basic (or 'pure') research conducted to satisfy scientific curiosity" he argued (1979, 33). The distinction between "curiosity driven" and "problem driven research" became something of a mantra for Alpers. While he continued to be committed to scientific research that might be respected internationally and would attract qualified scientists from abroad, he also organized the rapid growth of the institute around the diseases most affecting the health of Papua New Guineans, including programs on malaria (run out of a new branch established at Yagaum outside Madang Town), enteric diseases, malnutrition, pneumonia, and filariasis. The IMR's research programs continued to remain reliant on international scientists, but like Hornabrook before him, Alpers was wary of the extractive nature of their research. Based on his experience working with the Fore on kuru research, Alpers remained committed to the importance of interdisciplinary research and encouraged the IMR's researchers to take an anthropological and community-based approach to their projects (Alpers 1999).

In the 1990s, the institute faced a funding crisis when structural adjustment programs demanded cuts in public spending. In 1999 the government deleted its budgetary support to all its statutory institutions, including the IMR, and many of the institute's programs were cut or came to a standstill. Where the IMR had previously enjoyed a degree of autonomy vis-à-vis the Papua New Guinean state, now to get any kind of government support, it had to develop closer relations to the NDOH. Meanwhile, Papua New Guinean salaries were no longer attracting the foreign scientists that were still required to run many of the institute's programs in lieu of a substantial number of trained Papua New Guinean scientists. Medical research in Papua New Guinea had been an international endeavor since the beginning of the century, and Gadjusek's refusal to bow to the nationalist science of the Australian administration in the 1960s had arguably established an "open door" policy for foreign scientists ever since (Denoon 1989, 103; Anderson 2009), but now Alpers set out to reinstitutionalize those relationships in order to reflect new global health priorities and tap into the funding that accompanied them.

In 1999, Alpers established what he called a "buttressing coalition" of scientific collaborators from international institutions who would help to develop research programs aligned with IMR's own goals and participate in applications for funding (Alpers 2003). When Alpers left the IMR in 2000 he had built the institute up from five national and five Australian staff to a cohort of five Australian and 250 PNG staff spread across three branches.

Despite these changes the institute remained financially vulnerable and throughout the 2000s, radical changes were made to ensure a continued flow of international funding. At the heart of these institutional changes was a shift from institutional autonomy and an agenda set by the institute's charismatic director, to alignment with international discourses of development and scientific protocols. The institute had received funding from international development agencies in the past. In 1984, its malaria vaccine program was funded through USAID, and when that money was withdrawn in 1994, AusAID stepped into the breach. Now, in order to gain recognition as an institutional agent of development rather than purely medical research, a five-year strategic plan was developed under the new directorship of John

Reeder, which closely aligned the institute's goals with the national health plan and succeeded in attracting direct funding from AusAID.

Meanwhile, in order to secure international scientific research funding the institute began to align itself with the best management structures of international science, including the establishment of an Institutional Review Board and other procedural ethics. Alper's buttressing coalition was expanded to a whole network of international collaborations that tapped into increased funds for global medical research following the establishment of the health oriented Millennium Development Goals. Foreign scientists could now only conduct research in the country through the development of collaborations with the Institute of Medical Research, which would involve the provision of funding for the services provided by the institute inside the country. The IMR would provide local laboratories, offices, and staff. Foreign researchers would bring grants for investment in that infrastructure, would pay and train local staff, and would have the expertise to carry out the research. Crucially, the names of IMR partners would be on all the publications resulting from the research. While IMR still employed several foreign scientists to run their programs, the majority of foreign scientists in the country were now loosely affiliated with the IMR and did not come under its direct management.

It is with this development that hospitals have become increasingly important as sites of medical research. New research collaborations often align themselves with the agendas of global agencies and philanthropic organizations, which have sprung up in recent years following the collapse of public health institutions in many developing countries. These institutions are more often oriented toward the creation of internationally transferable, context independent technical solutions, such as pharmaceuticals, rather than community-based and locally tailored health-care projects (Kelly and Beisel 2011). IMR collaborations are dominated by individual projects that test specific pharmaceutical interventions or treatment protocols and address the narrow interests of particular funders. Hospitals have, by extension, become an important field laboratory in which to test such interventions through time bound, fly in–fly out clinical trials, the gold standard for evidence-based medicine. This has resulted in a network of research projects distributed across Papua New Guinea, including hospitals in Goroka and Port Moresby and rural health centers affiliated to IMR branches in East Sepik and other provinces.[8] With an increased focus internationally on malaria research Madang Hospital has become a particularly prominent research site in this new constellation of science collaborations and funding.

Where international scientists used to be employed by the IMR on national salaries, they are now more often employed by foreign universities or research consortiums and dispatched to Papua New Guinea for field research, with enormous implications for their relationships with the Papua New Guineans that they are working with and studying. In the early twentieth century the hospital was produced as a site of medical research because the town was an enclave of colonialism. Today Papuan New Guinea's towns are enclaves of cosmopolitanism that allow international scientists to conduct research while continuing to enjoy the lifestyles and living conditions to which they and their families are accustomed, rather than endure the comparative hardship of rural life.

As Fischer pointed out in relation to the Yanomami controversy in the 1990s: "1960s science and 1990s science are institutionally quite different enterprises" (2001, 9). The same can be said of Papua New Guinean medical research in the early, mid-, and late twentieth century, with important implications for ethics, representation ("who speaks for who"), and the kinds of human biology research projects that can be imagined, funded, and ventured (2001, 9). Old tensions between international science and Papua New Guinean public health are reproduced within this emergent research environment in new ways. The problem of ethical emplacement has emerged alongside new institutional arrangements for the production and governance of scientific research in the country. International science has become more explicitly geared toward the needs of "national development" rather than "pure science." Development claims are increasingly being made for science. The IMR now self-consciously styles itself as a national institution, contributing to the public health and development of Papua New Guineans. This agenda is reflected in the appointment of the first Papua New Guinean director of the IMR, Peter Siba, in 2006. Until 2011, Siba was the only Papua New Guinean doctor to gain a PhD. He graduated from Lae University of Technology with a BSc in Food Technology in 1984 and immediately took a position in the virology lab of IMR. He was awarded a PhD from Murdoch University in western Australia in 1997 and soon after began taking on administrative responsibilities. Siba was bequeathed a difficult challenge. On the one hand, he sought to emphasize the IMR's role as a national Papua New Guinean institution. On the other hand, the financial sustainability of the IMR has come to depend on the funding and resources that foreign scientists, usually funded by international organizations or consortiums, bring with them, and by association is driven in part by their research agendas.

In 2003, the location and institutional capacities of Madang Hospital were crucial in lending scientific credibility to the findings of Dr. Halland's clinical trial. In contrast to the scientific laboratory, which is valuable precisely because of its peculiar ability to artificially filter out the idiosyncrasies of a particular place—to operate as a "place-less place" (Livingstone 2003, 3; Kohler 2002; Knorr-Cetina 1999)—institutions like Madang Hospital are crucial for their real world authenticity and specificity. The controlled environment of the laboratory means that experimental findings can be replicated wherever those laboratory conditions are reproduced. The particular qualities of the laboratory as a placeless place are crucial for the ability of facts to travel and establishing links between situated experimental practices and universal truths. But precisely because the idiosyncrasies of everyday space have been excised from the artificial space of the laboratory, the knowledge produced within it is susceptible to accusations of irrelevance for the "real world" beyond its walls. This is exactly where scientific experiments conducted in the field gain their credibility.

Madang Province was a valuable site for Dr. Halland's clinical trial because it was deemed representative of the kinds of places where the resulting medical knowledge would be deployed. The trial needed to take place in a region with endemic malaria in order to recruit the right kind of sick patients. But the desirable patient-subject was not exclusively defined in biomedical terms. The trial was intended to provide knowledge about treatment for children in remote areas where the disease burden, difficult terrain, and widespread poverty contribute to a poor prognosis. As Dr. Halland's research group pointed out in a publication resulting from the trial: Most deaths from falciparum malaria occur in children living in remote tropical areas that have limited health-care facilities. A rapidly acting antimalarial suppository would be valuable in this setting. In contrast to oral therapy, it could be given to severely ill children with vomiting, prostration, and/or impaired consciousness, features associated with a poor prognosis. The alternative to rectal drug administration in this situation is intravenous (i.v.) or intramuscular (i.m.) injection, but this requires equipment and trained personnel that are often unavailable in the rural tropics.

The trial patient incorporated certain scientifically desirable infrastructural characteristics alongside biomedical ones. The infrastructural context for the trial was not screened out or externalized but was included in the rationale as a basic premise for its clinical significance. In this respect, the particularities of Madang Province and particularly its weak state infrastructure were crucial markers of the credibility of the knowledge produced (Gieryn 2006; Livingstone 2003; Shapin and Ophir 1991).

Madang Provincial Hospital was not of course located in the "rural tropics" but in the third largest town in Papua New Guinea. But for precisely the same reasons as it was considered by its staff to be failing in public health terms, it also replicated some of the characteristics of a rural health center. The infrastructural conditions of the hospital, and in particular the shortage of nurses to administer and properly supervise IV fluids, and the frequent absence of doctors, meant that in many ways the hospital's medical capacities reproduced those of rural health centers. In this regard, the institutional poverty of Madang Hospital was an asset in the production of scientific knowledge valid for all developing, tropical places. As a "real-life" example of the medical consequences of a development-tropics specific environment, the hospital was an ideal place in which to locate the trial.

Moreover, the hospital was an important gathering point for patients with severe malaria who were referred from rural health centers across the province. These patients were ideal research subjects because they were usually the most severe cases, referred because the patient had arrived at the health center when their condition was already advanced or because they had not responded to treatment. For these children, the chances of survival on conventional malaria treatment were already low. At the urban hospital Dr. Halland and Paul were able to recruit a statistically valid cohort of eligible patients in their limited time period of nine months. As a semi-remote "semi-field,"[9] the urban hospital effectively represented the state of remote health centers in the province, nation, and tropics without the need for the trial to be removed to an actual remote location.

EPISTEMIC DISPLACEMENT

How do you make knowledge that is embedded in the infrastructural limitations of Madang Hospital represent the rural tropics in general? The field, Livingstone notes, is "an inherently unstable scientific site" (2003, 45). The field trial bridges the "experimental gap" (Millo and Lezaun 2006) between experiment and world through contextualization in a specific field of application (Will 2007). But knowledge produced by Dr. Halland's clinical trial is not only meant to be about Madang Hospital, it also needs to represent the rural tropics in general. The trial must *represent* Madang Hospital but it cannot become *like* the hospital insofar as the biomedical knowledge produced within that institution for clinical purposes is construed as unreliable.

In order for the knowledge produced in the hospital to have any credibility beyond it, it was also necessary for certain conditions of control to be established; for certain aspects of the hospital to remain external to the study. While the knowledge produced needed to represent a resource-poor institution, it could not be tarnished by that poverty itself if it were to be able to move beyond it. Just as the field gives scientific knowledge authenticity, so it requires scientific conditioning in order for the knowledge produced to be recognized as generally valid. In the case of Dr. Halland's malaria trial, laboratory-produced pathology data was fundamental in ascertaining the relevance of the results for places beyond Madang Hospital. In other words, the relationships between this hospital and the "rural tropics" still needed to be mediated by a laboratory.

Patients were carefully screened at admission and only those with a blood slide result that tested positive for P. Falciparum parasite with a density of more than 500/ul were recruited to the trial. Unfortunately, the hospital's own pathology laboratory was unable to provide reliable results to this effect. As described in chapter 4, doctors at Madang Hospital constantly complained that the laboratory facilities at the hospital were deficient and that the test results were unreliable. Chemicals and equipment were said to be held up at ports, or delayed elsewhere in the supply chain; the frequent failure of the hospital back-up generator meant that steady temperatures could not always be maintained for fragile reagents; the machines in the laboratory were described as old and constantly breaking down and because there was no money to provide back-up machines the hospital could wait for months to receive spare parts from Australia or Port Moresby. The laboratory technicians were demoralized by the poor facilities and the lack of opportunities for promotion and often refused to carry out what doctors considered urgent tests.

The extractability of laboratory-produced pathology knowledge from the exigencies of place was crucial to the trial's scientific and instrumental value. The hospital laboratory was too contaminated by the institution's particular qualities (exactly those qualities that made the ward so valuable as a field site), to function as a "placeless" place of science. As another researcher for IMR explained, "If we use the hospital laboratory then we couldn't control it. We would have to use their workers and then we couldn't control the quality of the tests, then they would be worthless."

On admission Paul took two blood slides from each patient. One was sent to the hospital laboratory, which provided Dr. Halland with an immediate gauge of the severity of a patient's condition. The second was sent to the laboratory at the IMR, which is located seventeen kilometers south of the town. It was the IMR test result that determined inclusion in the trial and that was used as evidence in subsequent publications. Eligible patients were then given either artesunate suppositories or oral treatment. As they progressed through the trial, further drug assays were done to determine the efficacy of the drugs in reducing the number of parasites in the blood. Again, due to the unreliability of the hospital laboratory these blood samples were carefully packaged, labeled, and stored in the large freezer in the trial office before being sent to a private laboratory in Australia in large batches. A second set of tests carried out in the hospital laboratory gave Dr. Halland immediate feedback on how the patient was doing but was not deemed valid as scientific evidence. In fact, the need to use nearby facilities at IMR and to be able to courier samples to Australia was another reason for the trial to be located in the town rather than a rural health center.

The epistemic emplacement of the trial in the hospital was necessarily partial. On the one hand the dilapidated public health infrastructure of the hospital wards was crucial for establishing the authenticity and real world relevance of the knowledge produced. On the other hand, in order for this principle of representativeness to be enshrined as scientific fact, the trial had to be removed from the specificities of the "remote" and "tropical" altogether (Latour 1999) and emplaced instead within the infrastructure of IMR and Australian research laboratories. The urban hospital site was crucial for its capacity to convincingly represent all remote and resource short settings while at the same time having nearby access to laboratory resources that were anything but typical of such settings. The combined infrastructure of laboratory and ward linked the specificity of the hospital as a place to the ability of the facts produced within it to travel to other places. It was emplaced and displaced in the right proportions.

ETHICAL EMPLACEMENT

Alongside the epistemological challenges of field experimentation are the ethical challenges raised when scientists, participants, and health workers collide in places where health services are chronically underfunded and health workers struggle to carry out their daily tasks.[10] A defining feature of field science is that the wider ramifications of experimental action cannot be controlled or contained in the same way as they can in a bounded laboratory (Szerszynski 2000), creating new kinds of "ethical plateaus" for decision making (Fischer 2005). Medical anthropologists have paid particular attention to ethical problems raised in relation to the vulnerability of research subjects when clinical trials become entangled with public health in places beset by poverty and poor access to health facilities.[11] Petryna states that "experiments . . . are not only hypothesis-testing instruments; they are operative environments that redistribute public health resources and occasion new and often tense medical and social fields" (2009, 30). If this redistribution of resources has implications for patients seeking treatment, then it also has profound effects on the public health institutions where those trials are increasingly carried out (Geissler et al. 2008).

The location of trials in resource-poor hospitals, where the knowledge-production activities of scientists significantly overlap with those of doctors, raises important questions about the ways in which medical science redistributes institutional and expert capacities to produce knowledge and, indeed, what kinds of knowledge a public hospital should generate. How is global medical research experienced by the medical personnel who work in those institutions; people who have been trained in laboratory science or clinical medicine, but are often unable to make use of these capacities because of the limited health infrastructure?

Over the past decade, international research institutions and funding agencies have become increasingly aware of the global inequalities entailed by scientific research in low-income countries. Criticisms from both scientists' home countries, usually in America and Europe, and from the countries where such studies are carried out have led to the emergence of new kinds of reflexive institution (Fischer 2005) that interrogate research ethics protocols and emphasize the need for such studies to benefit publics in their host countries as well as multinational corporations and academic institutions in the West (Benatar et al. 2005; Bhutta 2002; Edejer 1999; Emmanuel et al. 2004). More recently, as concerns about aid effectiveness in countries such as Papua New Guinea have become focused on issues of "governance" and "capacity,"[12] the ethical elements of research protocols have also been assessed in terms of their direct investment in research or public health capacities (Binka 2005; Gaillard 1994; Lairumbi et al. 2008). In fact, the establishment of research governance systems in Papua New Guinea is itself portrayed as a way to enhance the state's managerial capacities. Research governance has become a crucial part of the way science relates to place through practices of "ethical" as well as "epistemic emplacement."

In Papua New Guinea the issue of foreign-funded medical research is particularly sensitive. In 1995, medical research in Papua New Guinea came to national and international attention when an IMR-employed American medical anthropologist, Carol Jenkins, collaborated with the U.S. National Institute of Health in the patenting of a virus called Human T-Lymphotropic Virus-1, which was derived from the blood of a man from the Hagahai tribe in the remote hills of Madang Province. The primary goal of the research was to explore the possibility of devising a diagnostic test for the virus in Melanesia, and the patent noted that, in the unlikely event that commercial value arose from the patent, the Hagahai would receive any royalties due to the researchers. Despite these provisions, a Papua New Guinean journalist and Canadian indigenous rights group published press releases and news reports on the internet, describing the scientists as "vampires" and "bio-prospectors" who were exploiting the world's vulnerable and remote peoples for commercial gain. A media storm ensued, resulting in the personal interviewing of Carol Jenkins by the PNG secretary of foreign affairs. Although no wrongdoing was found to have taken place, this incident led to public outcry within Papua New Guinea and the recognition by the IMR of the need to reevaluate the ethical codes for medical research in the country.

In Madang Hospital, anxieties about bioprospecting and the possibilities for exploitation entailed by scientific research are still fresh in people's minds: As one hospital doctor explained: "The Hagahai thing happened when I was at medical school so I remember it well. Everyone was talking about it. We were all thinking, 'How can this woman just come in and take our blood and go and make money from it in her own country?' that is very wrong."

As with low-income countries elsewhere (Binka 2005; Gaillard 1994), in Papua New Guinea increasingly provisions have been put in place to ensure that the IMR and the Papua New Guinean health system more generally would benefit from those partnerships. All medical researchers in Papua New Guinea have to be affiliated with and have a coinvestigator from the Institute of Medical Research. All medical research projects also have to go through the national level Medical Research Advisory Committee (MRAC). This is made up of medical professionals from IMR, and representatives from the country's medical schools and the Department of Health. In principle, the MRAC puts substantial emphasis on the ethical considerations addressed by the application and all applicants are expected to detail the contribution their research would make to the improvement of public health in the country.

For research gatekeepers in Papua New Guinea and international medical research funders, the production of capacity in persons and places is now an important consideration in giving permissions or funding to a research project. These ideas were integral to Dr. Halland's clinical trial. By comparison with the commercial "offshore" trials that anthropologists such as Adriana Petryna have described elsewhere, Dr. Halland's trial aimed to produce research with which government bodies in PNG and elsewhere in the "rural tropics" could improve the treatment of children with malaria. The employment of Paul was also crucial. Already trained as a health extension officer, Paul was now to acquire new skills in research design and practice and was included as an author on the project outputs. The research process was not only intended to contribute to future health developments in the country, but also to improve the knowledge, skills, and research capacities of a Papua New Guinean person.[13] The clinical trial was therefore organized so as to contribute both to future treatment protocols and to future research capacities in Papua New Guinea.

SCALAR MAGIC

For doctors working in Madang Hospital, however, the applied nature of scientific knowledge and the training of PNG's future researchers was less important than the immediate infrastructural disparities between research and public health. These were evidenced by the respective role of the hospital laboratory in the knowledge practices of scientists and doctors. The unreliability of the hospital laboratory was just as damaging to doctors' attempts to produce diagnostic knowledge as it was to the researchers' experimental knowledge practices. In contrast to the researchers, however, the hospital doctors were unable to bypass this problem by outsourcing investigations to foreign-funded research laboratories. Their work was emplaced in the hospital in a different, stickier way to that of the scientists.[14] In other words they were less able to control what was internal or external to their field of knowledge (and personhood) production.

Without reliable diagnostic facilities, doctors employed pragmatic clinical strategies to manage patients using the treatments available. As we saw in the previous chapter, doctors aligned clinical signs with "what we can do" in order to treat a patient, rather than attempting to identify specific pathogens or diseases. A very different kind of patient body and a different kind of medical expert was enacted by these practices than by the clinical trial. Patients were not individualized as biological entities whose internal processes were revealed by a penetrative medical gaze. In the crowded wards, patients accumulated into a mass of "generally sick," undifferentiated bodies that were being treated with variations of the same cocktail of drugs. Meanwhile the doctors claimed that being able to deal with these difficult conditions required a unique form of located expertise. The universal, standardized knowledge found in the Western textbooks they had read at university was, they claimed, often irrelevant. Instead they relied on clinical experience, and on building relationships with nurses, relatives, and laboratory workers who might assist them in "doing what we can." This was a world apart from the individualized biochemical bodies that were made visible through pathology investigations in the clinical trial, and the ability of Dr. Halland to act as an "international" scientist, whose expertise extended far beyond the local parameters of Madang Hospital.

Dr. Halland recognized that locating the trial in the hospital could lead to resentment from the hospital employees about disparities between the resources available for research and for public services. Fortunately, Dr. Halland was also uniquely well placed to negotiate the politics of research in the clinical spaces of the hospital. Prior to coming to Madang Hospital to conduct research in 2003, Dr. Halland had spent six months at the institution in 2000 as part of his training in infectious diseases. Confident, outgoing, and overwhelmingly genial, Dr. Halland had succeeded in building good professional relationships with the other doctors, who therefore knew him as a physician long before they knew him as a researcher. It was through the connections made on this prior visit that Dr. Halland was able to build a relationship with the hospital's managers and obtain institutional approval for research. Throughout the trial, Dr. Halland continually blurred his role as clinician and scientist by wandering around the hospital wards and assisting other doctors in their clinical work.

It was also fortuitous that Dr. Halland had only a very modest infrastructural set up located within the grounds of the hospital itself. Although he had access to laboratory facilities that were unavailable to hospital doctors or technicians, the fact these facilities were located off-site meant that this disparity was not materially visible within the institution. Moreover, Dr. Halland made a concerted effort to engage in interpersonal relationships with technicians in the hospital laboratory. Before he left the hospital he purchased a large comprehensive textbook of clinical microbiology worth several hundred Australian dollars for the laboratory. I walked with him to the laboratory in order to hand it over. As we entered the laboratory workers stopped what they were doing and crowded around us. Dr. Halland held up the two heavy books: "I want to thank you all for all the help that you have given me for this project. Your help with blood slides and other tests has enabled us to do a very important study. Our research shows that those patients with malaria who are treated with suppositories recover much quicker. The parasites die more quickly than those on arthemeter. These are very significant findings."

He then held up a graph showing his findings and pointed out the two different lines on the graph showing the results from the drug assay tests carried out in Australia, which demonstrated that the number of parasites in patients treated with suppositories declined faster than in those treated with arthemeter. "I will write a paper about this research" he said, "and it will be widely distributed and read around the world. These results are very significant, not just for Papua New Guinea but worldwide, particularly in African countries. The study would not have been able to happen without your help. I wanted to make a contribution to show you my appreciation and I thought that the best way was to give you some resources because I know you have had a difficult time here and that resources are scarce. So I have brought you these two volumes of a textbook on clinical microbiology from Melbourne."

Dr. Halland's gift was a success on many levels. He acknowledged the difficulties and challenges faced by the lab workers, where the doctors in the hospital only blamed them for doing a bad job. But more significantly, with the use of the textbooks and a few pieces of paper as props, he performed what might be deemed a feat of scalar magic. Where hospital workers often associated foreign researchers with a privileged "global" world of science and resources from which they were excluded, Dr. Halland both conjured the world of global science *in the laboratory*, and at once brought the laboratory *into global science*. His speech began with a reference to the very specific local work that the laboratory workers had done for his project. He then provided material evidence of the outcome of that work in the form of a graph, skillfully omitting to mention that the laboratory tests on which the graph was based were done in Australia and not in the hospital. Instead the graph appeared to be a direct result of the work that had been done by these laboratory workers in this specific hospital and laboratory. The graph also acted as a crucial intermediary between the hospital and global science. It was an outcome of work done in the hospital, it would be used by people in developing countries in the tropics, but it would also be seen and read about in many other countries worldwide. Through reference to the articles he would write, his recent trip to Melbourne, and his access to resources such as the textbook he gave the laboratory, Dr. Halland established himself as an international figure, an embodiment of the global connections that make up the world of scientific research. At the same time, his gift materialized the laboratory workers' relationship to him and through him to the wider scientific community.

Through the giving of the textbook, Dr. Halland met capacity building requirements for scientific research and symbolically overcame the binary oppositions between "Papua New Guinean medicine" and "global science," and between research subjects and objects that could have fueled resentments and anxieties about relationships with foreign scientists in the hospital. The "material politics" (Law and Mol 2008) of Dr. Halland's textbook presentation established a connection between wealthy places of science and poor objects of research by enacting the hospital clinical laboratory as an intrinsic part of the global scientific endeavor. The movement of the journal article through the networks of global science extended the capacities of laboratory workers in time and space (Munn 1986). Indeed Dr. Halland's presentation of the journal article as a composite of efforts by multiple persons departs significantly from a dominant model of scientific personhood as a form of individual encompassment which was described in chapter 6.

THE RESEARCH HOSPITAL

In 2003, Dr. Halland was the first researcher that hospital workers could remember carrying out research in the hospital. As described in chapter 7, hospitals in Papua New Guinea were under pressure from the government and from donors at this time to increase their revenues through independent partnerships with civil society, the private sector, and foreign donors rather than relying on the Papua New Guinean government for funds. While hospitals officially remained "public" institutions and a responsibility of the Department of Health, hospital managers were increasingly expected to compete with one another in economic efficiency and entrepreneurial fund-raising activities.

The Madang Hospital board chairman (who was also the president of Divine Word University, see chapter 7) saw in Dr. Halland's trial the opportunity to develop the hospital into a cutting edge hub for medical research and training in Papua New Guinea. With the link between health and poverty reinforced by the Millennium Development Goals, ever more funding for research into infectious diseases such as malaria and tuberculosis was making its way to Papua New Guinea.[15] The board chairman realized that the institution's location in a province with one of the highest rates of transmission for both malaria and tuberculosis would make it of special interest to medical scientists, and in 2006 he approached IMR with a proposal to turn Madang Hospital into a fully fledged "research hospital." Rather than depending on government funding, he envisaged the hospital prospering through its own partnerships with the Institute of Medical Research, Divine Word University, and other foreign donors.

When I returned to the hospital in 2009 I was struck by the proliferation of research projects in diverse clinical spaces of the hospital. The small side room that had once been used by Dr. Halland and Paul had been replaced by a full-blown research laboratory, which had been established in an unused building at the back of the pediatric ward. The laboratory was financed by a PhD project from Dr. Halland's old university that was looking into the genetic basis of immunity to malaria in the region alongside numerous side projects on malaria and meningitis treatment responses. Two research projects on malaria in pregnancy were being run simultaneously by different international funding consortiums in the obstetrics ward. The hospital's TB clinic was hosting a global-fund funded IMR project that looked at the efficacy of the DOTS (directly observed treatment short course) program in the region. Two European medical students were conducting research in the pediatric ward on the deviations of meningitis treatment practices from official protocols.

Dr. Halland's initial trial had paved the way for the rediscovery of Madang Hospital as a valuable "truth spot" (Gieryn 2008), while several young Australian researchers and medical consortiums had been able to build on his relationship to the IMR and the hospital in order to gain access to the institution. In 2009, the financial stability offered by ongoing international interest in Madang as a research site enabled the IMR to secure the title to a large piece of land located opposite Madang Hospital and in 2010 they were in the process of building a new research center on the site.

Researchers who have worked for IMR since the 1970s describe tensions between the institute and the hospital as long-standing. However, the pressures on relationships between doctors and researchers have today been increased by the rapid expansion and increase of funding for medical research in the province and the associated rise in value of the hospital as a "semi-field," by the current lack of overlap between research staff and clinical staff, and by the increasing expectation, attendant to the new discourse on ethics, that research should make a contribution to the provision of public health services.

In 2009, the capacity-building elements of the new projects had, if anything, become more pronounced. The IMR had established its own Institutional Review Board that interrogated the ethical protocols of prospective research projects in terms of processes of informed consent, confidentiality, risks, and benefits to participants and simultaneously emphasized the need for any externally led projects to contribute to "research capacity" in Papua New Guinea. For the first time a Papua New Guinean national had been appointed to the position of IMR Director, and he had made it clear that North-South research partnerships would now be more tightly regulated. Any researchers wanting to enter the country would need to show what contribution they would make to the IMR. The proliferation of research on HIV/AIDS that accompanied the growing epidemic in the country had also led to an increased emphasis on ethical processes such as informed consent, the provision of anonymity, and the need for research to address the public health priorities of a health system in "crisis."

In practice, however, the structure of research governance institutions in Papua New Guinea has opened up room for variability in the definition and application of ethics (Petryna 2009), especially with regard to how research is expected to contribute to the national health system. Criteria for approval by the MRAC are not made publicly available, even to those submitting a proposal, and there is no transparency over how the MRAC reaches its decisions. Some projects, often those without substantial backing from well-known foreign academic institutions or funding bodies, are rejected on the basis of minor technicalities (the requirements of which have not been made apparent prior to the application process). The research institutions represented on the MRAC continue to be dependent on foreign funds for their survival and prospective applicants are informally advised that successful proposals are usually backed by a member of the committee whose institution is involved in the research and stands to benefit from it financially. This has significant repercussions for the government health institutions in which research is carried out.

What kinds of places and what kinds of expert capacities do these research governance exercises and the discursive emphasis on capacity building produce? In Madang Hospital researchers made a concerted effort to contribute to institutional infrastructure. These efforts coalesced around the renovation of an unused and deteriorating building at the back of the pediatric ward into a new research laboratory.[16] This renovation project included the conversion of a room adjoining the laboratory into a hospital library and meeting room for hospital staff.

Despite these capacity-building endeavors, the growing visibility of research in the hospital had been accompanied by heightened tensions. Medical research continued to be perceived by hospital staff as a foreign, extractive endeavor. The research staff often used the library they had built as a quiet space to write up notes and input data. However, hospital staff expressed frustration that the researchers were using "hospital space" and "treating it as their own." Some complained that there had been plans to convert the space now being used as the laboratory into a staff tearoom, although these had never come to fruition, and there were lingering frustrations that the IMR had been able to acquire this building. Doctors complained that the "partnership" was a one-way arrangement and the IMR scientists were using the hospital facilities and patients to make their careers as international scientists, while the hospital and the doctors who worked in it did not benefit. Equipment was also an issue. The laboratory technicians complained that the researchers had up to date testing equipment, while theirs was old and unreliable. There was particular resentment from hospital laboratory workers that the IMR had established a separate laboratory and were usurping the hospital laboratory by providing testing facilities for some of the hospital wards. For example, the research laboratory was carrying out all the tests for the pediatric ward, where many of the IMR's research projects continued to be based. This both generated resentment among the doctors in other wards, who remained dependent on the main laboratory, and the laboratory workers who saw it as a sign of disrespect for their work.

The central role of the Institute of Medical Research in developing and regulating the research governance system in Papua New Guinea means that protocols focus on inequalities between foreign and Papua New Guinean "research capacities." In this regard the imagined benefits of research for the hospital were twofold. In the short term, contributions to infrastructure and training would transform the hospital into a research hospital. In the long term, that research was anticipated to contribute to improved treatment protocols relevant for a resource-poor context. "Development" was either spatially separated from the public hospital through its location in a space of research, or was temporally separated from the public hospital through its location in unspecified improvements for public health in the future.

The temporal distinction between hospital benefits and public health benefits were made evident when a European medical student, who was conducting research on meningitis treatment practices in the hospital, complained that results from her previous hospital site in Port Moresby had already been communicated to the Madang team by the Port Moresby pediatrician. She was concerned that this might make doctors in Madang improve their treatment practices and would bias her results. While it was hoped that her research project would eventually produce "useful knowledge" for the crafting of medical protocols, this usefulness was better situated in the future, after she had collected her data.

These spatiotemporal disjunctions were justified by the emphasis in re-search protocols on North-South inequalities in research capacity. None-theless hospital staff questioned the long-term opportunities for those, like Paul, who worked as research assistants at the IMR. They complained that there were few opportunities for promotion of nationals within the IMR structure, which still has expatriates heading up many of its research units. The kind of research training that Paul received is not incidental, and in some cases opened up future opportunities for employment. However one research assistant, Frank, who was working in Madang Hospital in 2009, and who had taken the job on a malaria research project soon after graduating from the Lutheran Nursing School in Madang, said he did not see any long-term opportunities in IMR because "nursing officers don't do the research in IMR, they just work as assistants for the foreign scien-tists." The IMR research assistants are paid at lower rates than government nurses and so several of those in employment in 2009 were planning to get a government nursing job as soon as possible and were hoping their stint at the IMR would improve their employment prospects in the public health sector. Others were hoping that their experience at IMR would assist them in developing a career path in the rapidly developing NGO sector. Very few saw long-term opportunities in research. In 2010, when I returned to PNG, Paul was working as an HEO in a Catholic-run health center a few kilometers outside Madang Town. Frank's contract at IMR had also come to an end, and he had managed to get a job as a Nursing Officer in the mission-run hospital on Karkar Island off the coast of Madang. For both men, their time at IMR had simply been a brief interlude in a nursing or HEO career rather than the beginning of a new research career.

For doctors in Madang Hospital, meanwhile, differences between north-ern and southern research capacities were less important than discrepancies between "research" and "medical" capacities. Doctors in Madang Hospital voiced anger that the presence of medical research in the hospital had not assisted them in their own medical work, nor provided opportunities for their own career advancement.

> IMR are one of our partners. They come in that way. They are front lin-ers for the government. They are advising the government on provin-cial health, on health trends. You should ask them that. Where is their research being used? You see the infectious diseases in this country are rising. So what are you giving to the government? You are getting money for research but what are you telling the government? I would like to do

research too. But I have so much work to do here. I cannot do it. (Laboratory Technologist, Madang Hospital)

People have a negative view of IMR because we see that no national doctors have made their way up through the organization. We just see a lot of white people coming in to do research. And we don't see that their work improves the situation. We cannot see the clinical benefits. (Emergency Medicine Physician, Madang Hospital)

Hospital doctors find themselves embedded in the sticky, messy infrastructural limitations of the PNG national health system where light-footed white scientists appear to be able to drop in and out, emplacing themselves in and displacing themselves from the hospital as they see fit. "White scientists," doctors complain, travel around the world presenting their results at international conferences, while the hospital doctors' expertise remains idiosyncratic to Madang Hospital and is often seen as bad practice from the perspective of international norms and standards. Their knowledge and their body remain firmly entrenched in the specificity of place (see also Sullivan 2012). From the perspective of hospital workers, research and public health are two different "places" in Madang Hospital, with different infrastructures and different spatiotemporal capacities built into them. Foreign scientists, it is assumed, bring to Madang Hospital more authoritative versions of biomedicine that are being practiced in the world's wealthy centers of science and garner international recognition. Like other scientific practitioners in the Global South, Papua New Guinean doctors have to navigate a route between their desire for their knowledge to be recognized as valid by scientists elsewhere and their investment in local forms of knowledge and expertise (Crane 2010, 845; Johnson 2013). It will be vital for responsible discussion about the future of medical science and public health in Papua New Guinea to follow the ways in which these tensions play out as the Institute of Medical Research continues to become simultaneously both more "nationalized" and more "internationalized" in the future.[17]

CONCLUSION

This chapter has explored relationships between the epistemic value that science derives from the places where it is done and what science does to those places. How has the place of the public hospital been transformed by the interventions of globally funded science and its international standards for research governance? In a context where ethical protocols increasingly substitute for state infrastructure, what kinds of public health institution do these moneys, practices, and protocols build? And what kinds of expert persons appear in their vicinity?

Scientific research in places like Madang Hospital is clearly extremely important. For example, Dr. Halland's trial eventually led to a rewriting of standard protocols for the treatment of children with severe malaria. But, in the making of knowledge that is relevant for underresourced places, there is a risk that continued underresourcing becomes taken for granted. The medical researchers I spoke to were clear that responsibility to improve the public health infrastructure lay with the state. They had an obligation to build capacity to carry out research in such places but not to change their institutional capacities as service providers. On one occasion, for example, an Australian researcher complained about the attitude of staff in the hospital. When I suggested that those tensions could be ameliorated if foreign research institutions invested in the hospital's own laboratory as a clinical and research space, rather than creating their own separate research laboratory, she replied that to invest in the hospital laboratory would be a waste of funds because "they will never have a working laboratory here. It is impossible because of the climate and lack of power infrastructure." This was despite the fact scientists affiliated with the IMR had established a fully functioning research laboratory within the hospital grounds. Such comments naturalized disparities in people's knowledge producing capacities by attributing to them very different kinds of embeddedness in Papua New Guinea as a place and demonstrated an "ethic of refusal" (Redfield 2005) to engage with the infrastructural particularities of health care in the country. On the one hand governance of "ethical emplacement" is intended to ensure science contributes to the places where it is done. On the other hand, ethical protocols disentangle the infrastructure of research from that of public health. This is particularly problematic for hospital workers, for whom infrastructure is deemed central to their capacities as expert persons.

This situation affords us a different perspective on the 2003 trial. Ironically, the fact the trial's superior pathology capacities were hidden offsite at IMR or an Australian laboratory meant the difference between the place of research and the place of public health was not made visible. Meanwhile, precisely because Dr. Halland did not have a separate isolated laboratory building or office his project was emplaced in the hospital in a different way to scientists working at the hospital in 2009. He was forced to occupy and move around the wards in a similar way to hospital doctors. He participated in the clinical practices of the hospital wards, and he built up close relationships with hospital laboratory workers to ensure that tests were done. In doing so, he recognized hospital workers as persons operating within the same spatiotemporal coordinates of knowledge production as himself, and acknowledged the infrastructural constraints that they faced. In other words, while the emplacement of the trial was partial, Dr. Halland, to some extent embraced everyday entanglements between hospital and research. In fact, Dr. Halland can be construed as pursuing the same strategies of pragmatic attachment that I have argued are central to everyday clinical medicine in the hospital.

In 2003, Dr. Halland was able to forge connections between the activities of hospital technicians and clinicians and the world of global science. This conceptual and concrete relationship was premised on proximity and exchange. As Geissler et al. pointed out in relation to a community response to a malaria vaccine trial in the Gambia, research ethics might be based on "material benefits, on substantial transactions and on immediate relations" rather than formal ethical protocols (2008, 700). By 2009, however, the growing regulation of "ethical emplacement" through such formal protocols had ironically led to a spatiotemporal disjuncture between research and clinic. Infrastructural investments were displaced to separate laboratories in the same compound and public health benefits were displaced to a future of regulations and standards, abstracted from everyday emplaced practices. The tensions between epistemic emplacement and displacement that are central to experimental field science were now mirrored in partial processes of "ethical emplacement," which engaged with inequalities between research capacities but not those between research and medical practice. Here ethical protocols that require the investment of funds in research capacity safeguards the epistemic and ethical value of scientific data but don't improve public health infrastructure (Petryna 2009).

The location of medical research in a struggling health institution creates ambiguities and tensions in relationships between the specificity of the hospital as a place and the kinds of knowledge that can be produced within it. The relationships between Papua New Guinean and foreign, public and private, universities, and research institutes that are in the process of transforming Madang Provincial Hospital into a global center for medical research do not only provide the material infrastructure for medical and scientific knowledge production but also partake in the production of powerful distinctions between persons and places.

From the perspective of hospital workers, research scientists are able to simultaneously embed themselves in the hospital and travel with their knowledge to other places. Their findings will be applied in other "tropical" places of "development," but they will also publish their findings in international journals, present at international conferences, and get jobs in universities around the world. Madang Hospital doctors and laboratory technicians, by contrast, are not able to establish the relevance of their knowledge and expertise beyond the hospital grounds. Their local know-how gives them a particular kind of "modest" authority, but this is an authority that is unrecognized beyond the confines of the institution. The disjuncture between the time-space parameters (Munn 1986) of the new "global" research hospital and that of the dilapidated, resolutely local public hospital, is experienced by doctors as a difference in personal capacities and professional visibility.

Biomedicine in a Fragile State

■ What is a public hospital in a fragile state? In Papua New Guinea, discourses of state failure are equated with the state's inability to provide basic public services such as health care and infrastructure. But state hospitals have not disappeared. They exist as layered landscapes, bearing the living traces of successive failed state-building and development programs. In a country where the private health sector is confined to the resource extraction industry and a scattering of urban clinics aimed at expatriates or the Papua New Guinean elite, the public hospital remains the only health-care option for the vast majority of patients and the only workplace for many trained medical and nursing professionals. It has also been the object of ongoing intervention for foreign governments, development agencies, and international organizations focused on improving national development through health. The public hospital lies at the technological heart of the public health system, but it is unable to operate as people (politicians, donor agencies, health workers, or patients) expect. How, this book has asked, do medical professionals, nurses, and patients experience this ambiguous space of modernity and development? What kinds of hopes for the future and what kinds of disappointments are generated within its walls? Perhaps most important, what kinds of lives does it make possible?

The public hospital has often been construed by anthropologists as a technology of governance, a place where the biological individual is made medically legible and amenable to classification and control, and where engagements with medical technologies shape both expert and patient subjectivities in ways that facilitate the monitoring and regulation of the body.

In Papua New Guinea, the state has been the primary provider of public health services since the establishment of the colonial administration over a century ago. But, as this book has shown, the public hospital in Papua New Guinea has never been a straightforward vehicle for the state's management and governing of biological life or the surveillance and disciplining of governable or self-governing subjects.

People's predominant experience of Madang Hospital is of its failure to render them visible to a clinical or governing gaze. Institutional confinement instead generates a *desire to be seen* by others (whether by the politicians, medical experts, or foreign scientists) and a hopefulness that institutional visibility will afford bodily and social transformations. Rather than an institutional locus for the distributed operations of state power, the Papua New Guinean hospital has provided a focus for ongoing attempts to consolidate biomedical and state technologies of knowledge production, control, and intervention against a backdrop of state fragility and biomedical failure. Significantly, attempts to "make the state see" have been pursued by those traditionally considered the objects of state knowledge (such as patients) as well as by those who are positioned to deploy its technologies of knowledge and legibility (such as managers, bureaucrats, or politicians).

Just as "the forms of illegibility, partial belonging, and disorder that seem to inhabit the margins of the state . . . constitute its necessary condition as a theoretical and political object" (Das and Poole 2004, 6), so, this book has argued, can uncertainty, failure, and invisibility tell us much about the way in which biomedicine is done and the state is imagined and constituted in majority places of poverty and infrastructural instability. Patients, nurses, and doctors alike experience the hospital as a place where they are rendered imperceptible to the gaze of others and, at the same time, where novel opportunities for experimentation with techniques of visibility emerge. This conclusion deals with the implications of this politics of visibility for the anthropology of biomedicine and its institutions in unstable places.

ANTHROPOLOGY OF UNCERTAINTY

This book has asked how biomedical technologies and rationalities travel to low-income settings in global locations, where the ability to effectively produce biomedical knowledge is severely curtailed by resource shortages and where biology may not be the only way of imagining and governing "life." Papua New Guinea is particularly significant in this regard. On the one hand, it offers a perspective on state-society relationships from a vantage point where the existence of neither can be taken for granted and where the state-run health system is widely considered to be in crisis. On the other hand, anthropologists have found the fiction of "Melanesia" a handy tool precisely because of the alternative ontological conditions for personhood and agency that are implied by people's kinship and exchange practices and the different knowledge operations and objects of knowledge that it brings into relief.

In Madang Hospital weak infrastructure places limitations on the authority and certainty of biomedical knowledge. Biomedical ways of knowing, and the objects biomedical practitioners seek to render visible, remain inherently unstable. In this space of uncertainty, different biological and nonbiological projects of bodily transformation collide. As I have shown, these interferences can be usefully described in terms of what Marilyn Strathern calls aesthetics: a constraint on the forms in which persons must appear in order to be recognized by others. Strikingly, both biomedical knowledge practices and Melanesian kinship and exchange practices depend on intrinsic connections between knowledge, personhood, and visibility. Patients in Madang Hospital dwell on their physical state as evidence for their ability to mobilize relationships. It is only through other's response to their visual appearance that they know their own social capacities: that they know what kind of a person they are. Their anxieties in relation to hospital technologies therefore often concentrate on their ability to harness those technologies in such a way that their body will appear in a guise that doctors consider appropriate. Meanwhile, techniques of visibility are similarly central to the knowledge practices of modern medicine. Learning to become a medical expert is often equated with the process of learning to see the body as a biological system (e.g., Good 1994) and of acquiring the skills to decode medical images such as the X-ray or ultrasound (Cartwright 1995; Crary 1990). Just as patients worry whether they have appeared in the appropriate visual form, so do doctors intensely examine X-ray or ultrasound images searching for signs of disease.

In Madang Hospital, then, biomedicine is not the only set of aesthetic conventions for making persons visible. Biological life is not the only form in which a body can be known and acted on. Persons are also made visible, and their bodies physically transformed, for example, through exchanges of food, intentions, and bodily substance with others. A person's body can appear as the materialization of social failure or accomplishment; their physical state provides evidence of their social efficacy rather than the presence of external disease agents. Moreover, nonbiomedical modes of personhood are sometimes reproduced through people's engagements with biomedical and bureaucratic technologies, as for example, when patients engage with X-rays as a relational technology.

The space of the public hospital destabilizes the conditions of possibility for both projects of visibility. The anthropologist can no longer take for granted that they are either in "Melanesia" or in a "Euro-American" hospital, with all the contextual associations of personhood, agency, and knowledge that such categorization entails. Patients in Madang Hospital do not know what kind of aesthetic criteria governs doctors' decisions about whether an X-ray will result in a "name." They do not know how they need to appear in order to be recognized as a patient and treated. Meanwhile, doctors find that the technologies that should visualize and represent unruly bodies and incorporate them into established norms for disease frequently fail to separate medical knowledge off from its object. The result is not a new set of conventions, classifications, or norms, but "generally sick" bodies that must be acted on in highly pragmatic and experimental ways. In each case, the aesthetic criteria for visualizing persons and bodies must be actively reconstructed and reimagined.

Studies of technological uncertainty in anthropology and science studies have tended to focus on new technologies in wealthy countries and the epistemological and ethical complexities generated in their wake (e.g., Strathern 1992; Mesman 2008; Jensen 2010; Rapp 1999. But see also Livingston 2012). By contrast, uncertainty in Madang Hospital proceeds from the limitations of both biomedical and kinship practices to make bodies visible in a form that can be recognized, responded to, and acted on. Frequently, bodies are not made visible to a clinical gaze. Nor are they made visible to the relational gaze of external kin. This raises fundamental questions for the hospital's inhabitants about what kind of person should or could be made visible in this space and what the aesthetic conventions for rendering them visible might be. Institutional uncertainty is not only epistemic (What are the conditions for knowledge?) but ontological (What are the conditions of viability for a person?).

For a doctor, a patient, a kinsperson, or a public servant, uncertainty raises the prospect of failure. Nonetheless, Madang Hospital is not only a place of failure. Ontological uncertainty provokes people to experiment with medical and bureaucratic technologies (Livingston 2012). Nurses, doctors, and patients alike improvise in the hope of eliciting a productive relationship with others (politicians, medical scientists, and doctors). Chapter 4 described how doctors improvise and adapt biomedical technologies like the medical record to generate pragmatic outcomes and new kinds of bodies; chapter 5 described how patients engage with biomedical technologies such as the X-ray in order to elicit the clinical gaze of the doctor; chapter 7 described how nurses seek to make themselves visible through bureaucratic documents and engagement with the law. It is this ethic of experimentation and improvisation that sustains the hospital as a space of hope as well as failure.

POLITICS OF VISIBILITY

The fieldwork on which this book is based began in 2003. In the decade since then, changes in the fields of international development and health financing have radically transformed the ways in which health services are delivered in developing countries. How does this book speak to those changes and how might it inform current anthropology? The politics of visibility encountered in Madang Hospital, I argue, reveal new dynamics of marginality and exclusion in the arena of global health. There people are not excluded from the rule of law, from state services, or from targeted programs for health and development. Rather this book highlights the sense of marginality and failure that is experienced by those who have gained access to public institutions in places of weak state infrastructure. This book draws attention to the everyday hospital, where international development and health interventions take their course, as a site of exclusion reproduced at the heart of the state.

A growing interest in relationships between health and poverty in developing countries has been accompanied in recent years by a substantial increase in global funding for health. With the millennium development goals targeting specific diseases and health risks, and growing international concern over the health security issues posed by existing and emergent infectious diseases, a plethora of global funding schemes for health programs has emerged. These include the involvement of established international organizations such as the WHO, new international financial bodies such as the Global Fund, and philanthrocapital organizations such as the Bill and Melinda Gates Foundation.

The emergence of these new funding programs has been accompanied by an emphasis on disease control, with the majority of programs targeted at specific diseases such as HIV. With a focus on value for money and performance targets, such programs have also tended to seek out technological "silver bullet" solutions, such as pharmaceuticals, mosquito nets, or rapid diagnostic tests, which are intended to bypass or substitute for depleted state infrastructures. By framing the disease burden of fragile states as a "crisis" the case is made for immediate action that draws attention away from state building and "good governance" and toward the need to save as many lives as is possible with as little money in the least amount of time.

This respatialization of international health governance has not escaped criticism. Public health analysts worry that the prevailing disease control model has led to the fragmentation of national health systems. As crisis discourse has coalesced around particular diseases, such as HIV, so medical researchers and public health experts have raised the specter of "neglected diseases," which are unlikely to attract research or donor funding because of their lack of market opportunity. Medical anthropologists have argued that the emphasis disease control programs place on biological causation ignores the social, economic, and political conditions through which health inequalities are produced (Harper 2014; Farmer 2005). Approaches from science and technology studies have shown how universal technocratic solutions neglect opportunities for the development of local pragmatic collaborations that incorporate medical technologies into emergent relationships between communities, disease vectors, and urban landscapes (Kelly and Biesel 2011). As Fischer has argued, the continued purchase of "problem-based" approaches to disease alongside new developments in technology and molecular biology invite us to think "of technologies as simple matters of implementation . . . rather [than] as constant negotiation and invention within social organizations and networks" (Fischer 2013).

Responding to such concerns, the WHO has highlighted "health systems strengthening" as a priority for international health governance. In 2007 their "Everybody's Business" report spelled out the need to improve capacity in such systemic areas as drug procurement, health financing, and human resources in order for disease control programs to have a lasting and sustainable impact on health systems in the developing world. The Global Fund now also incorporates a health systems strengthening component into its funding schemes. This can include "disease-specific" health systems strengthening activities "aimed at strengthening those aspects of the health system that are relevant for improving outcomes of a specific disease" or, crucially, stand alone "cross-cutting HSS proposals" that are intended to improve the capacity for disease control in relation to more than one disease (Global Fund 2011, 1).

This tension between disease control and health systems strengthening (or "vertical" versus "horizontal" programs) has been integral to the reshaping of the public health landscape in Papua New Guinea over the past decade. Chapter 8 described the increase in global medical research activities focused on high-profile diseases such as malaria in the hospital and, alongside this disease-focused approach, the emergence of governance frameworks to ensure those activities feed back into the public health system. Chapters 3 and 7 described the emphasis that international development agencies such as AusAID placed on "good governance" and health management in the 1990s and the early years of the twenty-first century. At the same time that it has invested in capacity-building programs, however, AusAID has continued also to operate in a "crisis" mode, circumnavigating the state and their own sectorwide funding mechanisms in order to fund projects that it hoped would directly deliver vital services. In 2009, for example, AusAID funded the roll-out of specialist STI clinics across the country, including a stand-alone clinic built in the grounds of Madang Hospital.

These issues have become the source of widespread public debate in Australia following the publication of a series of damning reports about the expensive failure of a technical assistance model to achieve any change in health indicators (e.g., AusAID 2009; Janovsky et al. 2010). As the largest donor to PNG's health sector, AusAID is under increasing pressure to directly fund, and possibly administer, health services, and to produce quantitative results in terms of lives saved. As I described in chapter 7, these tensions are often ameliorated through a model of good "health management" that entails the outsourcing of basic services to nonstate organizations and the development of "partnerships" with international organizations, faith-based organizations, and the private sector. "Health systems strengthening" is here equated with public-private partnership. Ironically, this often leads to the further fragmentation of health into a series of "projects" run by different organizations, further depleting the public spaces and systems that exist at their interstices.

Amidst these transformations in international health and development, anthropologists have tended to follow the money by examining the social implications of national and international disease control programs, medical research programs, and pharmaceutical marketing. Anthropologists have concentrated on the ways in which these interventions have transformed social identities and people's relationship to the state. The rollout of ARVs by global philanthropic and international organizations in many African countries, for example, has led to the construction of the diseased body as a valuable resource capable of securing access to health-care services and employment possibilities that the state does not otherwise provide (Cassidy and Leach 2009; Nguyen 2005). Just as patients in Madang Hospital focus on the acquisition of particular "names," such as malaria or tuberculosis, so in the context of disease control, have specific diseases become the dominant biological "aesthetic" governing recognition of health citizenship rights. "Disease" has become the means by which states and statelike actors transform generic populations into specific, knowable populations and targets for intervention. Chapter 4, for example, described how between 2003 and 2009, the "generally sick" body in the medical ward was transformed into a target for a new series of strict protocols and guidelines surrounding HIV and TB.

These new forms of biolegitimacy generate new exclusions in their wake (Fassin 2009). As people become incorporated into the architecture of welfare that grows up around disease-based crises, so gaps in the gaze (Gibson 2004) open up around the bodies that fall outside these medical clearings. The substitution of disease control programs or clinical trials for state-provided health care raises questions about what kinds of health pathways remain possible for those who fail to conform to the correct biological aesthetic or state and nonstate expectations of citizenship behavior. Joao Biehl (2005b), for example, describes how persons who are unable to fulfill expectations of the self-actualizing pharmaceutical consumer within the Brazilian pharmaceutical economy are consigned to zones of abandonment outside the public health system. He describes how the restructuring of state, civil society, and pharmaceutical markets that enabled the highly successful rollout of ARVs in Brazil in the 1990s and an acceleration of human rights and citizenship claims, coincided "with a continuous local production of social death that remains by and large unaccounted for" (2005b, 3). These are the deaths of the poor, homeless, mentally ill, and destitute, who are treated at state hospitals for AIDS symptoms, but who remained unregistered in official government statistics. These exclusions, Biehl argues, are systematic. Homosexual men are less likely to be registered. The unemployed and uneducated poor are less likely to be registered. The fragmentation of the health system prevents communication and creates omissions. So does confusion over diagnostic criteria. Medical and bureaucratic systems for "life extension" simultaneously operate as "technologies of invisibility" that allow a hidden population to die in abandonment.

Rather than focus on new disease programs or systems of health financing, this book has concentrated on the spaces of the public hospital, which continue to exist at their interstices. Here processes of exclusion are far more murky. Madang Hospital is not a "zone of abandonment" for those excluded from a health care system that, as in Brazil, can otherwise boast huge success rates. Patients confined to the medical ward of this hospital have not been excluded from a state-based public health service but have gained access to the buildings, technologies, and experts that lie at its heart. This is not a select population of homeless, drug abusers, the mentally ill, and vagrants who the state chooses not to see. The bodies that inhabit Madang Hospital are not exceptional. They are not constituted as "killable" by the law (following Agamben) or as disposable bodies that can be "allowed to die" (following Foucault). The patients who inhabit the public wards of Madang Hospital are the so-called "poor majority" that successive National Health Plans and international health policies have consistently identified as the prime target for public health policy and legitimate recipients of state services.

And yet patients experience the public ward as a place of invisibility—they are unseen by medical experts, by the state, and by kin. They are not only rendered invisible as a population by epidemiological "technologies of invisibility" that fail to properly register disease incidence and deaths (Biehl 2005a). The sense of social failure that is generated through patients' social interactions in the institution structures invisibility into their very experience of illness. Moreover, it is not only patients who experience the hospital as a space of invisibility. Doctors and nurses working in the public wards similarly fear they are not seen by those from whom they seek professional recognition or citizenship rights. If people in the hospital feel themselves to lie at the unseen margins of the state, it is unclear where the center might be.

Logics of inclusion and exclusion have been written into colonial and postcolonial public health policy in Papua New Guinea, but "inclusion" has not necessarily entailed either state visibility or access to vital services. In early prewar colonial health policy, as chapter 2 discussed, a focus on hospitals, racial segregation, and the prioritization of the white or colored laborer population specifically excluded the rural indigenous population from the gaze of the medical state. But even then colonial hospitals were renowned for their inability to diagnose and treat Europeans, while colored laborers tended to be nursed ineffectively as an opaque mass of dark bodies, rather than examined as individual repositories of biological truth. Biomedical technologies produced generic "generally sick" bodies rather than specific objects of knowledge and intervention.

Meanwhile, new partnerships and structures of health financing in Papua New Guinea have led to the emergence of isolated spaces in the hospital, such as those of medical research or tuberculosis patient monitoring, where the resources to make individual biologies visible are available. But the majority of patients still wait in the public wards with uncertain diagnoses and hospital doctors still feel condemned to work in underresourced medical spaces where they are unable to perform as global professionals. Donations for buildings, vehicles, or medical technologies pour in from international donors. But these only amplify nurses' sense of their exclusion from international networks of development and capital. The respatialization of the hospital through international "partnerships" has only generated new spaces of exclusion and landscapes of inequality within the institution. In the public places of the state hospital the absence of the state and other statelike actors continues to be felt. Not only have biopolitical technologies of inscription, legibility, and visibility failed to operate as intended. Through the course of successive colonial and postcolonial public health policies the hospital has been systematically reproduced as a place where bodies are made unknown and where Papua New Guinean publics are rendered unseen.

LIVES AT STAKE

Social studies of biomedical technologies and the anthropology of Melanesia have tended to concentrate on the technologies and implicit aesthetic conventions by which persons and bodies are made knowable and visible (whether through molecular models of biological life or gendered notions of relational personhood). The ontological uncertainty that pervades Madang Hospital, by contrast, challenges us to focus on everyday struggles to mobilize techniques of visibility and, crucially, what is at stake in the capacity to conform to those conventions. The question is not only how "life" is defined but rather, to paraphrase Didier Fassin (2009), how "lives" are lived. The possibility of failure that hangs over the inhabitants of Madang Hospital, and which has profound implications for the physical transformation of patients' bodies, demands attention to the enactments of personhood and agency that are possible when biomedical technologies and institutions travel to places of infrastructural instability.

In Madang Hospital doctors sense their marginality to global science and its publishing networks. Here nurses become aware of their own irrelevance to managers, politicians, bureaucrats, and to international donor agencies. Meanwhile patients come to see themselves as peripheral in relation to a world of white people's knowledge and expertise. One could say that such forms of invisibility are experienced as a failure to be particular kinds of persons with particular kinds of social capacities. It is only by being seen and recognized by others, elsewhere, for example, that patients know they have become legitimate patients, that nurses are able to know themselves as central participants in the postcolonial nation-building process, or that doctors are able to know themselves as global professionals.

One effect of these experiences is that people internalize a responsibility to make themselves seen. Perceptions of the state's failure to fulfill its responsibilities toward its citizens in Madang Hospital has not given rise to a sense of self-reliance, resilience, and personal responsibility for care among staff and patients. Instead, patients, nurses, and doctors iterate a desire to be seen, monitored, and rendered legible to statelike others. In this regard, technologies of subjectification take a very different course from that suggested in recent social science literature on governmentality and the neoliberal self. Nurses attempt to elicit recognition from politicians by conforming to bureaucratic and legal conventions. Patients attempt to elicit an expert clinical gaze through their engagements with medical technologies. Doctors desire the recognition of international medical scientists who they feel perceive them as second-rate medics. The failure to be recognized in these ways is experienced as a personal failing and might be described as a form of internalized responsibility. But this is not so much as responsibility *for* the already individualized self as it is a sense that individual capacities and their very social existence as a person are at stake in their ability to mobilize relationships with others. To be seen and recognized by others is for those others to be drawn into an ongoing relationship, and for personal efficacy in mobilizing those relationships to be made apparent.

The anxiety that attends people's attempts to make themselves visible, recognizable, and knowable in Madang Hospital indicates that there is much at stake in the aesthetics of personhood. For patients invisibility entails the potential for physical and social death. At the same time the hospital technologies offer opportunities for patients to make themselves visible within new kinds of relationships and knowable as new "kinds" of person. For doctors and nurses, the hospital provides opportunities for transformation into modern, expert professionals. But the possibility that they may not be regarded as such by bureaucrats, politicians, donors, or foreign scientists generates anxiety that, as part of an undifferentiated Papua New Guinean population, they will continue to exist at the margins of global science, medical and international development agendas.

What happens to biomedical technologies and what effects do they have in the shadow of a fragile state? Clearly, in contexts like this, technologies of visibility do not entail a straightforward process of subjectification. One of the central arguments of this book has been that we need to pay closer attention to the ways in which bureaucratic and medical regimes of visibility are experienced as a source of personal agency and empowerment for people living in contexts of economic marginality, health inequality, and weak state infrastructure. The capacity to make oneself visible in the appropriate medical or bureaucratic form has crucial implications for the realization of professional identities and for physical and social survival.

■ Stories of life in the "big hospital" circulate around the small hamlets and villages that are dotted across Papua New Guinea's largely rural landscape. On a wet green-shadowed afternoon in early December 2010, a group of women sat around the floor of a bamboo lean-to kitchen, cooking dry taro on the fire in the center. They live in a hamlet called Wokaisor in the Begasin Hills, fifty miles southwest of Madang Town. There are no roads here and a journey to the town entails a five-hour walk over the hills to the highway before spending several long hours waiting in the sun for a bus to pick them up and drive them a further two hours into town. One of the women, Wali, comes from Amele, a village on the highway near to the town. Wali is often the source of stories about town life, urban employment, and interactions with government institutions. Today she is telling the other women the story of her uncle who, when she was only a girl, chopped off his legs with a chainsaw.

Wali explains how they wrapped him up and put him on a bus. She was sent with him to act as his guardian at the big hospital. "What was it like?" The other women asked. "Did they take a picture [X-ray]?" "Did they sew the legs back on?" "When I first arrived, I was terrified," Wali replied. "There are security guards everywhere. They stop you going outside. You have to ask to go to the toilet. You can't smoke or chew betel nut or they will fine you money. You can't speak when the doctor is there. All the nurses stand there, watching what you are doing. The security stand there, watching what you are doing." Some of the other women nodded, they had heard similar stories from others. They stayed there for weeks, Wali said. She had to look after her uncle, collect his food and water at the right times, watch while the doctors checked his legs. They had a time for everything. A time for the doctors to come to the ward and a time for getting medicine. They took pictures. Then they attached false legs. With the new legs he could learn to walk again and they left the hospital.

From the perspective of the village, the hospital is imagined as a place of rules, law, and government, on the one hand, and white people's knowledge on the other. Wali's story prompted the other women to tell their own stories: of a man who was carried to the hospital on a stretcher but died when he got there, of the operating theater where they send you to sleep and then cut you open, of seeing the hospital from the windows of the bus when visiting town but being too scared to go inside. Such stories, and the opposition they set up between hospital and village, depict the former as a place of exception in a rural landscape from which the state and modern services are otherwise absent. "We have no government here," people in Wokaisor regularly complain. The "big hospital," meanwhile, is imagined precisely as that "place of government."

The public hospital is indeed a crucial space of encounter with the state in Papua New Guinea. But this does not necessarily make it a place of efficient modern governance and surveillance where the state imposes rules but also serves up "development" in the form of white people's technologies, knowledge, and expertise. For the women in Wokaisor, a "place of government" is envisaged as a place where the state, in the form of politicians and public servants, recognizes and serves its publics, where Papua New Guineans might successfully tap the medical and development knowledge of white people, which is otherwise seen to be monopolized by an educated elite. But this vision generated within the village, of a landscape of neglect punctuated by enclaves of government, looks very different from within the government hospital itself.

What, this book has asked, are the places and infrastructures through which biomedicine is done? In Papua New Guinea, the public hospital has emerged as a place of invisibility and failure but also of improvisation and hope. It is an institution in which people continue to anticipate the arrival of "development," but where an everyday sense of marginalization and neglect prevails. It is, in this regard, an archetypal modern institution.

CHAPTER 1. MAKING A PLACE FOR BIOMEDICINE

1. The official name for the institution is "Modilon Hospital." However, people in Madang Province commonly refer to the hospital as "Madang Hospital." I follow this common usage here in order to convey the association of the hospital with the province that it serves.

2. See NSO, "National Census." This is widely considered to be a vast underestimate of Madang's population. The projected population of Madang Province for 2010 was 476,561.

3. World Bank Urbanization Data 2011: http://data.worldbank.org/indicator/SP .URB.TOTL.IN.ZS. Retrieved August 2013. It should be noted that these figures do not reflect the transience of the urban population and the frequent movement of young men to and from town.

4. These concerns have been repeatedly reflected in the five-year National Health plans developed since independence.

5. See Street and Coleman ("Real and Imaginary Spaces") for an elaboration of this argument and its implications for the theorization of space and society and the growing field of hospital ethnography.

6. In his definition of "heterotopic spaces" as spaces where different kinds of social ordering, which can be either transgressive or hegemonic, are tried out, Hetherington uses the notion of "orderings" rather than orders to draw attention to the incompleteness and contingency of any sociospatial arrangement (Hetherington, *The Badlands of Modernity*, 9). See also Law, *Organizing Modernity*.

7. The meaning of "form" here is taken from both Marilyn Strathern's account (*The Gender of the Gift*) of reification as the limited aesthetic that persons or things have to take in order to be recognized, and from Bruno Latour's definition as "simply

something which allows something else to be transported from one site to another" (Latour, *Reassembling the Social*, 223).

8. See Berg and Mol, *Differences in Medicine*. Foucault is not alone in locating the birth of modern medicine in the Paris hospitals for the late eighteenth century. For a perhaps more historically accurate account of this period, see Ackerknecht, *Medicine at the Paris Hospital*. However, it was Foucault's peculiar attention to the spatiality of modern medicine and the way this related to the emergence of the human subject as an object of knowledge and governance that has made him such a significant figure in medical anthropology and deserving of attention here.

9. See also Byron Good (*Medicine, Rationality, and Experience*) on biomedical practices of writing and speaking and their role in the production of bodily objects.

10. See Jones and Porter "Introduction"; and Harrison "Introduction."

11. "This lapse in Foucault's medical geography is ironic considering he set out in *The Birth of the Clinic* to write an account of the spatiality of medicine at the level of the nation-state, the institution, and the body.

12. See Mol (*The Body Multiple*; *Logics of Care*). Mol pays particular attention to the ways in which ontological differences in disease might be distributed across institutional space. Atherosclerosis enacted in the pathology laboratory as the thickening of the vessel wall can coexist with very different material ontologies enacted in the consultation room, where it is enacted as pain when walking. Each version enables patients, relatives, and biomedical practitioners to take located pragmatic action rather than producing universal scientific truths. Mol, *The Body Multiple*.

13. Livingston, *Improvising Medicine*, chapter 3.

14. There is a substantial literature on technology transfer in development studies, much of it on agricultural technologies and techniques. The approach I take here follows the smaller number of contributions to this field from science and technology studies, including most notably the work of Madeleine Akrich ("The De-scription of Technical Objects"), De Laet (*Research in Science and Technology Studies*), and De Laet and Mol ("The Zimbabwe Bush Pump").

15. The capacity of sociomaterial networks, such as those making up scientific facts or technological artefacts, to hold stable as they move has been central to sociologists' understandings of relationships between science, technology, and power (Latour, *Science in Action*; Law, "On the Methods of Long Distance Control"). However, Mol argues that what is interesting about biomedicine is precisely the *mutability* of its technologies, bodies, and facts, which afford different kinds of efficacy (Mol, *The Body Multiple*). In underresourced and hot African laboratories the network of technicians and machines that enables the diagnosis of anemia as a numerical value of haemoglobin in the blood in the Netherlands might cease to hold together. But technicians can instead use clinical observation of the patients' eyelids to identify the presence of anemia; a practice that is possible in Africa precisely because anemia is often severe enough to have clear clinical symptoms (Mol and Law, "Regions, Networks and Fluids"). Neither the sociotechnical assemblages of biomedicine nor the materiality of anemia remain the same in these two settings, and yet they both continue to be successfully assembled or enacted. Biomedicine

(or the hospital) is able to travel so effectively, they suggest, precisely because it has a distinctly fluid topology.

16. The sign of otherness accorded postcolonial biomedicine has been discussed by a number of anthropologists and historians dealing with issues of biomedicine, science, nationalism, and indigenous politics. See especially Prakash (*Another Reason*), Adams (*Doctors for Democracy*), and more recently Crane ("Adverse Events and Placebo Effects") and Anderson and Pols ("Scientific Patriotism").

17. Hospital ethnography is a growing field and a full review of the literature cannot be done justice to here. Most significant edited volumes and collections in recent years include those by van der Geest and Finkler ("Hospital Ethnography"), Long et al. ("When the Field Is a Ward or a Clinic"), and Finkler et al. ("What Is Going On"). Hospital ethnography is an increasingly varied field, and the authors cited here do not necessarily conceptualize the hospital in the way I have done here. In a backlash against earlier sociological accounts of the hospital as an island (Coser, *Life in the Ward*) there is today a tendency to consider the hospital as a reflection of the society in which it is located (van der Geest and Finkler, "Hospital Ethnography"; Zaman, *Broken Limbs, Broken Lives*) and to neglect the standardized systems of biomedical discipline and control that make the hospital such a unique site of power and contestation.

18. For literature on conceptions of the body as an index of social relations in the Papua New Guinea Highlands, see Biersack ("Ginger Gardens for the Ginger Woman"), Strathern ("The Self in Self-Decoration"), and Clark ("The Incredible Shrinking Men"). For Madang, see Leach on kinship practices and initiation ("Drum and Voice"; *Creative Land*); and Keck (*Social Discord and Bodily Disorders*) on concepts of sickness and the body.

19. This is to some extent explored in studies of indigenous knowledge, especially in the work of David Turnbull and Helen Watson-Verran (Turnbull, "Local Knowledge and Comparative Scientific Traditions"; Turnbull and Watson-Verran, "Science and Other Indigenous Systems"), and James Fairhead and Melissa Leach ("Fashioned Forest Pasts"), who argue that we should study all knowledges as local knowledges and not privilege one kind of knowledge epistemologically. However, these studies usually compare different kinds of knowledge practices rather than explore how they become involved with one another in their everyday reformation.

20. Anderson points out in relation to actor network theory: "Often a sort of semiotic formalism seems to supervene on the analysis of . . . local sites: the 'local' can seem quite abstract, depleted of historical and social specificity. The structural features of the network become clear, but often it is hard to discern the relations and the politics engendered through it. A postcolonial study of science and technology might offer new, and more richly textured, answers to many of the questions posed in actor-network theory" ("Postcolonial Technoscience," 649).

21. Indeed Harrison argues that "some of the features of what Michel Foucault dubbed clinic-anatomical medicine were flourishing in the European colonies some years before they appeared in revolutionary Paris" (Harrison 2009, 6). This postcolonial critique has also been made in relation to metropolitan-centric histories of tropical medicine more generally (e.g., Anderson, "Disease, Race and Empire"; Arnold,

Colonizing the Body; Cussins, "Producing Reproduction"; Palladino and Worboys, "Science and Imperialism"). Dipesh Chakrabarty (*Provincializing Europe*) calls on historians to "Provincialise Europe" and to review its central positioning in the making of modernities more widely. In relation to hospitals, see Anderson's account ("Modern Sentinel and Colonial Microcosm") of the emergence of the modern hospital in the Philippines.

22. With the growing interest in hospital ethnography, the African hospital has become the subject of several recent ethnographic studies. See, for example, Sullivan ("Enacting Spaces of Inequality") on the relations of global governance in a hospital in Tanzania, Brown (*Living with HIV/AIDS*) on practices of care in a hospital in Kenya, and Hull ("Paperwork and the Contradictions of Accountability in a South African Hospital") on audit cultures in a Tanzanian hospital.

23. For perceptions of the state in Papua New Guinea, see Clark ("Imagining the State"), Douglas ("Weak States and Other Nationalisms"), and Foster ("Introduction"). Robbins (*Becoming Sinners*) describes how people from Papua New Guinea's more remote areas describe themselves as living in its "last place."

24. On desire for the state, see Aretxaga, "Maddening States."

25. Foucault, *The Birth of the Clinic*; Good, *Medicine, Rationality, and Experience*.

26. Foucault (*Power/Knowledge*: 166–182). In this sense the hospital is a place that makes it possible for governing actors to "see like a state" (Scott, *Seeing Like a State*). See also Joao Biehl ("Technologies of Invisibility") on statistical practices and visibility in hospitals.

27. Prior, "The Architecture of the Hospital"; Casey, "The Place of Space in the Birth of the Clinic."

28. For relationships between visibility, technology, and the formation of expert subjects, see Crary, *Techniques of the Observer*; Barry, "Reporting and Visualising"; Casey, "The Place of Space in the Birth of the Clinic."

29. Foucault's writings on hospitals span his work on incarceration and governance in *Discipline and Punish*; his writings about the relationship between postrevolutionary notions of liberty, the emergence of new forms of urban policing, and the development of the human sciences in *The Birth of the Clinic*; and essays on public health as a field of nineteenth-century government in *Power/Knowledge*. Foucault's analysis of hospitals as spaces of discipline and surveillance (Foucault, *Discipline and Punish*, 190; "Of Other Spaces"; *The Birth of the Clinic*; "The Incorporation of the Hospital into Modern Technology") have been widely taken up by social scientists interested in processes of subjectification and relationships between space and power (e.g., Elden, "Plague, Panopticon, Police"; Rhodes, *Emptying Beds*; Philo, "The Birth of the Clinic"; Prior, "The Architecture of the Hospital"; Gibson, "The Gaps in the Gaze in South African Hospitals"). Like earlier functionalist accounts of hospital space, however, Foucault's view of the hospital as a space of scientific order, cleanliness, and rationality existing in opposition to and separation from the messy reality of everyday social space can be said to overemphasize the efficacy of regimes of spatial control (Gibson, "The Gaps in the Gaze in South African Hospitals"; Elden, "Plague,

Panopticon, Police") and overlook the contested and multiple nature of hospital space (see Street and Coleman, "Real and Imaginary Spaces").

30. Rapp also draws on the ethnographic detail of her study to qualify Rabinow's notion of "biosociality." Some women, she points out, reject the support groups that develop around amniocentesis and perceive other class-based identities as more significant (Rapp, *Testing Women, Testing the Fetus*).

31. Strathern writes: "For a body or mind to be in a position of eliciting an effect from another, to evince a power or capability, it must manifest itself in a particular concrete way, which then becomes the elicitory trigger. This can only be done through the appropriate aesthetic" (Strathern, *The Gender of the Gift*, 1988, 180–181). In *The Gender of the Gift* Strathern argued that personification and reification are both modes of objectification; they are both ways of making persons and things known to ourselves: "The commodity logic of Westerners leads them to search for knowledge about things (and persons as things); the gift logic of Melanesians to make known to themselves persons (and things as persons)" (Strathern, The *Gender of the Gift*, 177).

32. In processes of personification an implicit limited "aesthetic" determines the forms in which a person must appear in order to be recognized by others. "Establishing attributes, the nature of things, is not the explicit focus of these symbolic operations, but it is present as an implicit technique of operation. . . . There is a very small number of (conventional) forms that will do as evidence that relations have been thus activated" (Strathern, *The Gender of the Gift*, 180).

33. In the decade between the publications of *The Gender of the Gift* and *Property, Substance, and Effect*, Strathern's analysis shifts significantly. In *Property, Substance, and Effect*, Strathern reflects on the ways in which her earlier work established comparative symmetry between Melanesia and Euro-America through the rendering of both personification and reification as modes of knowledge. This, she reflected, presumes that Melanesians are motivated by a desire for knowledge. But this analysis is itself driven by the Euro-American conflation of visibility and knowledge: "I re-read the passages in *The Gender of the Gift* [M. Strathern 1988, 180–182] which deal directly with reification, and am struck by a question that troubled me at the time but that I did not allow to appear as a question: what was the underlying motive for making relations visible? I had no account (description) of the apparent need I imputed to these Melanesians to make relations visible. It did not have to be asked because the desire to know seemed self-sufficient, the counterpart to the anthropologists' analysis, as the end of the book suggests (1988, 309). It was a blind spot. For it seemed a kind of self-evident fact of social and cultural life that people make themselves explicit to themselves in various ways for which visibility itself is a powerful metaphor. . . . What I now think is mistaken is the axiomatic assumption that visibility is somehow for the sake of knowledge, and that knowledge addresses, and thus gathers information about, the larger world in which one lives" (Strathern 1999, 257–258). In this later work she suggests that relations are made visible in Melanesian exchange not *for* knowledge (of the world, or of relationship/persons) but for effect (1999, 255).

34. This anxiety may well be generic to the biomedical encounter. Cussins, for example, describes the ways in which IVF patients actively seek to "objectify" themselves so as to appear as good candidates for the procedure. In such circumstances, Cussins argues "it is quite reasonable to expect the patient to take an active interest in her own presentation as an object of study" (Cussins, "Producing Reproduction," 178).

35. Most notable for this comparative genre are the works by Strathern (*The Gender of the Gift*; *Reproducing the Future*; *Property, Substance and Effect*; *Kinship, Law, and the Unexpected*) and Wagner (*The Invention of Culture*). For a contemporary rendering of this debate, see Bamford, *Biology Unmoored*.

36. See especially Gewertz and Errington, *Emerging Class in Papua New Guinea*; Foster, *Social Reproduction and History in Melanesia*; Josephides, "Metaphors, Metathemes, and the Construction of Sociality"; Knauft, *Exchanging the Past*; Li Puma, *Encompassing Others*.

37. "New Melanesian Ethnography" is a phrase coined by Lisette Josephides in 1991, "Metaphors, Metathemes, and the Construction of Sociality." Strathern borrows the notion of the "dividual" from Mariott's account of South Asian notions of personhood and their contrast with Western individualism. Reviewing the notion of "dividuality" in Melanesian and South Asian anthropology Busby ("Permeable and Partible Persons") describes the difference as substance as flow from a person compared with substance objectified as part of a person (in Melanesia); and a person who is internally whole and permeable in South Asia as opposed to a person who is internally divided and partible (in Melanesia).

38. Strathern makes this point herself in a little-cited interview (Simoni et al., "Pigs and mobile phones").

39. Latour similarly points out that we should not presume that microbes *always* existed before Pasteur developed techniques for making them visible, or that they currently exist *everywhere*. Instead he calls for the historical study of "partially existing objects" (Latour, "On the Partial Existence of Existing and Nonexisting Objects").

CHAPTER 2. LOCATING DISEASE

1. German New Guinea Annual Report (GNGAR) 1886–87, 4.

2. Irregularities in the purchase of land from Papua New Guineans, often with only a few stone axes for payment, caused numerous problems for subsequent colonial governments, and led to a foiled uprising against the colonial administration in 1904.

3. GNGAR 1890–91, 66.

4. GNGAR 1889–90, 53.

5. There is an extensive literature charting the emergence of tropical medicine and the notions of place and race that it reinforced and produced. There is no space to provide a comprehensive overview of this field here; however, key texts include Anderson (*Colonial Pathologies*), Arnold (*Colonizing the Body*; *Warm Climates and Western Medicine*), Curtin (*Disease and Empire*), Livingstone ("Race, Space, and Moral Climatology"), and Stepan (*Picturing Tropical Nature*). Tropical medicine in Papua

New Guinea features far less frequently in this literature than histories of medicine in India, Brazil, and African countries.

6. See especially Curtin (*Disease and Empire*) on Africa. In the south of the island, which was partitioned by Britain in 1886, debates raged over the possibilities for establishing a white settler society, akin to that of neighboring Australia. Eves ("Unsettling Settler Colonialism") describes the debates that took place in the British press at this time.

7. GNGAR 1886–87, 18.

8. GNGAR 1886–87, 18.

9. GNGAR 1891–92, 73.

10. GNGAR 1891–92, 77.

11. GNGAR 1911–12.

12. The role of the missions in the provision of medical services in Papua New Guinea is central to the history of biomedicine in the country and has been documented well elsewhere (Barker, "Christian Bodies"; Eves, "In God's Hands"; Li Puma, *Encompassing Others*). In accord with the focus of this book, I here emphasize the less-frequently analyzed role of government hospitals in state building in the country.

13. GNGAR 1898–99, 157.

14. Worboys has described how the limited influence of Ross's public health approach by comparison with Patrick Manson's treatment of tropical medicine as a science greatly affected the development of nineteenth-century imperial medicine (Worboys, "Germs, Malaria and the Invention of Mansonian Tropical Medicine").

15. Historians of medicine have pointed out that the discipline of tropical medicine did not simply emerge in the metropolis and spread to the colony through imperial encounter. Western medicine was not simply a "tool of empire" (MacLeod and Lewis, *Disease, Medicine and Empire*, x). Rather, the research that emerged out of "peripheral" sites such as India and Papua New Guinea was crucial in the shaping of institutional and conceptual parameters for European medical science (Palladino and Worboys, "Science and Imperialism"; Baber, "Colonizing Nature"; Arnold, *Colonizing the Body*; Haynes, *Imperial Medicine*). The experiences of scientists in the colonial south were also instructive in the formulation of notions of whiteness, national identity, and imperial purpose.

16. This chapter deals with the northern half of the island, first colonized by the German Nui Guinea Compagnie. However, hospitals were also central to the prewar policy of British and later Australian administrations in the south of the island, and I provide a brief summary here for those interested. The New Guinea territory remained better funded than its Papuan counterpart because of the established plantation industry and, later, the highlands resources boom. In Papua, annexed by the British in 1885 as a response to the German acquisition of the north side of the island, and taken over by an Australian in 1906, no hospitals at all were built in the first years of colonial administration. The British regime's medical officers, who usually held several administrative positions, attended to the European population in their homes and made occasional patrols into the rural areas surrounding the administrative centers. It was only when an epidemic of dysentery broke out in

1898 following the discovery of gold and an influx of Australian miners on Woodlark Island that the British administration was forced to consider building hospitals for the European and native laborer populations. The British administration passed the Public Hospital Ordinance in 1898, which gave the administrator power to establish hospitals in the territory and to recruit all paid hospital workers. However, a lack of government funding meant that the first "government" hospitals were built by private subscription, and the European Hospital built in Port Moresby in 1898, which consisted of the local gaol premises and two temporary tents, was forced to close a year later due to lack of funds (British New Guinea Annual Report [BNGAR] 1898–99). During the next decade the administration and miners who paid subscriptions jointly funded the construction of European hospitals in the main administrative and mining centers. Gradually, the colonial administration's contributions to building costs and hospital supplies increased under the Australian administration, but the notion that hospitals should be built by the state with taxpayers' money was slow to materialize.

17. Vicky Luker has suggested that the vilification of colonial public health in PNG has been overstated and that some good, at least, was done and has been ignored. See Luker, "Papua New Guinea."

18. Historians of colonial medicine have emphasized its implication in the establishment of the colonial state. MacLeod argued that medicine became "an agency of western expansionism" and that medical regimes were "participants in the expansion and consolidation of political rule" (MacLeod and Lewis, *Disease, Medicine and Empire*, 1–2). Arnold argued that

> medicine was one of the ways in which imperialism sought to "know" the people and establish its authority over them—through the vast quantities of information about diseases and health that began to be amassed in statistical and scientific form and through the development of medical agencies, themselves often branches of the state structures itself, that began to reach out into the countryside as well as the towns. . . . Medical intervention impinged directly upon the lives of the people, assuming an unprecedented right (in the name of medical science) over the health and over the bodies of its subjects (Arnold, "Introduction," 18).

But this was only true where colonial powers touched local lives. Largely in hospitals rather than villages.

CHAPTER 3. PUBLIC BUILDINGS, BUILDING PUBLICS

1. The role of Papua New Guineans in the war effort became captured in the Australian imagination by the "fuzzy wuzzy angels" who assisted Australian troops as they fought the Japanese along the Kokoda trail. Historians have begun to unpick this harmonious picture of relationships between the Australian administration and its Papua New Guinean helpers (Connell, "Health in Papua New Guinea"; Robinson, *Villagers at War*; Nelson, "Taim Bilong Pait"). Papua New Guineans who were found

to have cooperated with the Japanese were accused of treason and some were hung or executed. There were also repercussions for villages that supported the Japanese in terms of reduced assistance from the state in the postwar period and fewer reparations for war damage to homes and land. Yet villagers often had little choice over who they could cooperate with. They worked as carriers, laborers, couriers, and scouts for those troops who arrived in their area. They were forced to use their gardens to grow food for the soldiers, which combined with the recruitment of young able men, contributed to food shortages. Participation in the war effort was construed by the administration as a form of self-improvement—through participation in the military campaign Papua New Guineans would learn about sanitation, hygiene, and self-discipline. But treatment by Australian soldiers and labor conditions were often harsh.

For Papua New Guineans who saw black American soldiers fighting alongside whites, participation in the war had a major impact on ideas of inequality and expectations of postwar life. As Peter Lawrence has described in his monograph about the Yali cargo movement in Madang Province, the Australian administration exploited people's interest in the technologies and material goods (vehicles, planes, weaponry, knapsacks, cameras, and water bottles) that the war made visible to Papua New Guineans by making promises of "development" in return for their support during the war (Lawrence, *Road Belong Cargo*).

2. See, for example (Bonneuil, "Experiment") and (Prakash, *Another Reason*).

3. "Report on Proposed Expansion of Department of Public Health," NAA: Department of Postwar Reconstruction; correspondence files, 1943–1950.

4. "Report to the Inter-departmental Committee on Health Services in Papua New Guinea," NAA: A4940 C522.

5. "Report to the Inter-departmental Committee on Health Services in Papua New Guinea," NAA: A4940 C522.

6. Warick Anderson makes a similar point in relation to colonial hospitals in the Philippines. He writes: "Charles E. Rosenberg has described the dominant 'inward vision' of North American hospitals during this period, contrasting this introspection with their mere 'outward glance' toward surrounding communities and environment. No doubt this remains an apt assessment of the interests of the medical and nursing staffs of major Philippines hospitals, but for the colonial health service, these institutions also became appealing symbols of progress and benevolence, lighthouses throwing into sharp relief otherwise obscure features of their settings. They made all sorts of novel views and interventions possible" (Anderson, "Modern Sentinel and Colonial Microcosm," 2).

7. "European and Native Hospital–Madang–Papua New Guinea," NAA: A452 1960/1897.

8. "European and Native Hospital–Madang–Papua New Guinea," NAA: A452 1960/1897.

9. "European and Native Hospital–Madang–Papua New Guinea," NAA: A452 1960/1897.

10. "European and Native Hospital–Madang–Papua New Guinea," NAA: A452 1960/1897.

11. "European and Native Hospital–Madang–Papua New Guinea," NAA: A452 1960/1897.

Menzies was the liberal prime minister at the time.

12. This ambivalence in Australian public culture about Papua New Guineans has continued today. It is now expressed most clearly in the contrast between depictions of the Papua New Guinean "fuzzy wuzzy angels" who aided the Australian soldiers on their horrific but ultimately successful trek across Kokoda in 1942 and widespread fears about the savage, untamed violence of the "uncivilised" Papua New Guinea. See Foster, *Materializing the Nation*, 131–150.

13. The Chinese population in New Guinea grew first through the German New Guinea Company indentured labor scheme and later as free immigration was encouraged to increase the supply of plantation labor and then to promote international trade and enterprise. Early on, many of the Chinese immigrants set up companies and trade stores in town, using their links with China to source imports. By 1913 the Chinese population was 1,427 (Wu, "Chinese in Papua New Guinea," 710). By 1946, the Chinese population stood at around 2,000 (Jones, "*Chinese-Australian Journeys*," 233).

14. "European and Native Hospital–Madang–Papua New Guinea," NAA: A452 1960/1897.

15. The correspondence files for the Port Moresby, Lae, and Madang base hospitals are full of telegrams and letters from the Port Moresby administration requesting previously approved funds. NAA: A452 1960/1897; NAA: A452 1960/1079 ; NAA: A452 1962/8043; NAA: A518 C241/3/5.

16. "European and Native Hospital–Madang–Papua New Guinea," NAA: A452 1962/80843. A further letter from Dr. Gunther, the director of public health in PNG, pointed out that the local people had given Knowles the nickname "muruk" (cassowary) a large bird known for its clumsiness and stupidity.

17. "Health services general–Papua New Guinea," NAA: Department of Territories 1899–1983; Correspondence files; Health services general–Papua and New Guinea 1951–1954.

18. "Territory of Papua New Guinea–Health Services-Hospital Building Programme–Decision 450," NAA: A4905 278; "Development of External Territories Committee–Papua New Guinea–Hospital Construction Programme," NAA: A4933 DET/1; "Report to the Inter-departmental Committee on Health Services in Papua New Guinea," NAA: A4940 C522.

19. The model of the integrated hospital was also useful in requisitioning funds from an ever-reluctant Canberra. When the secretary of territories suggested that Madang Hospital should be built in two stages, the European Hospital first, Cleland, administrator in Port Moresby refused, stating that "the engineering and mechanical services of both hospitals are so integrated into each design that any cleavage would render both useless." "European and Native Hospital–Madang–Papua and New Guinea," NAA: A452 1960/1897.

20. "Report to the Inter-departmental Committee on Health Services in Papua New Guinea," NAA: A4940 C522.

21. "Lae Native Hospital–Papua New Guinea," NAA: A452 1960/1079.

22. "Lae Has a Modern Hospital Which Is Not Being Run on Modern Lines," *New Guinea Times Courier*, September 9, 1959.

23. "Not Enough Food in Lae Hospital," *South Pacific Post*, November 3, 1961.

24. "Visit of Fellow of Royal College of Surgeons to Papua and New Guinea for Assessment of Port Moresby Hospital," NAA: A452 1959/2867.

25. "Modilon to Open Up to Public," *PNG Post Courier*, September 5, 2003.

26. The phrase comes from the influential and highly controversial comment piece by Susan Windybank and Michael Manning of the Australian Centre for Independent Studies (Windybank and Manning, "Papua New Guinea on the Brink").

27. This policy was strongly influenced by a report produced by the East Anglia Overseas Development Group in 1973 (Overseas Development Group, "A Report on Development Strategies for Papua New Guinea") and was encapsulated in the Eight-Point Plan commissioned by the new prime minister, Michael Somare.

28. National Department of Health, "National Health Plan 1979."

29. World Bank, *Structural Adjustment Loan Agreement Papua New Guinea*.

30. See Iliffe (*East African Doctors*) for a similar account of the transformations undergone by Tanzanian hospitals following structural adjustment programs in the country. Ironically, Tanzania provided the model for the earlier Papua New Guinean policy of self-reliance and localization written by the Overseas Development Group, University of East Anglia (*A Report on Development Strategies for Papua New Guinea*).

31. Curtin challenges the notion that PNG's public service was too big. "On a persons per bureaucrat basis, there were 100 Papua New Guineans per public servant in 1973, and 245 in 1998, far more than in Australia, New Zealand, or Singapore. This would suggest that the country is very lightly governed, as even casual acquaintance with Papua New Guinea's rural areas shows" (Curtin, "Public Sector Reform in Papua New Guinea and the 1999 Budget," 9).

32. The impact of decentralization on the Papua New Guinean health services has become a dominant narrative in consultant and donor accounts of health system failure in the country (see Thomason et al., "User Charges for Rural Health Services in Papua New Guinea"). This is today reflected in the introductory comments to the 2001–2011 National Health Plan (NDOH, "National Health Plan 2001–2010"). While the administrative separation of hospitals and rural health services was certainly important, such narratives effectively place the blame on nationalist politics and underplay the role of international funding and structural adjustment policies.

33. See World Bank, *Financing Health Services in Developing Countries*.

34. These proved to be poorly administered and to act as a deterrent for those from rural areas (Thomason et al., "User Charges for Rural Health Services in Papua New Guinea").

35. Following the perceived increase in government corruption and bureaucratic inefficiency, donors such as AusAID had shifted their funding model from support for the recurrent budget to project-based aid over which they had increased control and for which institutions like hospitals now had to compete.

1. In traditional medical systems, Nichter (*Anthropology and International Health*) has argued, for example, healers are concerned with "taskonomies" that will safeguard the well-being of the patient in the future. In biomedicine doctors attempt to search for causes and on that basis allocate the case a place in disease "taxonomy."

2. In 2003 the Accident and Emergency Department did not have a consultant doctor overseeing it. By 2009, however, a Papua New Guinean doctor had become fully qualified in emergency medicine and had taken over this department. This meant there were trainee doctors, studying under the consultant, to see the incoming patients as well as health extension officers.

3. As Livingston argues, in resource poor contexts "one must lead with unbracketing" (*Improvising Medicine*, 109).

4. Mol (*The Body Multiple*) describes how different "versions" of atherosclerosis are given different hierarchical values in the Dutch hospital where she carried out research.

5. I am not sure why the registrar claimed the laboratory was unable to do lumber punctures. It is possible he was referring to the unreliability of the lumber punctures, or that the laboratory had briefly claimed it could not run that test.

6. The growing resistance of the hemophilis influenza strand of meningitis led to a change in this protocol in 2009.

7. I was not able to find out why supplies of Chloramphenicol would reach the hospital and not other drugs. This raises questions about the ways in which medical suppliers in the country are determining what kinds of drugs are used, with potentially lethal consequences for patients.

8. The hospital operates on a replacement blood donation system. See Street, "Failed Recipients."

9. In the terminology of actor network theory, the doctor could not establish himself as a "centre of calculation" (Latour, *Science in Action*) that could use inscription technologies to delegate to other parts of the network, but had to be present at every point on the network to get things done.

10. The effects of relational exposure that proceed from people's failure to enroll others to their cause has been widely observed and discussed in STS (e.g., Callon, "Some Elements of a Sociology of Translation"; Law, "On the Methods of Long Distance Control"; Shapin, "The Invisible Technician," 558).

11. Ira Bashkow (*The Meaning of Whitemen*) has described the potency of the figure of the white man in Papua New Guinea as an absent observer and potential critic of the activities and lifestyle of Papua New Guineans.

12. Wendland similarly describes how medical students in Malawi envied visiting medical students from abroad for being able to practice the medicine learned in textbooks, but simultaneously made claims to practicing "real medicine" themselves, based on their ability to improvise and be flexible with minimal resources (Wendland, *A Heart for the Work*, chapter 6).

13. De Laet and Mol ("The Zimbabwe Bush Pump") describe a comparable case of a "modest engineer" in the design, manufacture, and distribution of bush water pumps in Africa. Biagioli ("Documents of Documents") has discussed the significance of giving up or distributing authorship in scientific publishing.

14. See Rhodes (*Emptying Beds*) on hospital work as a process of "emptying beds."

15. In anthropological and STS studies of Euro-American hospitals the medical record has often featured as an archetypal artefact of biomedical knowledge production (e.g., Good, *Medicine, Rationality, and Experience*; Berg and Bowker, "The Multiple Bodies of the Medical Record"; Rees, "Records and Hospital Routine"). As with the Australian medical student described here, the value placed on the medical record in these institutions appears to be related to its capacity to provide a conclusive account of a patient's condition, transforming them into a manageable case. For example, Robert Barrett has described the intricate processes of editing and omission by which complex and often contradictory interactions with patients and relatives in an Australian psychiatric institution are transformed into coherent psychiatric "cases" in the medical record (Barrett, "Clinical Writing and the Documentary Construction of Schizophrenia"). Both Barrett (in Australia) and Byron Good (in the United States) describe how trainee doctors are judged by their peers and supervisors on the basis of their ability to create a convincing and consistent argument in the medical record.

16. Julie Livingston describes similar challenges surrounding the diagnosis of cancer in Botswana. Here cancer remains "a fuzzy sort of cancer, one that is hard to bring into the kind of sharp focus that PCR, MRI, mammography, colonoscopy, and other such technologies enable" (Livingston, *Improvising Medicine*, 106).

17. This is not true for the surgeons, who do not have to play the same waiting game as internists precisely because they can open the body up to see what is inside.

18. There is a substantial literature related to the aid industry that surrounds HIV in Papua New Guinea and the Pacific region. Much of this relates to responses to HIV-related interventions in rural areas (e.g., Eves and Butt, *Making Sense of Aids*; Hammar, "Epilogue") and cultural conceptions of HIV and AIDS (e.g., Lepani, "Mobility, Violence, and the Gendering of HIV in Papua New Guinea"; Wilde, "Turning Sex into a Game"). Less attention has been given to the impact of these interventions on the public health infrastructure and institutional practices and relationships.

19. Harper ("Extreme Condition, Extreme Measures?") describes the problems of exclusion generated by this protocol in rural Nepal.

CHAPTER 5. THE WAITING PLACE

1. A broad-spectrum antibiotic. See more on chloramphenicol and why it is used so commonly in Papua New Guinea's hospitals in chapter 4.

2. The biomedical version of Michael's story can be followed in Street ("Artefacts of Not-Knowing").

3. The connections drawn here between physical mobility and social exchange resonate with ethnographic material from across the Melanesia region. See, for example, Hirsch ("Between Mission and Market"; "A Landscape of Powers in Highland Papua"), Leach (*Creative Land*), Munn (*The Fame of Gawa*), and Rumsey and Weiner (*Emplaced Myth*).

4. See Keck (*Social Discord and Bodily Disorders*) for an in-depth account of people's conceptions of the body and sickness in a Madang village.

5. See more on the leaving hospital at own risk form in chapter 6.

6. There are several villages on the outskirts of the town, and many of the households in these areas include people who are both engaged in subsistence farming and wage labor. These villages might be referred to by patients and health workers in the hospital as both *ples* (village) and *taun* (town) in different contexts.

7. Of course, money is highly visible in the rural context and exchanges hands regularly, including both traditional ceremonial events (Akin and Robbins, "An Introduction to Melanesian Currencies") and interactions with government, such as the payment of health clinic fees or school fees (Sykes, "Paying a School Fee Is a Father's Duty"). But the notion that "everything in the town costs money" and "everything in the village is free" has become a common trope through which people position themselves in relation to the urban economy and articulate their felt exclusion from it.

8. Garden food consists of the main staples grown in the Madang area, including taro, sweet potato, yams, plantains, and various leafy greens.

9. The symbolic and potent qualities of garden food have been well documented in Papua New Guinea; most famously by Malinowski (*Coral Gardens and Their Magic*). For an analysis of gardens as the basis for establishing relatedness in a Madang context see Leach, *Creative Land*.

10. In his famous account of sorcery and sickness in Dobu Reo, Fortune described how the Dobu separate good men from bad men not on ethical grounds but in terms of what the health of their bodies indicates about their social capacities and magical strength. A good man has achieved prestige in the form of women and yams without suffering at the hands of sorcerers acting out of revenge or envy. They are both successful and healthy. A bad man is one who has suffered revenge and therefore evidently disrupted social relations in the past (Fortune, *Sorcerers of Dobu*).

Bodily aesthetics and the presentation of the bodily surface have featured prominently in Melanesian ethnography. Literature on initiation rituals from across Papua New Guinea describes how returning initiates will smother their bodies with pig fat in order to look shiny, strong and fatter. Biersack describes how the beauty of Paiela boys' bodies displays the internal growth accomplished through transactions with a female spirit in the bush (Biersack, "Ginger Gardens for the Ginger Woman"). Clark gives an account of how for the Wiru the effects of colonialism, leading to the denigration of male ceremonial practices, are revealed in the shrinkage of Wiru male bodies (Clark, "The Incredible Shrinking Men"). Marilyn Strathern describes how, for Hageners, wealth, assets, and skills are said to lie on the skin, and bodily well-being is perceived as a sign of the regard of ancestral spirits and of strength and prestige.

While internal intentions and desires can only be known to that person, what lie on the skin, she argues, are ones public transactions and relationships with others (Strathern, "The Self in Self-Decoration"). Andrew Strathern further notes that the Melpa of Mount Hagen claimed to wear shame on their skin (Strathern, "Why Is Shame on the Skin?"). Although for the Melpa sickness usually results from internal anger, shame is an external response to others seeing them when they have done wrong or displayed their social inadequacy. In the hospital shame is similarly connected to the patient's visibility in the eyes of their relatives and other patients, but it is also connected to their sickness in the sense that their physical state displays their social inadequacies to others.

11. Adam Reed remarks that in Bonmana Prison prisoners talk positively of the fact the government provides food for free (pers. comm.). In the hospital patients see the poor provision of food as further evidence of the government's refusal to care for them. However, this devaluation of Western foodstuffs is not universal. *Taun kai kai* such as rice, tinned fish, or corned beef are often purchased for special occasions, including funerals or the birth of a child. It was also common knowledge that people living in the town for long periods of time often suffered from *sik bilong rais* (rice sick), whereby they felt weak and ill if they did not eat rice for some days. Town dwellers who returned to the village to visit family often complained of this sickness. But food in the hospital did not merit these positive associations.

12. On the "good" and "bad" death in Papua New Guinea see Counts and Counts, "The Good, the Bad, and the Unresolved Death in Kaliai."

13. Patients who did not receive an immediate diagnosis were often subject to repeated investigations. For example, white blood cell counts could tell doctors if an infection was improving or getting worse; repeating malaria tests was a safeguard against the possibility the laboratory had got the previous tests wrong. For anemic patients requiring several blood transfusions multiple blood tests were necessary, first to check the hemoglobin levels and second to enable cross-matching with the donated blood.

14. Patient accounts of hospital medicine as occupying a parallel universe to that of sorcery and kinship provides a stark contrast with other contexts of engagement with modern institutions where the latter have been explicitly likened to sorcerers (Kirsch, *Reverse Anthropology*; Anderson, "Modern Sentinel and Colonial Microcosm"). On the notion of parallel as opposed to involved moralities see Strathern, "Binary License."

15. For a more detailed account of blood donation and transfusion practices in the hospital, see Street, "Failed Recipients."

16. In this sense the names of Western medicine might be compared to the significance of names as sources of power across the region. In the Begasin area, where I conducted rural fieldwork, the names of spirits are breathed into taro and yam seeds in order to make them grow. These names are highly secret, their powers tightly controlled, and only certain initiated men have access to them, see Lawrence (*The Garia*) and Harrison (*Stealing People's Names*). Weiner writes "names are part of things they label, and the similarities between labels, the resemblances between

the sounds of words, are also part of these names; language is laid out in the world as a property of it and not as a result of an artificial imposition of semantic value onto such a world" (Weiner, "Technology and Techne," 36).

17. On the partible body in Melanesia and elsewhere, see Gell, *Art and Agency*; Strathern, *The Gender of the Gift*; Konrad, *Nameless Relations*.

18. Social scientists have tended to analyze imaging practices in terms of relationships between visibility and knowledge rather than social relationships and personhood. However, for a sociological account of the role of MRI scanning in the production of professional identities and boundary work, see Burri ("Doing Distinctions"). For an account of the social effects and meanings of ultrasound in Tanzania see Rockstroh (*Ultrasound Travels*).

19. By contrast, Heather Leslie writes of doctor-patient relationships in Tonga that patients "did not need a translator at the hospital. They did not fear that their doctor would ask for something culturally inappropriate. They were not surprised that their doctor spoke their language. Moreover, medical school scholarships were not considered quota-driven handouts. In short, Tongans had almost none of the problems dealing with the medical profession reported by indigenous people elsewhere" (Leslie, "Tongan Doctors and a Critical Medical Ethnography," 280).

20. Mattingly discusses the difference between popular American conceptions of hope, associated with the individualism of the American dream, and the "blues hope" of African Americans who hope to overcome the social borders generated in the course of "othering" practices (Mattingly, *The Paradox of Hope*). See also Delvecchio Good et al. ("American Oncology and the Discourse on Hope") on the cultural specificity of hope within American oncology practices.

21. See also Julie Livingston on the ways in which the advanced technologies of medical oncology generate hope for patients and the attempts by clinicians to mediate and manage those hopes. Livingston writes: "Novel technologies burst onto complicated political and economic landscapes generating new desires and hopes. But as these technologies become normative and embedded in complex and often dysfunctional infrastructural fields their ambiguities are revealed, and the challenges of practice become more burdensome, spawning both political critique and individual creativity" (*Improvising Medicine*, 235). By contrast with the technologies imported to the Botswana cancer ward, the technologies employed in Madang Hospital are old and basic. And yet, as I have shown, such mundane technologies are part of complex social relationships and still have the potential to generate surprises and spur improvisation.

22. The irony of the structural aesthetic of concealment and revelation is that patients also perceive the hospital to be a highly visible place. Where inmates in Bomana Prison describe the prison as a dark place, like a men's ceremonial house, where they cannot be seen by kin (Reed, *Papua New Guinea's Last Place*, 26), patients constantly refer to the eyes of other patients, carers, and visitors and their total exposure within the ward. Reed uses these descriptions of darkness to counter a Foucauldian view of prisons, which sees them as places of surveillance and visual

control (Foucault, *Discipline and Punish*). But when patients refer to the hospital as a place where "plenti ai lukim yumi" (many eyes are looking at us) this does not necessarily indicate the modern objectifying gaze that Foucault describes as characterizing modern institutions including both prisons and hospitals, but rather the inability to either avoid or engage effectively in the kind of gaze of reciprocity that, following Strathern, Reed describes as characterizing Melanesian sociality (Reed, "Anticipating Individuals"), and which enables social recognition.

23. Accounts of medical pluralism in Papua New Guinea have tended to emphasize Papua New Guinean's acceptance of multiple explanations of disease (Feinberg, "Spiritual and Natural Etiologies"; Frankel and Lewis, *A Continuing Trial of Treatment*; Hamnet and Connell, "Diagnosis and Cure"; Jilek, *Traditional Medicine and Primary Health Care in Papua New Guinea*; Lepowsky, "Sorcery and Penicillin"; Lewis, "A Failure of Treatment"; Haiveta, "Health Care Alternatives in Maindroin"; Romanucci-Schwartz, "The Hierarchy of Resort in Curative Practices"; Welsch, "Traditional Medicine and Western Medical Options among the Ningerum of Papua New Guinea"). But patients in Madang Hospital seemed less inclined to *explain* their sickness in either social or biomedical terms than to engage, through improvisation, with the relational possibilities for bodily transformation that kinship and biomedicine offered. For a similar argument made in relation to a Ugandan hospital, see Mogensen, "Finding a Path through the Health Unit."

24. See also Mattingly on the ways in which the scepticism of social scientists blinds them to the hope with which their interlocutors engage with terrible circumstances (Mattingly, *The Paradox of Hope*, 17–24).

CHAPTER 6. TECHNOLOGIES OF DETACHMENT

1. A mind/body distinction is central to this concept of personhood. As Shapin ("The House of Experiment in Seventeenth-Century England") described for relationships between scientists and their technicians in seventeenth-century Britain, creativity is taken to inhere in the mind of the scientist rather than the everyday technical practicalities of scientific work.

2. Such notions of creativity have implications for property law. Individual scientific creativity dovetails with the models of possessive individualism that lie at the heart of Euro-American property law and which have formed the basis for a new era of cultural property claims (Leach, "Creativity, Subjectivity, and the Dynamic of Possessive Individualism") and bioprospecting (Hayden, *When Nature Goes Public*).

3. It is in this sense that Strathern's theorization of the gift in Melanesia departs significantly from that of Mauss (*The Gift*).

4. The one non–Papua New Guinean doctor was a Polish surgeon who had come to Papua New Guinea with the Society of the Divine Word Missionary Society in 1996 and who since 2001 had been employed as lecturer at the Divine Word University in Madang Town. He was on a government salary in the hospital, another sign of the difficulty entailed in attracting Papua New Guinean doctors to provincial specialist positions.

5. Between 1964 and 1970 there were 36 graduates from the Papuan Medical College. By 1999, 463 Papua New Guineans, 97 Pacific Islanders, and 51 other nationalities had graduated from UPNG (Vince, "Medical Postgraduate Education in Child Health in Papua New Guinea," 55). In 2003 an average of 40 medical doctors were graduating each year. By 1990, national doctors comprised two-thirds of the doctors in the country, with estimates that by 1995 more than 80 percent of the specialists in the country would be nationals (Biddulph, "Twenty-five Years of Medical Graduates in Papua New Guinea"). Nonetheless, in 2003, there was still a shortage of national doctors available within the public health system. This was because graduates and experienced doctors saw greater opportunities in administrative roles, other countries, urban private practice, or increasingly, with development agencies and NGOs. It was also because hospital-employed doctors were very expensive and the Department of Health was unable to increase the number on their payroll.

6. Some doctors in the hospital, such as Doctor Nabik, described how their fathers had worked in the colonial health services as native medical assistants, had worked as government interpreters, or were among the first generation of Papua New Guinean church leaders. The privileged status given to particular families by virtue of their association with government or church therefore became consolidated over consecutive generations through the education opportunities it gave them.

7. See full biographical portrait in Steinbauer (1974, 23–30).

8. Anderson and Pols ("Scientific Patriotism") describe how, following earlier periods of anticolonial activism, national medics in the Philippines and the Dutch East Indies became reconciled to the importance of the late colonial state in guiding their nations toward development.

9. Interestingly, however, the motivation for going to medical school was also often described as economic—medical students were offered generous study grants and graduates were more likely to get a job afterward) rather than moral.

10. Iliffe argues that in East Africa a kind of deprofessionalization took effect in the postindependence years. "What chiefly damaged the power and status of East African doctors after independence was not the power of the state but the weakening of the state in the face of population growth, economic crisis, commercialisation, and (in Uganda) political collapse" (Iliffe, East African Doctors, 5).

11. A new dual salary scale had been put in place in 1962, which paid national doctors at a level deemed appropriate for the Papua New Guinean economy but maintained expatriate salaries at Australian rates. See Denoon, A Trial Separation, 47.

12. The image of the heroic, autonomous, rural doctor who is loved and appreciated by the surrounding community has been historically reproduced in Papua New Guinea through the medical and promotion work of the country's many Western missionary societies. This is an image also frequently invoked by European doctors working in Papua New Guinea and circulated in missionary society newsletters, which emphasize the values of self-sacrifice and humble living espoused by figures such as Edwin Tscharke and the famous German missionary doctor, Albert Schweitzer. These aspects of rural medicine are also present in the version presented by Papua New Guinean doctors but more prominent are the desire for autonomy, the

possibility of being the "only boss," and the awe of the community that they antici-pate their presence engendering.

13. It is a government policy that health centers should have a health extension officer as the officer in charge. However, the Catholic Health Service does not com-ply with this requirement due to lack of funds. The officer in charge of Catholic-run facilities is usually a nursing officer.

14. Corruption in drug procurement became national news in 2011: "Drug Scam Latest Revelation of PNG Corruption," *Post Courier*, May 31, 2011.

15. In late 2010, AusAID provided funding for consultants to work in the Depart-ment of Health to overhaul the tendering and procurement processes. This was very controversial because the "drug tsar" was not to act in an advisory role. Questions were raised by public servants and in the press over whether it was appropriate for foreigners to occupy "in-line positions" in government institutions.

16. Moreover, they claimed, it was the "village level" patient care provided by family and nurses, including the provision of food, the checking and changing of the IV line, or the turning of the body to prevent bed sores, which was most important in preventing deaths, not the intellect and skills of the doctor.

17. This modernist notion of "belief" has been crucial to the formation of insti-tutional policies and attitudes toward traditional healers elsewhere. See Stacy Pigg's work on Nepal (Pigg, "The Credible and the Credulous").

18. Recent hospital ethnography has emphasized processes of localization, by which "global" biomedicine is adapted to local cultural concepts and values (Van der Geest and Finkler, "Hospital Ethnography"). Such approaches respond to and challenge assumptions about the globalization and universality of biomedicine.

19. Joel Robbins makes a similar argument in relation to Papua New Guineans' claims to Christian conversion. Anthropologists, Robbins argues, always seek to explain away the "Christianity" of Papua New Guinean Christian practices by em-phasizing their assimilation into "traditional" cosmologies. The people he works with in Urapmin, he argues, have not hybridized the propositions of traditional and Christian culture, but have adopted Christian "belief" (as a set of values rather than propositions) wholesale (Robbins, *Becoming Sinners*).

20. Ethnographies of biomedical work in non-Western countries frequently ex-plore the conflicts and uncertainties that arise from encounters between local cos-mologies and biomedical knowledge (e.g., Wendland, *A Heart for the Work*; Sanal, *New Organs within Us*; Lock, *Twice Dead*). Aslihan Sanal, for example, describes transplant surgeons in Turkey who are uncomfortable about the cadavers they receive and cre-ate new social rituals in order to humanize the dead and turn them into appropri-ate donors. See also Adams (*Doctors for Democracy*) and Prakash (*Another Reason*).

21. For work on evidence, traditional medicine, and its institutionalization within biomedical systems, see for example the work of Wahlberg ("Bio-politics and the Promotion of Traditional Herbal Medicine in Vietnam").

22. See by contrast, Ian Harper's account of the hospital as a biomedical space barricaded by its high walls, which keep out multiple other medical practices and ways of knowing (Harper, "Translating Ethics").

23. The Papua New Guinean hospital is different in this respect from other hospitals in the Pacific, where indigenous categories have become institutionalized within the medical system. Heather Leslie writes about Tonga for example: "At the tertiary care hospital, the operating theatre has been Tonganised: people who have a classificatory brother–sister relationship will not be scheduled to work in the same surgery if it entails exposure of the patient's genitalia, because brothers and sisters should not witness such sights while together" (Leslie "Tongan Doctors and a Critical Medical," 280).

24. The subtitle I've used above is borrowed from a book of the same name, based on postindependence life in Port Moresby (Levine and Levine, *Urbanization in Papua New Guinea*). Levine and Levine describe townsmen's derogation of city life in comparison to the village, and yet their continued desire to live in Port Moresby because of the perceived freedoms from kinship obligations that it enables.

CHAPTER 7. THE PARTNERSHIP HOSPITAL

1. "On the Road to Failure," PNG *Post-Courier*, March 24, 2004. These media debates were fueled by political events, such as the visit by the Australian foreign secretary, Alexander Downer, in September 2003. The purpose of that visit was to finalize a new set of conditions for Australian aid under the "Enhanced Cooperation Program," which would include the installation of Australian "experts" in the Papua New Guinean bureaucracy and police forces in a bid to improve governance and ensure aid effectiveness. At his meetings with government ministers, Downer made comments suggesting that Papua New Guinea might become a "failed state" overrun by criminals and terrorists if Australia reduced its aid budget and that the country should be "grateful" for Australian Aid. This "big-stick diplomacy approach" (*The Australian*, September 20, 2003) was reported favorably in Australia. Giving directive orders to Papua New Guinea was, political commentators argued, only right when "Australia is about all there is stopping Papua New Guinea from becoming a failed state" (*The Australian*, October 25, 2003). In Papua New Guinea, meanwhile, politicians quickly struck back with claims that Australia was acting like a colonial power and threats that they would turn instead to China for assistance. Although the government eventually accepted the terms of the program, in 2005 the PNG Supreme Court found that the ECP's declaration of legal immunity for Australian police in Papua New Guinea was constitutionally invalid. All Australian police were sent home within the week.

2. "Modilon Tops Debt," PNG *Post Courier*, August 11, 2003.

3. "Madang Nurses Plan Strike over Back Payment Petition," PNG *Post Courier*, February 13, 2004.

4. See PNG Exposed, "President Clinton's Support for Super-hospital Locked in Says Paki."

5. "US Embassy Clears Air on New Hospital," PNG *Post Courier*, October 29, 2010.

6. "PM Stops Funds for Super Hospital," PNG *Post Courier*, November 1, 2010.

7. "Zibe Told to Come Clean," PNG *Post Courier*, September 3, 2010.

8. "Malau Awaits Evidence," *PNG Post Courier*, September 9, 2010.

9. "Malau Awaits Evidence," *PNG Post Courier*, September 9, 2010.

10. See Cross (*Dream Zones*).

11. The kind of gaze they desired and which they sought to elicit through their actions, does not belong to an abstract state, existing on another plane from everyday relationships, but is exchanged between persons (see Reed "Anticipating Individuals" and Reed "Number One Enemy"). Strathern ("Discovering Social Control") argues that people in Melanesia do not conventionally imagine power as a "second order" external force acting on society but as an innate force released by the appropriate elicitation of exchange relationships.

CHAPTER 8. RESEARCH IN THE CLINIC

1. Derivative of artemesinin.

2. Laboratory ethnography became increasingly popular in science and technology studies throughout the 1980s and 1990s. For example, Latour and Woolgar, *Laboratory Life*; Latour, *Science in Action*; Knorr-Cetina, *Epistemic Cultures*; Lynch, "Laboratory Space and the Technological Complex"; Pinch, "Art and Artifact in Laboratory Science"; and Shapin, "The House of Experiment in Seventeenth-century England."

3. While there is an extensive history of the Euro-American research hospital, the historical analysis of research in non-Western medical institutions is extraordinarily limited. Debates over the ethics of medical research in developing countries began to surface in medical arenas in the late 1990s. See Angell, "The Ethics of Clinical Research in the Third World"; Benatar, "Imperialism, Research Ethics, and Global Health"; Benatar and Singer, "A New Look at International Research Ethics"; Varmus and Satcher, "Ethical Complexities of Conducting Research in Developing Countries."

4. See also Henke ("Making a Place for Science") on farm advisors in the United States. Farm advisors, he argues were not only trying to produce credible knowledge, but were also trying to transform and improve the places where trials were carried out. The power of science derived from local demonstration as much as universal truth.

5. See recent collections on postcolonial technoscience, including Anderson ("Postcolonial Technoscience") and McNeil ("Introduction").

6. Aranova et al. ("Big Science and Big Data in Biology") note that "a belief in the prospects for human control of nature and enthusiasm for cybernetics on the one hand, and public enthusiasm for ecology during the age of growing environmentalism on the other, contributed to the sense that ecology was the most important new science of the day."

7. As Michael Fischer ("In the Science Zone") suggests, these projects can be seen as a precursor to the Big Data projects that are driving Big Science in today's information technology age.

8. For an up-to-date list of current IMR research projects and collaborations, see http://www.pngimr.org.pg/Research/research.htm (accessed February 2014). Projects are divided into international collaborations that are often driven by outside

research interests and funding and ongoing local public health surveys, which are driven by the IMR and ultimately funded by core AusAID provided grants.

9. On the semi-field Gieryn writes: "In some scientific specialities, knowledge claims gain legitimacy by preserving and drawing on simultaneously—and in a complementary way—the assumed distinct virtues of both lab and field" (Gieryn, "Laboratory Design for Post-Fordist Science," 6). Henke writes: "Standing between the standardized space of the lab and the messiness of the field, advisors use field trials to 'make a place for science,' controlling the field through experimentation but also trying to maintain the particular, 'authentic' character of a given field. Advisors need to strike a tricky balance between making a place for science and making the place seem like a regular field" (Henke, "Making a Place for Science," 484).

10. There is an extensive literature on north-south collaboration in medical research. See for example Angell, "The Ethics of Clinical Research in the Third World"; Bhutta, "Ethics in International Health Research"; Binka, "Editorial"; Geissler and Pool, "Popular Concerns about Medical Research Projects in Sub-Saharan Africa"; and Petryna, "Ethical Variability."

11. Adriana Petryna has described the ethical issues involved when the provision of drugs by private-sector funded clinical trials begins to substitute for a public health system. She argues that ethical guidelines in such places fail to account for the "cost-effective variability" (Petryna, *When Experiments Travel*, 32) through which ethics are put into practice. When the standard of care provided by a health system is already so low, what standard of care do clinical trials need to be held to? Petryna argues that ethical protocols are in fact far more effective at facilitating access to poor research populations and safeguarding data rather than the welfare of patients. Informed consent becomes a process for ensuring that the data is seen as useable and credible rather than ensuring that patients know what they are agreeing to and that they receive the best standard of care (Petryna, *When Experiments Travel*, 32).

12. The concern with "capacity" reflects a much broader shift in development discourse and practice, captured in the replacement of the time-limited, goal specific aid "project" with investments in "capacity building," "sector-wide approaches," and "systems strengthening." As described in the concluding chapter of this book, however, the emerging sense of crisis surrounding specific diseases has also put development agencies such as AusAID under increasing pressure to provide direct services rather than invest in government systems in order to generate evidence of success.

13. As Ann Kelly states in relation to similar policies regarding entomology field trials in Tanzania: "The [experiments] generate, then, not only entomological data but amateur entomologists as well" (Kelly, "Entomological Extensions").

14. On stickiness see Bill Maurer's description of capital flows (Maurer, "A Fish Story"). Capital is sticky, but so is science. A focus on stickiness goes further than a focus on material networks—it foregrounds the relationships of *friction* between persons, things, and places that produce scientific knowledge (Tsing, *Friction*).

15. Funding came from philanthropic conglomerates such as the Bill and Melinda Gates Foundation; the Global Fund, or GAVI; and from Medical Research Councils in Australia, the United States, and the United Kingdom.

16. The building was originally constructed as an extension to the pediatric ward. However, the hospital had not had enough doctors or nurses to open up the beds for several years, leading to the building's deterioration.

17. See also Celia Lowe (*Wild Profusion*) on the nationalization of biodiversity science in Indonesia's Togean Islands and the attempts by Indonesian scientists to mediate the access of a growing body of interested international scientists to the region.

Ackerknecht, E. (1967). *Medicine at the Paris Hospital, 1794–1848*. Baltimore, MD: Johns Hopkins University Press.

Adams, V. (1998). *Doctors for Democracy: Health Professionals in the Nepal Revolution.* Cambridge: Cambridge University Press.

Akin, D., and J. Robbins. (1999). "An Introduction to Melanesian Currencies: Agency, Identity, and Social Reproduction." In D. Akin and J. Robbins (Eds.), *Money and Modernity: State and Local Currencies in Melanesia* (1–40). Pittsburgh: University of Pittsburgh Press.

Akrich, M. (1994). "The De-scription of Technical Objects." In W. E. Bijker and J. Law (Eds.), *Shaping Technology/Building Society: Studies in Sociotechnical Change* (205–224). Cambridge, MA: MIT Press.

Alpers, M. (1979). "Delivery of Health Care in Papua New Guinea." *Papua and New Guinea Medical Journal* 22 (3), 159–162.

Alpers, M. (1999). "Past and Present Research Activities of the Papua New Guinea Institute of Medical Research." *Papua New Guinea Medical Journal* 42 (March), 32–51.

Alpers, M. (2003). "The Buttressing Coalition of the PNGIMR: An Example of International Collaborative Research." *Trends in Parasitology* 19 (6), 278–280.

Amarshi, A., K. Good, and R. Mortimer. (1979). *Development and Dependency: The Political Economy of Papua New Guinea.* Melbourne, AU: Oxford University Press.

Anders, G. (2005). "Good Governance as Technology: Towards an Ethnography of the Bretton Woods Institutions." In D. Mosse and D. Lewis (Eds.), *The Aid Effect: Giving and Governing in International Development* (37–60). London: Pluto Press.

Anderson, H. R., J. A. Anderson, H. O. M. King, and J. E. Cotes. (1978). "Variations in the Lung Size of Children in Papua New Guinea: Genetic and Environmental Factors." *Annals of Human Biology* 5 (3), 209–218.

Anderson, W. (1996). "Disease, Race, and Empire." *Bulletin of the History of Medicine* 70 (1), 62–67.

Anderson, W. (2002). "Postcolonial Technoscience." *Social Studies of Science 32* (5), 643–658.

Anderson, W. (2005). *The Cultivation of Whiteness: Science, Health and Racial Destiny in Australia.* Carlton, AU: Melbourne University Press.

Anderson, W. (2006). *Colonial Pathologies: American Tropical Medicine, Race, and Hygiene in the Philippines.* Durham, NC: Duke University Press.

Anderson, W. (2008). *The Collectors of Lost Souls: Turning Kuru Scientists into Whitemen.* Baltimore, MD: Johns Hopkins University Press.

Anderson, W. (2009). "Modern Sentinel and Colonial Microcosm: Science, Discipline, and Distress at the Philippine General Hospital." *Philippine Studies 57* (2), 153–177.

Anderson, W., and H. Pols. (2012). "Scientific Patriotism: Medical Science and National Self-Fashioning in Southeast Asia." *Comparative Studies in Society and History 54* (1), 93–113.

Angell, M. (1997). "The Ethics of Clinical Research in the Third World." *New England Journal of Medicine 337* (12), 847–849.

Anghie, A. (2002). "Colonialism and the Birth of International Institutions: Sovereignty, Economy, and the Mandate System of the League of Nations." *New York University Journal of International Law and Politics 34* (3), 513.

Aranova, E., K. Baker, and N. Oreskes. (2010). "Big Science and Big Data in Biology: From the International Geophysical Year through the International Biological Program to the Long Term Ecological Research (LTER) Network, 1957–Present." *Historical Studies in the Natural Sciences 40* (2), 183–224.

Aretxaga, B. (2003). "Maddening States." *Annual Review of Anthropology 32* (1), 393–410.

Arnold, D. (1988). "Introduction: Disease, Medicine and Empire." In D. Arnold (Ed.), *Imperial Medicine and Indigenous Societies* (1–26). Manchester: Manchester University Press.

Arnold, D. (1993). *Colonizing the Body: State Medicine and Epidemic Disease in Nineteenth-Century India.* Berkeley: University of California Press.

Arnold, D. (1996). *Warm Climates and Western Medicine: The Emergence of Tropical Medicine, 1500–1900.* Amsterdam, Neth.: Rodopi.

Arnold, D. (2004). "Race, Place, and Bodily Difference in Early Nineteenth-century India." *Historical Research 77* (196), 254–273.

ASPI. (2004). *Strengthening our Neighbour: Australia and the Future of Papua New Guinea.* Canberra, AU.

AusAID. (2009). *Evaluation of Australian Aid to Health Service Delivery in Papua New Guinea, Solomon Islands and Vanuatu.* Canberra.

AusAID. (2013). "Overview of Australian Aid in Fragile and Conflict-affected States." Available at http://www.ausaid.gov.au/aidissues/fragility-conflict/Pages/over view.aspx.

Baber, Z. (2001). "Colonizing Nature: Scientific Knowledge, Colonial Power, and the Incorporation of India into the Modern World-System." *British Journal of Sociology 1* (52), 37–58.

Bamford, S. C. (2007). *Biology Unmoored: Melanesian Reflections on Life and Biotechnology*. Berkeley: University of California Press.

Barker, J. (2003). "Christian Bodies: Dialectics of Sickness and Salvation among the Maisin of Papua New Guinea." *October* 27 (3), 99–118.

Barrett, R. J. (1988). "Clinical Writing and the Documentary Construction of Schizophrenia." *Culture, Medicine and Psychiatry* 12 (3), 265–299.

Barry, A. (1995). "Reporting and Visualising." In C. Jenks (Ed.), *Visual Culture* (42–57). London: Routledge.

Bashkow, I. (2006). *The Meaning of Whitemen: Race and Modernity in the Orokaiva Cultural World*. Chicago, IL: University of Chicago Press.

Benatar, S. R. (1998). "Imperialism, Research Ethics, and Global Health." *British Medical Journal* 24 (4), 221–222.

Benatar, S. R., A. S. Daar, and P. A. Singer. (2005). "Global Health Challenges: The Need for an Expanded Discourse on Bioethics." *PLoS Medicine* 2 (7), 587–589.

Benatar, S. R., and P. A. Singer. (2000). "A New Look at International Research Ethics." *British Medical Journal* 321 (7264), 824–826.

Berg, M. (1997). *Rationalizing Medical Work: Decision-Support Techniques and Medical Practices*. Cambridge, MA: MIT Press.

Berg, M., and G. Bowker. (1997). "The Multiple Bodies of the Medical Record: Toward a Sociology of an Artifact." *Sociological Quarterly* 38 (3), 513–537.

Berg, M., and A. Mol. (1998). "Differences in Medicine: An Introduction." In M. Berg and A. Mol (Eds.), *Differences in Medicine: Unraveling Practices, Techniques, and Bodies* (1–12). Durham, NC: Duke University Press.

Bhutta, Z. A. (2002). "Ethics in International Health Research: A Perspective from the Developing World." *Bulletin of the World Health Organization* 80 (2), 114–120.

Biagioli, M. (2006). "Documents of Documents: Scientists' Names and Scientific Claims." In Annalise Riles (Ed.), *Documents: Artefacts of Modern Knowledge* (127–157). Ann Arbor: University of Michigan Press.

Biddulph, J. (1990). "Twenty-five Years of Medical Graduates in Papua New Guinea." *Papua and New Guinea Medical Journal* 33 (1), 43–49.

Biehl, J. (2005a). "Technologies of Invisibility: Politics of Life and Social Inequality." In J. X. Inda (Ed.), *Anthropologies of Modernity: Foucault, Governmentality, and Life Politics* (248–271). London: Blackwell.

Biehl, J. (2005b). *Vita: Life in a Zone of Social Abandonment*. Berkeley: University of California Press.

Biehl, J. (2007). *Will to Live: AIDS Therapies and the Politics of Survival*. Princeton, NJ: Princeton University Press.

Biersack, A. (1982). "Ginger Gardens for the Ginger Woman: Rites and Passages in a Melanesian Society." *Man* 17 (2), 239–258.

Binka, F. (2005). "Editorial: North–South Research Collaborations: A Move towards a True Partnership?" *Tropical Medicine and International Health* 10 (3), 207–209.

Bonneuil, C. (2000). "Experiment: Science and State Building in Late Colonial and Postcolonial Africa, 1930–1970." *Osiris* 15, 258–281.

Bowker, G. C., and S. L. Star. (2000). *Sorting Things Out: Classification and Its Consequences*. Cambridge, MA: MIT Press.

Brasier, A. (2010). "Prisoners' Bodies: Methods and Advances in Convict Medicine in the Transportation Era." *Health and History* 12 (2), 18–38.

Brighenti, A. (2007). "Visibility: A Category for the Social Sciences." *Current Sociology* 55 (3), 323–342.

British New Guinea Administrator. *Annual Report on British New Guinea 1898–99.* Victoria, AU: Government Printer.

Brown, H. (2010). *Living with HIV/AIDS: An Ethnography of Care in Western Kenya*. Manchester, UK: Manchester University.

Burri, R. V. (2008). "Doing Distinctions: Boundary Work and Symbolic Capital in Radiology." *Social Studies of Science* 38 (1), 35–62.

Burton-Bradley, B. G. (1990). *A History of Medicine in Papua New Guinea: Vignettes of an Earlier Period*. Kingsgrove, AU: Australian Medical Publishing.

Busby, C. (1997). "Permeable and Partible Persons: A Comparative Analysis of Gender and Body in South India and Melanesia." *Journal of the Royal Anthropological Institute* 3 (2), 261–278.

Butler, A. G. (1938). *The Official History of the Australian Army Medical Services in the War of 1914–1918*. Melbourne, AU: Australian War Memorial.

Callon, M. (1986). "Some Elements of a Sociology of Translation: Domestication of the Scallops and the Fishermen of St Brieuc Bay." In John Law (Ed.), *Power, Action, and Belief: A New Sociology of Knowledge*, Vol. 32 (196–233). London: Routledge.

Cameron-Smith, A. (2010). "Australian Imperialism and International Health in the Pacific Islands." *Australian Historical Studies* 41 (1), 57–74.

Carroll, P. (2006). *Science, Culture, and Modern State Formation*. Berkeley: University of California Press.

Cartwright, L. (1995). *Screening the Body: Tracing Medicine's Visual Culture*. Minneapolis: University of Minnesota Press.

Casey, E. S. (1987). "The Place of Space in the Birth of the Clinic." *Journal of Medicine and Philosophy* 12 (4), 351–356.

Cassidy, R., and M. Leach. (2009). "Citizenship and Global Funding: A Gambian Case Study." Working Paper 325. Institute of Development Studies. Brighton, UK.

Chakrabarty, S. D. (2000). *Provincializing Europe: Postcolonial Thought and Colonial Difference*. Princeton, NJ: Princeton University Press.

Clark, J. (1989). "The Incredible Shrinking Men: Male Ideology and Development in a Southern Highlands Society." *Canberra Anthropology* 12, 120–143.

Clark, J. (1997). "Imagining the State, or Tribalism and the Arts of Memory in the Highlands of Papua New Guinea." In N. Thomas and T. Otto (Eds.), *Narratives of Nation in the South Pacific* (65–90). London: Routledge.

Comaroff, J. (2007). "Beyond Bare Life: AIDS, (Bio)Politics, and the Neoliberal Order." *Public Culture* 19 (1), 197–219.

Connell, J. (1997). "Health in Papua New Guinea: A Decline in Development." *Australian Geographical Studies* 35 (3), 271–293.

Connell, J., and J. Lea. (1995). "Distant Places, Other Cities? Urban Life in Contemporary Papua New Guinea." In *Postmodern Cities and Spaces*, edited by S. Watson and K. Gibson, 165–186. Oxford: Blackwell.

Coser, R. L. (1962). *Life in the Ward*. East Lansing: Michigan State University Press.

Counts, D., and D. Counts. (2004). "The Good, the Bad, and the Unresolved Death in Kaliai." *Fortune* 58, 887–897.

Crane, J. (2010). "Adverse Events and Placebo Effects: African Scientists, HIV, and Ethics in the 'Global Health Sciences.'" *Social Studies of Science* 40 (6), 843–870.

Crapanzano, V. (2011). "Reflections on Hope as a Category of Social and Psychological Analysis." *Cultural Anthropology* 18 (1), 3–32.

Crary, J. (1990). *Techniques of the Observer: On Vision and Modernity in the Nineteenth Century*. Cambridge, MA: MIT Press.

Cross, J. (2014). Dream Zones: Capitalism and Development in India. London: Pluto.

Cueto, M. (2013). "A Return to the Magic Bullet? Malaria and Global Health in the Twenty-First Century." In *When People Come First: Critical Studies in Global Health*, edited by Joao Biehl and A. Petryna, 30–53. Princeton, NJ: Princeton University Press.

Curtin, P. D. (1998). *Disease and Empire: The Health of European Troops in the Conquest of Africa*. Cambridge: Cambridge University Press.

Curtin, T. (2000). "Public Sector Reform in Papua New Guinea and the 1999 Budget." *Labour and Management in Development* 1 (4), 1–26.

Cussins, C. (1998). "Producing Reproduction: Techniques of Normalization and Naturalization in Infertility Clinics." In S. Franklin and H. Ragone (Eds.), *Reproducing Reproduction: Kinship, Power and Technological Innovation*. Philadelphia: University of Pennsylvania Press.

Dalton, D. M. (1996). "The Aesthetic of the Sublime: An Interpretation of Rawa Shell Valuable Symbolism." *American Ethnologist* 23 (2), 393–415.

Das, V., and D. Poole. (2004). *Anthropology in the Margins of the State*. New Delhi, India: Oxford University Press.

De Laet, M. (2002). *Research in Science and Technology Studies: Knowledge and Technology Transfer*. Amsterdam, Neth.: JAI Press.

De Laet, M., and A. Mol. (2000). "The Zimbabwe Bush Pump: Mechanics of a Fluid Technology." *Social Studies of Science* 30 (2), 225–263.

Denoon, D. (1989). *Public Health in Papua New Guinea: Medical Possibility and Social Constraint*. Public Health. Cambridge: Cambridge University Press.

Denoon, D. (1991). "The Idea of Tropical Medicine and Its Influence on Papua New Guinea." In D. Denoon and R. Macleod (Eds.), *Health and Healing in Tropical Australia and Papua New Guinea* (12–22). Townsville, AU: James Cook University.

Denoon, D. (2002). *Public Health in Papua New Guinea: Medical Possibility and Social Constraint, 1884–1984*. Cambridge: Cambridge University Press.

Denoon, D. (2005). *A Trial Separation: Australia and the Decolonisation of Papua New Guinea*. Canberra, AU: Pandanus Books.

Dinnen, S. (2004). "Aid Effectiveness and Australia's New Interventionism in the Southwest Pacific." *Australian National University Development Studies Network Development Bulletin 65* (1), 76–80.

Dobbes, M.-A., and C. R. Hofman. (1999). *The Social Dynamics of Technology: Practice, Politics, and World Views.* Washington, DC: Smithsonian Institution Press.

Douglas, B. (2000). "Weak States and Other Nationalisms: Emerging Melanesian Paradigms. State Society and Governance in Melanesia Discussion Paper 00/3. Australian National University. Canberra." Available at: https://digitalcollections .anu.edu.au/bitstream/1885/41823/3/nationalism_in_weak_states.pdf.

Duffield, M. (2002). "Social Reconstruction and the Radicalization of Development: Aid as a Relation of Global Liberal Governance." *Development and Change 33* (5), 1049–1071.

Edejer, T. (1999). "North-South Research Partnerships: The Ethics of Carrying Out Research in Developing Countries." *British Medical Journal 319* (7207), 438.

Elden, S. (2003). "Plague, Panopticon, Police." *Surveillance and Society 1* (3), 240–253.

Elyachar, J. (2012). "Next Practices: Knowledge, Infrastructure, and Public Goods at the Bottom of the Pyramid." *Public Culture 24* (1), 109–130.

Emanuel, E. J., D. Wendler, J. Killen, and C. Grady. (2004). What Makes Clinical Research in Developing Countries Ethical? The Benchmarks of Ethical Research. *Journal of Infectious Diseases 189* (5), 930.

Englund, H., and J. Leach. (2000). "Ethnography and the Meta-Narratives of Modernity." *Current Anthropology 41* (2), 225–248.

Eves, R. (2005). "Unsettling Settler Colonialism: Debates over Climate and Colonization in New Guinea, 1875–1914." *Ethnic and Racial Studies 28* (2), 304–330.

Eves, R. (2010). "'In God's Hands': Pentecostal Christianity, Morality, and Illness in a Melanesian Society." *Journal of the Royal Anthropological Institute, n.s. (16)*, 496–514.

Eves, R., and L. Butt. (2008). *Making Sense of Aids.* Honolulu: University of Hawaii Press.

Ewers, W. H. (1972). "Malaria in the Early Years of German New Guinea." *Journal of Papua and New Guinea Society 6* (1), 3–30.

Farmer, P. (2001). *Infections and Inequalities.* Berkeley: University of California Press.

Farmer, Paul. (2005). *Pathologies of Power: Health, Human Rights, and the New War on the Poor.* Berkeley: University of California Press.

Fassin, D. (2009). "Another Politics of Life Is Possible." *Theory, Culture, and Society 26* (5), 44–60.

Feinberg, R. (1990). "Spiritual and Natural Etiologies on a Polynesian Outlier in Papua New Guinea." *Social Science and Medicine 30* (3), 311–23.

Ferguson, J. (1990). *The Anti-Politics Machine: Development, Depoliticisation, and Bureaucratic Power in Lesotho.* Minneapolis: University of Minnesota Press.

Finkler, K., C. Hunter, and R. Iedema. (2008). "What Is Going On: Ethnography in Hospital Spaces." *Journal of Contemporary Ethnography 37* (2), 246–250.

Firth, S. (1982). *New Guinea under the Germans.* Melbourne, AU: Melbourne University Press.

Fischer, M. (2001). "In the Science Zone: The Yanomami and the Fight for Representation." *Anthropology Today* 17 (4), 9–14.

Fischer, M. (2005). "Technoscientific Infrastructures and Emergent Forms of Life: A Commentary." *American Anthropologist* 107 (1), 55–61.

Fischer, M. M. J. (2011). "In the Science Zone II: The Fore, Papua New Guinea, and the Fight for Representation." *East Asian Science, Technology and Society* 5 (1), 87–102.

Fischer, M. M. J. (2013). "Afterword—The Peopling of Technologies." In João Biehl and Adriana Petryna (Eds.), *When People Come First: Critical Studies in Global Health* (347–374). Princeton, NJ: Princeton University Press

Fortune, R. (1931). *Sorcerers of Dobu: The Social Anthropology of the Dobu Islanders of the Western Pacific*. London: Routledge.

Foster, R. J. (1995a). "Introduction." In Robert Foster (Ed.), *Nation-Making: Emergent Identities in Postcolonial Melanesia* (1–33). Ann Arbor: University of Michigan Press.

Foster, R. (1995b). *Social Reproduction and History in Melanesia: Mortuary Ritual, Gift Exchange, and Custom in the Tanga Islands*. Cambridge: Cambridge University Press.

Foster, R. J. (1995c). "Print Advertisements and Nation-making in Metropolitan Papua New Guinea." In Robert Foster (Ed.), *Nation-Making: Emergent Identities in Postcolonial Melanesia* (151–184). Ann Arbor: The University of Michigan Press.

Foster, R. J. (1999). "Melanesianist Anthropology in the Era of Globalization." *Contemporary Pacific* 11 (1), 140–159.

Foster, R. J. (2002). *Materializing the Nation: Commodities, Consumption, and Media in Papua New Guinea*. Bloomington: Indiana University Press.

Foucault, M. (1975). *Discipline and Punish: The Birth of the Prison*. London: Penguin.

Foucault, M. (1980). *Power/Knowledge: Selected Interviews and Other Writings 1972–1977*. Ed. Colin Gordon. New York: Pantheon Books.

Foucault, M. (1986). "Of Other Spaces." Trans. J. Miskowiec. *Diacritics* 16 (1), 22–27.

Foucault, M. (2003). *The Birth of the Clinic*. London: Routledge.

Foucault, M. (2007). "The Incorporation of the Hospital into Modern Technology." In J. W. Crampton and S. Elden (Eds.), *Space, Knowledge and Power: Foucault and Geography* (141–152). London: Ashgate.

Frankel, S., and G. Lewis. (1989). *A Continuing Trial of Treatment: Medical Pluralism in Papua New Guinea. The Journal of Nervous and Mental Disease*. London: Kluwer Academic.

Frerichs, A., and S. Frerichs. (1957). *Anutu Conquers in New Guinea: A Story of Mission Work in New Guinea*. Minneapolis: Augsburg.

Fukuyama, F. (2004). *State-Building: Governance and World Order in the 21st Century*. Ithaca, NY: Cornell University Press.

Fukuyama, F. (2006). "Observations on State-Building in the Western Pacific." Washington, DC.

Fukuyama, F. (2007). "Governance Reform in Papua New Guinea." Washington, DC.

Fukuyama, F. (n.d.). "Governance Reform in Papua New Guinea." Available at http://www.sais-jhu.edu/faculty/fukuyama/Governance_PNG.doc.

Gaillard, J. F. (1994). "North-South Research Partnership: Is Collaboration Possible between Unequal Partners?" *Knowledge and Policy* 7 (2), 31–63.

Gawande, A. (2003). *Complications: A Surgeon's Notes on an Imperfect Science*. New York: Picador.

Geest, S. Van Der, and K. Finkler. (2004). "Hospital Ethnography: Introduction." *Social Science and Medicine*, 59 (10), 1995–2001.

Geissler, P. W., and R. Pool. (2006). "Popular Concerns about Medical Research Projects in Sub-Saharan Africa: A Critical Voice in Debates About Medical Research Ethics." *Tropical Medicine and International Health* 11 (7), 975–982.

Geissler, P., A. Wenzel, B. Kelly, B. Imoukhuede and R. Pool. (2008). "'He Is Now Like a Brother, I Can Even Give Him Some Blood'—Relational Ethics and Material Exchanges in a Malaria Vaccine 'Trial Community' in The Gambia." *Social Science and Medicine* 67 (5), 696–707. doi:10.1016/j.socscimed.2008.02.004.

Gell, A. (1988). *Art and Agency: An Anthropological Theory*. Oxford: Clarendon Press.

Gewertz, D., and F. Errington. (1999). *Emerging Class in Papua New Guinea: The Telling of Difference*. Cambridge: Cambridge University Press.

Gibson, D. (2004). "The Gaps in the Gaze in South African Hospitals." *Social Science and Medicine* 59, 2013–2024.

Gieryn, T. F. (2006). "City as Truth-Spot: Laboratories and Field-Sites in Urban Studies." *Social Studies of Science* 36 (1), 5–38.

Gieryn, Thomas F. (2008). "Laboratory Design for Post-Fordist Science." *Isis* 99 (4), 796–802.

Global Fund. (2011). *The Global Fund's Approach to Health Systems Strengthening*. Geneva.

Good, B. (1994). *Medicine, Rationality, and Experience: An Anthropological Perspective*. Cambridge: Cambridge University Press.

Good, Mary-Jo Delvecchio, B. J. Good, C. Schaffer, and S. E. Lind. (1990). "American Oncology and the Discourse on Hope." *Culture, Medicine, and Psychiatry* 14 (1), 59–79.

Good, Mary-Jo Delvecchio, S. Hyde, S. Pinto, and B. Good. (2008). *Postcolonial Disorders*. Berkeley: University of California Press.

Greenhouse, C. (2002). "Introduction: Altered States, Altered Lives." In C. Greenhouse, E. Mertz, and K. Warren (Eds.), *Ethnography in Unstable Places: Everyday Lives in Contexts of Dramatic Political Change* (1–34). Durham, NC: Duke University Press.

Guntner, M. W. (2006). *Doctors in Paradise: Challenges and Rewards in Medical Service New Guinea 1958–1970*. Belair, AU: Crawford House.

Hacking, I. (2007). "Making Up People." In M. M. Lock and J. Farquhar (Eds.), *Beyond the Body Proper: The Anthropology of Material Life* (150–163). Durham, NC: Duke University Press.

Hage, G. (2003). *Against Paranoid Nationalism: Searching for Hope in a Shrinking Society*. Annandale, New South Wales, AU: Pluto Press.

Haiveta, C. (1990). "Health Care Alternatives in Maindroin." In N. Lutkehaus (Ed.), *Sepik Heritage: Tradition and Change in Papua New Guinea*. Durham, NC: Carolina Academic Press.

Hammar, L. (2007). "Epilogue: Homegrown in PNG-Rural Responses to HIV and AIDS." *Oceania* 77 (1), 72–94.

Hamnet, M. P., and J. Connell. (1981). "Diagnosis and Cure: The Resort to Traditional and Modern Medical Practitioners in the North Solomons, Papua New Guinea." *Social Science and Medicine* 15 (4), 489–498.

Harloe, L. (1991). "Anton Breinl and the Australian Institute of Tropical Medicine." In D. Denoon and R. MacLeod (Eds.), *Health and Healing in Tropical Australia and Papua New Guinea* (35–46). Townsville, AU: James Cook University.

Harper, I. (2007). "Translating Ethics: Researching Public Health and Medical Practices in Nepal." *Social Science and Medicine* 65 (11), 2235–2247.

Harper, I. (2010). "Extreme Condition, Extreme Measures? Compliance, Drug Resistance, and the Control of Tuberculosis." *Anthropology and Medicine* 17 (2), 201–214.

Harper, I. (2014). *Development and Public Health in the Himalaya*. London: Routledge.

Harrison, G. A., A. J. Boyce, C. M. Platt, and S. Serjeantson. (1975). "Body Composition Changes during Lactation in a New Guinea Population." *Annals of Human Biology* 2 (4), 395–398.

Harrison, M. (2009). "Introduction." In M. Harrison, M. Jones, and H. Sweet (Eds.), *From Western Medicine to Global Medicine: The Hospital beyond the West* (1–32). HyderabadOrient BlackSwan.

Harrison, S. (1990). *Stealing People's Names: History and Politics in a Sepik River Cosmology*. Cambridge: Cambridge University Press.

Hayden, C. (2003). *When Nature Goes Public: The Making and Unmaking of Bioprospecting in Mexico*. Princeton, NJ: Princeton University Press.

Haynes, D. M. (2001). *Imperial Medicine: Patrick Manson and the Conquest of Tropical Disease*. Philadelphia: University of Pennsylvania Press.

Henke, Christopher, R. (2000). "Making a Place for Science: The Field Trial." *Social Studies of Science* 30 (4), 483–511.

Hetherington, K. (1997). *The Badlands of Modernity: Heterotopia and Social Ordering*. London: Routledge.

Hirsch, E. (1994). "Between Mission and Market: Events and Images in a Melanesian Society." *Man* 29 (3), 689–711.

Hirsch, E. (2001). "Making Up People in Papua." *Journal of the Royal Anthropological Institute* 7 (2), 241–256.

Hirsch, E. (2003). "A Landscape of Powers in Highland Papua, C. 1899–1918." *History and Anthropology* 14 (1), 3–22.

Hobbins, P., and K. Hillier. (2010). "Isolated Cases? The History and Historiography of Australian Medical Research." *Health and History* 12 (2), 1–17.

Holbraad, M., and M. A. Pedersen. (2010). "Planet M: The Intense Abstraction of Marilyn Strathern." *Anthropological Theory* 9 (4), 371–394.

Hongoro, C., and B. McPake. (2004). "How to Bridge the Gap in Human Resources for Health." *The Lancet 364* (9443), 1451–1456.

Hornabrook, R. W. (1970). "The Institute of Human Biology of Papua-New Guinea Japan (II): University Turmoil Is Reflected in Research." *Science,* 146–147.

Hornabrook, Richard W., S. Serjeaston, and J. M. Stanhope. (1977). "The Relationship between Socioeconomic Status and Health in Two Papua New Guinean Populations." *Human Ecology 5* (4), 369–382.

Hughes, H. (2003). *Aid Has Failed in the Pacific* (Vol. 33). Centre for Independent Studies Sydney.

Hull, E. (2012). "Paperwork and the Contradictions of Accountability in a South African Hospital." *Journal of the Royal Anthropological Institute 18* (3), 613–632.

Iliffe, J. (1998). *East African Doctors: A History of the Modern Profession.* Cambridge: Cambridge University Press.

Jackman, H. H. (1990). "Malaria in German New Guinea." In B. G. Burton-Bradley (Ed.), *A History of Medicine in Papua New Guinea: Vignettes of an Earlier Period* (119). Sydney, AU: Australasian Medical Publishing.

Janovsky, K., J. Tulloch, J. and J. Piel. (2010). *PNG Health SWAp Review: The Missing Middle.* AusAID, Unpublished Paper.

Jay, M. (1994). *Downcast Eyes: The Denigration of Vision in Twentieth-century French Thought.* Berkeley: University of California Press.

Jensen, C. B. (2010). *Ontologies for Developing Things: Making Health Care Futures through Technology.* Rotterdam, Neth.: Sense Publishers.

Jilek, W. (1985). *Traditional Medicine and Primary Health Care in Papua New Guinea.* Port Moresby: University of Papua New Guinea Press.

Johnson, A. (2013). "Measuring Fatigue: The Politics of Innovation and Standardization in a South African Lab." *BioSocieties, (Online First).*

Jones, C., and R. Porter. (1994). "Introduction." In C. Jones and R. Porter (Eds.), *Reassessing Foucault: Power, Medicine and the Body* (1–16). London: Routledge.

Jones, P. (2005). *Chinese–Australian Journeys: Records on Travel, Migration, and Settlement, 1860–1975.* National Archives of Australia Research Guide. Available at: http://guides.naa.gov.au/content/Guide021_tcm48-54599.pdf.

Josephides, L. (1991). "Metaphors, Metathemes, and the Construction of Sociality: A Critique of the New Melanesian Ethnography." *Man 26* (1), 145–161.

Keck, V. (2005). *Social Discord and Bodily Disorders: Healing among the Yupno of Papua New Guinea.* Durham, NC: Carolina Academic Press.

Kelly, A. (2011). "Entomological Extensions: Model Huts and Fieldworks." In J. Edwards and M. Petrović-Šteger (Eds.), *Recasting Anthropological Knowledge: Inspiration and Social Science* (70–87). Manchester, UK: Manchester University Press.

Kelly, A., and U. Beisel. (2011). "Neglected Malarias: The Frontlines and Back Alleys of Global Health." *BioSocieties 6,* 71–87.

Kirsch, S. (2006). *Reverse Anthropology: Indigenous Analysis of Social and Environmental Relations in New Guinea.* Stanford, CA: Stanford University Press.

Kleinman, A. (1986). "Some Uses and Misuses of Social Science in Medicine." In D. Fiske and R. Shweder (Eds.), *Methodology in Social Science* (222–224). Chicago, IL: University of Chicago Press.

Knauft, B. (2002). *Exchanging the Past: A Rainforest World of Before and After.* Chicago, IL: University of Chicago Press.

Knorr-Cetina, K. (1999). *Epistemic Cultures: How the Sciences Make Knowledge.* Cambridge: Harvard University Press.

Kohler, R. E. (2002). *Landscapes and Labscapes: Exploring the Lab-Field Frontier in Biology.* Chicago, IL: University of Chicago Press.

Konrad, M. (2005). *Nameless Relations: Anonymity, Melanesia, and Reproductive Gift Exchange between British Ova Donors and Recipients.* Oxford: Berghahn Books.

Lairumbi Mbaabu, G., S. Molyneux, R. W. Snow, K. Marsh, N. Peshu, and M. English. (2008). "Promoting the Social Value of Research in Kenya: Examining the Practical Aspects of Collaborative Partnerships using an Ethical Framework." *Social Science and Medicine* 67 (5), 734–747.

Latour, B. (1987). *Science in Action: How to Follow Scientists and Engineers through Society.* Cambridge, MA: Harvard University Press.

Latour, B. (1999). "Give Me a Laboratory and I Will Raise the World." In M. Biagioli (Ed.), *The Science Studies Reader* (257–279). New York: Routledge.

Latour, B. (2000). "On the Partial Existence of Existing and Nonexisting Objects." In L. Daston (Ed.), *Biographies of Scientific Objects* (247–269). Chicago, IL: University of Chicago Press.

Latour, B. (2005). *Reassembling the Social: An Introduction to Actor-Network-Theory.* Oxford: Oxford University Press.

Latour, B., and S. Woolgar. (1986). *Laboratory Life: The Construction of Scientific Facts.* Princeton, NJ: Princeton University Press.

Law, John. (1986). "On the Methods of Long Distance Control: Vessels, Navigation, and the Portuguese Route to India." In John Law (Ed.), *Power, Action, and Belief: A New Sociology of Knowledge* (234–263). London: Routledge.

Law, John. (1994). *Organizing Modernity.* Oxford: Blackwell.

Law, J., and A. Mol. (2008). "Globalisation in Practice: On the Politics of Boiling Pigswill." *Geoforum* 39 (1), 133–143.

Lawrence, P. (1964). *Road Belong Cargo: A Study of the Cargo Movement in the Southern Madang District, New Guinea.* Manchester, UK: Manchester University Press.

Lawrence, P. (1984). *The Garia: An Ethnography of a Traditional Cosmic System in Papua New Guinea.* Manchester, UK: Manchester University Press.

Leach, J. (2002). "Drum and Voice: Aesthetics and Social Process on the Rai Coast of Papua New Guinea." *Journal of the Royal Anthropological Institute* 8 (4), 713–734.

Leach, J. (2003). *Creative Land, Place and Procreation on the Rai Coast of Papua New Guinea.* Oxford: Berghahn Books.

Leach, J. (2005). "'Being in Between': Art-Science Collaborations and a Technological Culture." *Social Analysis* 49 (1), 141–160.

Leach, J. (2007). "Creativity, Subjectivity, and the Dynamic of Possessive Individualism." In E. Hallam and T. Ingold (Eds.), *Creativity and Cultural Improvisation* (99–116). Oxford: Berg.

Leach, M., and J. Fairhead. (2000). "Fashioned Forest Pasts, Occluded Histories? International Environmental Analysis in West African Locales." *Development and Change 31* (1), 35–59.

Lepani, K. (2008). "Mobility, Violence, and the Gendering of HIV in Papua New Guinea." *The Australian Journal of Anthropology 19* (2), 150–164.

Lepowsky, M. (1990). "Sorcery and Penicillin: Treating Illness on a Papua New Guinea Island." *Social Science and Medicine 30* (10), 1049–1063.

Leslie, H. Y. (2005). "Tongan Doctors and a Critical Medical Ethnography." *Anthropological Forum 15* (3), 277–286.

Levine, H., and M. Levine. (1979). *Urbanization in Papua New Guinea: A Study of Ambivalent Townsmen.* Cambridge: Cambridge University Press.

Lewis, G. (2000). *A Failure of Treatment.* Oxford: Oxford University Press.

Li Puma, E. (2001). *Encompassing Others: The Magic of Modernity in Melanesia.* Ann Arbor: University of Michigan Press.

Livingston, J. (2012). *Improvising Medicine: An African Oncology Ward in an Emerging Cancer Epidemic.* Durham, NC: Duke University Press.

Livingstone, D. N. (2002). "Race, Space, and Moral Climatology: Notes toward a Genealogy." *Journal of Historical Geography 28* (2), 159–180.

Livingstone, D. N. (2003). *Putting Science in Its Place: Geographies of Scientific Knowledge.* Chicago, IL: University of Chicago Press.

Lock, M. (2002). *Twice Dead: Organ Transplants and the Reinvention of Death.* Berkeley: University of California Press.

Logan, C., and J. Willis. (2010). "International Travel as Medical Research: Architecture and the Modern Hospital." *Health and History 12* (2), 116–133.

Long, D., C. Hunter, and S. van der Geest. (2008). "When the Field Is a Ward or a Clinic: Hospital Ethnography." *Anthropology and Medicine 15* (2), 71–78.

Lowe, C. (2006). *Wild Profusion: Biodiversity Conservation in an Indonesian Archipelago.* Princeton, NJ: Princeton University Press.

Luker, V. (2007). "Papua New Guinea: Epidemiological Transition, Public Health, and the Pacific." In J. Lewis, Milton and K. L. Macpherson (Eds.), *Public Health in Asia and the Pacific: Historical and Comparative Perspectives* (250–275). London: Routledge.

Lynch, M. (1991). "Laboratory Space and the Technological Complex: An Investigation of Topical Contextures." *Science in Context 4* (1), 51–78.

MacLeod, R., and M. Lewis. (1988). *Disease, Medicine, and Empire: Perspectives on Western Medicine and the Experience of European Expansion.* London: Routledge.

Malinowski, B. (2002). *Coral Gardens and Their Magic: The Language of Magic and Gardening.* London: Routledge.

Marsland, R., and R. Prince. (2012). "What Is Life Worth? Exploring Biomedical Interventions, Survival, and the Politics of Life." *Medical Anthropology Quarterly 26* (4), 453–469.

Mattingly, C. (2010). *The Paradox of Hope: Journeys through a Clinical Borderland*. Berkeley: University of California Press.

Maurer, B. (2000). "A Fish Story: Rethinking Globalization on Virgin Gorda, British Virgin Islands." *American Ethnologist* 27 (3), 670–701.

Mauss, M. (1966). *The Gift: Forms and Functions of Exchange in Archaic Societies*. Trans. Ian Cunnison. London: Cohen and West.

McNeil, M. (2005). "Introduction: Postcolonial Technoscience." *Science as Culture* 14 (2), 105–112.

Mesman, J. (2008). *Uncertainty in Medical Innovation: Experienced Pioneers in Neonatal Care*. Basingstoke, UK: Palgrave Macmillan.

Millo, Y., and J. Lezaun. (2006). "Regulatory Experiments: Genetically Modified Crops and Financial Derivatives on Trial." *Science and Public Policy* 33 (3), 179–190.

Mitchell, T. (2002). *Rule of Experts: Egypt, Techno-Politics, Modernity*. Berkeley: University of California Press.

Miyazaki, H. (2005). "From Sugar Cane to Swords: Hope and the Extensibility of the Gift in Fiji." *Journal of the Royal Anthropological Institute* 11 (2), 277–295.

Miyazaki, H. (2007). *The Method of Hope: Anthropology, Philosophy, and Fijian Knowledge*. Stanford, CA: Stanford University Press.

Miyazaki, H. (2010). "The Temporality of No Hope." In C. Greenhouse (Ed.), *Ethnographies of Neoliberalism* (238–250). Philadelphia: University of Pennsylvania Press.

Mogensen, H. O. (2005). "Finding a Path through the Health Unit: Practical Experience of Ugandan Patients." *Medical Anthropology* 24 (3), 209–236.

Mol, A. (2002). *The Body Multiple: Ontology in Medical Practice*. Durham, NC: Duke University Press.

Mol, A. (2008). *The Logic of Care: Health and the Problem of Patient Choice*. London: Routledge.

Mol, A., and J. Law. (1994). "Regions, Networks and Fluids: Anaemia and Social Topology." *Social Studies of Science* 24 (4), 641–671.

Mola, G. D. L. (2010). "Super Hospital" Could Jeopardise Entire PNG Hospital Sector." Working Paper, *Spotlight with National Research Institute* 4 (7). National Research Institute, Port Moresby. Available at: http://www.nri.org.pg /publications/spotlight/Volume%204/Spotlight%20with%20NRI%20Vo1.4 %20No.7.pdf.

Morgan, M. G., and A. McLeod. (2006). "Have We Failed our Neighbour?" *Australian Journal of International Affairs* 60 (3), 412–428.

Mosse, D., and D. Lewis. (2005). *The Aid Effect: Giving and Governing in International Development*. London: Pluto Press.

Munn, N. (1986). *The Fame of Gawa: a Symbolic Study of Value Transformation in a Massim (Papua New Guinea) Society*. Cambridge: Cambridge University Press.

Nachman, S. R. (1993). "Wasted Lives: Tuberculosis and Other Health Risks of Being Haitian in a U.S. Detention Camp." *Medical Anthropology Quarterly* 7 (3), 227–259.

Nandy, A. (1983). *The Intimate Enemy: Loss and Recovery of Self under Colonialism.* New Delhi, India: Oxford University Press.

National Academy of Science. (1975). "NAS Report on International Biological Program." *Science 187* (4177), 633.

National Archives of Australia. Cabinet Secretary; Fourth and Fifth Menzies Ministries–Folders of Cabinet Committee Papers, 1949–circa. 1955; A4940 C522, Report to the Inter-departmental Committee on Health Services in Papua New Guinea 1947–48.

National Archives of Australia: Department of Post-War Reconstruction; CA 49 correspondence files, 1943–1950; Report on Proposed Expansion of Department of Public Health, 1947.

National Archives of Australia: Department of Territories, A4933 DET/1, Development of External Territories Committee–Papua New Guinea–Hospital Construction Program.

National Archives of Australia: Department of Territories, A4940 C522, Hospital Building Programme–Territory of Papua New Guinea.

National Archives of Australia; Department of Territories 1899–1983; A452 1962/8043, Correspondence files; Public works–Papua and New Guinea–hospital–Port Moresby 1946–1956.

National Archives of Australia: Department of Territories; A452 1960/1897 Correspondence files, 1901–1981; European and Native Hospital–Madang–Papua and New Guinea, 1949–1961.

National Archives of Australia: Department of Territories 1899–1983; A518 C241/3/5, Correspondence files; Public Works–Papua and New Guinea–Lae Hospital, 1949–1956.

National Archives of Australia: Department of Territories 1899–1983; Correspondence files; Health services general–Papua and New Guinea 1951–1954.

National Archives of Australia: Department of Territories; Fifth Menzies Ministry–folders of Cabinet Submissions (first system) 1951–1954; A4905 278, Territory of Papua New Guinea–health services–hospital building programme–decision 450, 1952–1952.

National Archives of Australia: Department of Territories, A452 1960/1079, Correspondence Files, Lae Native Hospital–Papua New Guinea, 1960–1964.

National Archives of Australia: Department of Territories, A452 1959/2867, Correspondence Files 1951–1975, Visit of Fellow of Royal College of Surgeons to Papua and New Guinea for assessment of Port Moresby Hospital, 1959.

National Archives of Australia: Department of Territories, A4933 DET/1, Development of External Territories Committee–Papua New Guinea–Hospital Construction Programme, 1950.

National Department of Health. (1979). *National Health Plan 1979–1984.* Port Moresby, Papua New Guinea.

National Department of Health. (1991). *National Health Plan 1991–1995.* Port Moresby, Papua New Guinea.

National Department of Health. (2001). *National Health Plan 2001–2010*. Port Moresby, Papua New Guinea.

Nelson, H. (1980). "Taim Bilong Pait: The Impact of the Second World War on Papua New Guinea." In A. McCoy (Ed.), *Southeast Asia under Japanese Occupation*. New Haven, CT: Yale University Press.

Neu Guinea Compagnie. (1887). "German New Guinea Annual Report (GNGAR) 1886–87." In Clark and Dymphna (Eds.), *German New Guinea: The Annual Reports* (1979). Canberra, AU: Australia National University Press.

Neu Guinea Compagnie. (1890). "German New Guinea Annual Report (GNGAR) 1889–90." In Clark and Dymphna (Eds.), *German New Guinea: The Annual Reports* (1979). Canberra, AU: Australia National University Press.

Neu Guinea Compagnie. (1891). "German New Guinea Annual Report (GNGAR) 1890–01." In Clark and Dymphna (Eds.), *German New Guinea: The Annual Reports* (1979). Canberra, AU: Australia National University Press.

Neu Guinea Compagnie. (1892). "German New Guinea Annual Report (GNGAR) 1891–92." In Clark and Dymphna (Eds.), *German New Guinea: The Annual Reports* (1979). Canberra, AU: Australia National University Press.

Neu Guinea Compagnie. (1912). "German New Guinea Annual Report (GNGAR) 1886–87. In Clark and Dymphna (Eds.), *German New Guinea: The Annual Reports* (1979). Canberra, AU: Australia National University Press.

Nguyen, V. K. (2005). "Antiretroviral Globalism, Biopolitics, and Therapeutic Citizenship." In A. Ong and S. Collier (Eds.), *Global Assemblages: Technology, Politics, and Ethics as Anthropological Problems* (124–144). Oxford: Blackwell.

Nichter, M. (1996). *Anthropology and International Health: Asian Case Studies*. Amsterdam, Neth.: Gordon and Breach.

Norgan, N. G., A. Ferro-Luzzi, and J.V.G.A. Durnin. (1982). "The Body Composition of New Guinean Adults in Contrasting Environments." *Annals of Human Biology* 9 (4), 343–353.

NSO. (2000). *National Census*. National Statistics Office of Papua New Guinea. Available at http://www.spc.int/prism/country/pg/stats/2000_Census/census.htm.

Overseas Development Group. (1973). *A Report on Development Strategies for Papua New Guinea*. Port Moresby, Papua New Guinea.

Packard, R. M. (2007). *The Making of a Tropical Disease: A Short History of Malaria*. Baltimore, MD: Johns Hopkins University Press.

Palladino, P., and M. Worboys. (1993). "Science and Imperialism." *Isis* 84 (1), 91–102.

Petryna, A. (2002). *Life Exposed: Biological Citizens after Chernobyl*. Princeton, NJ: Princeton University Press.

Petryna, A. (2005). "Ethical Variability: Drug Development and Globalizing Clinical Trials." *American Ethnologist* 32 (2), 183–197.

Petryna, A. (2009). *When Experiments Travel: Clinical Trials and the Global Search for Human Subjects*. Princeton, NJ: Princeton University Press.

Philo, C. (2000). "The Birth of the Clinic: An Unknown Work of Medical Geography." *Area* 32 (1), 11–19.

Pigg, S. L. (1992). "Investing Social Categories through Place: Social Representations and Development in Nepal." *Comparative Studies in Society and History* 34 (03), 491–513.

Pigg, S. L. (1996). "The Credible and the Credulous: The Question of 'Villagers' Beliefs' in Nepal." *Cultural Anthropology* 11 (2), 160–201.

Pinch, T. (1987). "Art and Artifact in Laboratory Science: A Study of Shop Work and Shop Talk in a Research Laboratory." *Sociology of Health and Illness* 9 (2), 219–220.

Pinch, T. J., and W. E. Bijker. (1984). "The Social Construction of Facts and Artefacts: or How the Sociology of Science and the Sociology of Technology might Benefit Each Other." *Social Studies of Science* 14 (3), 399–441.

PNGExposed. (2010). "President Clinton's Support for Super-hospital Locked in Says Paki." Available at http://pngexposed.wordpress.com/2010/09/15/president -clintons-support-for-super-hospital-locked-in.

Porter, D. (1999). *Health, Civilization and the State: A History of Public Health from Ancient to Modern Times.* London: Routledge.

Porter, R. (2002). *Blood and Guts: A Short History of Medicine.* London: Allen Lane.

Prakash, G. (1999). *Another Reason: Science and the Imagination of Modern India.* Princeton, NJ: Princeton University Press.

Pratt, M. (1991). "Arts of the Contact Zone." *Profession* 91, 33–40.

Prior, L. (1988). "The Architecture of the Hospital: A Study of Spatial Organization and Medical Knowledge." *British Journal of Sociology* 39 (1), 86–113.

Rabinow, P., and N. Rose. (2006). "Biopower Today." *BioSocieties* 1 (2), 195–217.

Rapp, Rayna. (1999). *Testing Women, Testing the Fetus: The Social Impact of Amniocentesis in America.* London: Routledge.

Rapp, R. (2007). "Real-Time Fetus: The Role of the Sonogram in the Age of Monitored Reproduction." In *Beyond the Body Proper: The Anthropology of Material Life* (608–622). Durham, NC: Duke University Press.

Redfield, P. (2002). "The Half-Life of Empire in Outer Space." *Social Studies of Science* 32 (5–6), 791–825.

Redfield, P. (2005). "Doctors, Borders and Life in Crisis." *Cultural Anthropology* 20 (3), 328–361.

Reed, A. (1999). "Anticipating Individuals: Modes of Vision and Their Social Consequence in a Papua New Guinean Prison." *Journal of the Royal Anthropological Institute* 5 (1), 43–56.

Reed, A. (2003). *Papua New Guinea's Last Place: Experiences of Constraint in a Postcolonial Prison.* London: Berghahn Books.

Reed, A. (2011a). "Number-One Enemy: Police, Violence, and the Location of Adversaries in a Papua New Guinean Prison." *Oceania* 81 (1), 22–35.

Reed, A. (2011b). "Hope on Remand." *Journal of the Royal Anthropological Institute* 17 (3), 527–544.

Rees, C. (1981). "Records and Hospital Routine." In P. Atkinson and C. Heath (Eds.), *Medical Work: Realities and Routines* (55–70). Farnborough, UK: Gower.

Reilly, B. (2004). "State Functioning and State Failure in the South Pacific." *Australian Journal of International Affairs* 58 (4), 479–493.

Rheinberger, H. (1997). *Toward a History of Epistemic Things: Synthesizing Proteins in the Test Tube*. Stanford, CA: Stanford University Press.

Rhodes, L. A. (1995). *Emptying Beds: The Work of an Emergency Psychiatric Unit*. Berkeley: University of California Press.

Riles, Annelise. (1998). "Infinity within the Brackets." *American Ethnologist* 25 (3), 378–398.

Robbins, J. (2004). *Becoming Sinners: Christianity and Moral Torment in a Papua New Guinea Society*. Berkeley: University of California Press.

Robins, S. (2006). "From 'Rights' to 'Ritual': AIDS Activism in South Africa." *American Anthropologist* 108 (2), 312–323.

Robinson, N. K. (1979). *Villagers at War: Some Papua New Guinean Experiences of World War II*. Canberra: Australia National University.

Rockstroh, B. I. M. (2007). *Ultrasound Travels: The Politics of a Medical Technology in Ghana and Tanzania*. Maastricht, Neth: Maastricht University.

Rollason, W. (2011). "We Are Playing Football: Seeing the Game on Panapompom, PNG." *Journal of the Royal Anthropological Institute* 17 (3), 481–503.

Romanucci-Ross, L., L. R. Tancredi, and D. E. Moerman. (1997). "The Extraneous Factor in Western Medicine." In Lolo Romanucci-Ross, D. E. Moerman, and L. R. Tancredi (Eds.), *The Anthropology of Medicine: From Culture to Method* (351–368). London: Bergin and Garvey.

Romanucci-Schwartz, L. (1969). "The Hierarchy of Resort in Curative Practices: The Admiralty Islands, Melanesia." *Journal of Health and Social Behavior* 10 (3), 201–209.

Rose, N. (1999). *Governing the Soul*. London: Free Association Books.

Rose, N. (2007). *The Politics of Life Itself: Biomedicine, Power, and Subjectivity in the Twenty-First Century*. Princeton, NJ: Princeton University Press.

Ross, R. (1910). *The Prevention of Malaria*. London: J. Murray.

Rotberg, R. I. (2004). *When States Fail: Causes and Consequences*. Princeton, NJ: Princeton University Press.

Rumsey, A., and J. F. Weiner. (2001). *Emplaced Myth: Space, Narrative, and Knowledge in Aboriginal Australia and Papua New Guinea*. Honolulu: University of Hawaii Press.

Sanal, A. (2011). *New Organs within Us: Transplants and the Moral Economy*. Durham, NC: Duke University Press.

Scott, J. C. (1998). *Seeing Like a State: How Certain Schemes to Improve the Human Condition Have Failed*. New Haven, CT: Yale University Press.

Shapin, S. (1988). "The House of Experiment in Seventeenth-Century England." *Isis* 79 (3), 373–404.

Shapin, S. (1989). "The Invisible Technician." *American Scientist* 77 (6), 554–563.

Shapin, S., and A. Ophir. (1991). "The Place of Knowledge: A Methodological Survey." *Science in Context* 4 (1), 3–21.

Simoni, A., G. Cardoso, L. Oliveira, and R. Bulamah. (2010). "Pigs and Mobile Phones: A Conversation with Marilyn Strathern." Available at http://www.ifch.unicamp .br/proa/EntrevistasII/pdfs/strathern_en.pdf.

Sinclair, J. P. (2005). *Madang*. Madang, Papua New Guinea: Divine Word University Press.

Spielman, A., and M. D'Antonio. (2001). *Mosquito: A Natural History of our Most Persistent and Deadly Foe*. London: Faber and Faber.

Stanhope, J. M., and R. W. Hornabrook. (1974). "Fertility Patterns of Two New Guinea Populations: Karkar and Lufa." *Journal of Biosocial Science* 6 (04), 439–452. doi:10.1017/S002193200000986X.

Stasch, R. (2010). *Society of Others: Kinship and Mourning in a West Papuan Place*. Berkeley: University of California Press.

Stepan, N. L. (2001). *Picturing Tropical Nature*. London: Reaktion Books.

Stoler, A. L. (2008). "Imperial Debris: Reflections on Ruins and Ruination." *Cultural Anthropology* 23 (2), 191–219.

Strathern, A. J. (1975). "Why Is Shame on the Skin?" *Ethnology* 14 (4), 347–356.

Strathern, M. (1979). "The Self in Self-Decoration." *Oceania* 49 (4), 241–257.

Strathern, M. (1985). "Discovering Social Control." *Journal of Law and Society* 12 (2), 111–134.

Strathern, M. (1988). *The Gender of the Gift*. Berkeley: University of California Press.

Strathern, M. (1992). *Reproducing the Future: Essays on Anthropology, Kinship, and the New Reproductive Technologies*. New York: Routledge.

Strathern, M. (1996). "Cutting the Network." *Journal of the Royal Anthropological Institute* 2 (3), 517–535.

Strathern, M. (1999). *Property, Substance, and Effect: Anthropological Essays on Persons and Things*. London: Athlone Press.

Strathern, M. (2000). "Introduction: New Accountabilities." In M. Strathern (Ed.), *Audit Cultures: Anthropological Studies in Accountability, Ethics and the Academy* (1–18). London: Routledge.

Strathern, M. (2004). *Partial Connections*. Walnut Creek, CA: Altamira Press.

Strathern, M. (2005). *Kinship, Law, and the Unexpected: Relatives Are Always a Surprise*. Cambridge: Cambridge University Press.

Strathern, M. (2009). "Afterword." *Body and Society* 15 (2), 217–222.

Strathern, M. (2011). "Binary License." *Common Knowledge* 17 (1), 87–103.

Street, A. (2009). "Failed Recipients: Extracting Blood in a Papua New Guinean Hospital." *Body and Society* 15 (2), 193–215.

Street, A. (2010). "Belief as Relational Action: Christianity and Cultural Change in Papua New Guinea." *Journal of the Royal Anthropological Institute, n.s. (16)*, 260–278.

Street, A. (2011). "Artefacts of Not-Knowing: The Medical Record, the Diagnosis and the Production of Uncertainty in Papua New Guinean Biomedicine." *Social Studies of Science* 41 (6), 815–834.

Street, A. (2012). "Affective Infrastructure: Hospital Landscapes of Hope and Failure." *Space and Culture* 15 (1), 44–56.

Street, A., and S. Coleman. (2012). "Real and Imaginary Spaces." *Space and Culture* 15 (1), 4–17.

Sullivan, N. (2012). "Enacting Spaces of Inequality: Placing Global/State Governance within a Tanzanian Hospital." *Space and Culture* 15 (1), 57–67.

Sykes, K. (2001). "Paying a School Fee Is a Father's Duty: Critical Citizenship in Central New Ireland." *American Ethnologist* 28 (1), 5–31.

Szerszynski, B. (2000). "Beating the Unbound: Political Theatre in the Laboratory without Walls." In G. Giannachi and N. Stewart (Eds.), *Performing Nature: Explorations in Ecology and the Arts* (181–197). New York: Peter Lang.

Thomason, J., N. Mulou, and C. Bass. (1994). "User Charges for Rural Health Services in Papua New Guinea." *Social Science and Medicine* 39 (8), 1105–1115.

Tsing, A. (2005). *Friction*. Princeton, NJ: Princeton University Press.

Turnbull, D. (1993). "Local Knowledge and Comparative Scientific Traditions." *Knowledge, Technology, and Policy* 6 (3), 29–54.

Turnbull, David, and H. Watson-Veran. (1995). "Science and Other Indigenous Knowledge Systems." In S. Jasanoff, G. Markle, J. Peterson, and T. Pinch (Eds.), *Handbook of Science and Technology Studies* (115–139). Thousand Oaks, CA: Sage.

Varmus, H., and D. Satcher. (1997). "Ethical Complexities of Conducting Research in Developing Countries." *New England Journal of Medicine* 337 (14), 1003–1005.

Vince, J. (2000). "Medical Postgraduate Education in Child Health in Papua New Guinea." *Papua New Guinea Medical Journal* 43, 54–59.

Wagner, R. (1975). *The Invention of Culture*. Englewood Cliffs, NJ: Prentice-Hall.

Wahlberg, A. (2006). "Bio-Politics and the Promotion of Traditional Herbal Medicine in Vietnam." *Health* 10 (2), 123–147.

Wardlow, H. (2006). *Wayward Women: Sexuality and Agency in a New Guinea Society*. Berkeley: University of California Press.

Weiner, J. (1995). "Technology and Techne in Trobriand and Yolngu Art." *Social Analysis* 38 (S), 32–46.

Weiner, J. (2003). *Tree Leaf Talk: a Heideggerian Anthropology*. New York: Berg.

Welsch, R. (1983). "Traditional Medicine and Western Medical Options among the Ningerum of Papua New Guinea." In Lola Romanucci-Ross, D. E. Moerman, and L. R. Tancredi (Eds.), *The Anthropology of Medicine: From Culture to Method* (32–53). New York: Praeger.

Wendland, C. L. (2010). *A Heart for the Work: Journeys through an African Medical School*. Chicago, IL: University of Chicago Press.

Whyte, S. R. (1997). *Questioning Misfortune: The Pragmatics of Uncertainty in Eastern Uganda*. Cambridge: Cambridge University Press.

Whyte, S. R. (2009). "Health Identities and Subjectivities: The Ethnographic Challenge." *Medical Anthropology Quarterly* 23 (1), 6–15.

Wilde, C. (2007). " 'Turning Sex into a Game': Gogodala Men's Response to the AIDS Epidemic and Condom Promotion in Rural Papua New Guinea." *Oceania* 77 (1), 58–71.

Will, C. M. (2007). "The Alchemy of Clinical Trials." *Biosocieties* 2 (1), 85–99.

Windybank, S., and M. Manning. (2003). "Papua New Guinea on the Brink." *Issue Analysis* 30, 1–7.

Worboys, M. (1996). "Germs, Malaria and the Invention of Mansonian Tropical Medicine: From 'Diseases in the Tropics' to 'Tropical Diseases.'" In D. Arnold (Ed.), *Warm Climates and Western Medicine: The Emergence of Tropical Medicine, 1500–1900*. Vol. 35 (181–207). Amsterdam, Neth.: Rodopi.

World Bank. (1987). *Financing Health Services in Developing Countries: An Agenda for Reform*. Washington, DC.

World Bank. (1990). *Structural Adjustment Loan Agreement, Papua New Guinea*. Washington, DC.

World Bank. (1995). *Loan Agreement (Economic Recovery Program Loan) Between the Independent State of Papua New Guinea and the International Bank for Reconstruction and Development*. Port Moresby, Papua New Guinea.

World Bank. (2000). *Papua New Guinea: Country Assistance Evaluation*. Washington, DC.

World Bank. (2011). "Urbanization Data." Available at http://data.worldbank.org /indicator/SP.URB.TOTL.IN.ZS.

Wu, D. (2005). "Chinese in Papua New Guinea." In I. Ember, Melvin Ember, and Carol R. Skoggard (Ed.), *Encyclopedia of Diasporas* (706–715). New York: Springer.

Yarwood, A. (1991). "Sir Raphael Cilento and 'The White Man in the Tropics.'" In D. Denoon and R. Macleod (Eds.), *Health and Healing in Tropical Australia and Papua New Guinea*. Townsville, AU: James Cook University.

Zaman, S. (2005). *Broken Limbs, Broken Lives: Ethnography of a Hospital Ward in Bangladesh*. Amsterdam, Neth.: Het Sphnuis.

Page numbers in italics refer to figures.

abandonment, 142, 191
Abel, Tei, 147
Accident and Emergency room, 93–94
admission forms, 92–93
aesthetic qualities, 26
agency, 28–29, 105, 145, 189
aid, 171–72, 173, 175, 177, 192, 209
AIDS, 24, 113, 124, 216
Akrich, M., 96
Alpers, Michael, 201, 202
anatomical body, 92–93
anatomy, pathological, 14–15
Anderson, Warwick, 50–51, 52, 145,
    147, 166, 201; on Gadjusek, 144, 198,
    199; on kuru, 28
anesthetists, 150
Ann, 93–94
Anna, 5
antibiotics, broad-spectrum, 101, 102,
    103, 106
antimalarials, 102, 103
antiocularcentrism, 27
antiretroviral treatment, 112
anxiety, 127, 161, 233; institutional, 25, 27
Arnold, D., 20, 43

arthemeter, 213
Asians, 76
AusAID, 171–72, 173, 177, 181, 192, 202,
    203, 229; workers, 78
Australia: aid, 171–72; medical re-
    search, 198, 199
Australian administration, 49–58,
    59–77, 198
authoritative gaze, 15
authority: of CEO, 185, 193; compari-
    son with pig meat, 180; doctors', 83,
    106, 107, 112, 154, 157, 158, 160, 161,
    166, 222; medical, 13, 64, 90, 150, 225
autonomous agents, 105

beds, hospital, 94–95, 98–100
Beisel, U., 46–47
belief, 106, 156, 157
benefits of research, 217
Berg, M., 92, 105
Biehl, Joao, 142, 230
bifurcation, 29
Big Science, 200
biology, 200–201
Biomed Experts, 143–44

biomedical gaze, 23, 93, 97, 141
biomedical knowledge, 16, 22, 25, 106, 131; nonconventional, 114, 161; and Papua New Guinean beliefs, 157; and uncertainty, 111; and unreliability, 207; and weak infrastucture, 225
biopower, 17
Birth of the Clinic (Foucault), 14
black bodies, 43, 48, 49, 51, 52, 57
black market, 152
blood, shortages, 2, 102, 127–28
bodies, 48; anatomical, 92–93; black, 43, 48, 49, 51, 52, 57; dead, 115–16; decline, 125, 135, 148; deterioration, 18; diagnosis difficulties, 97; generally sick, 16–17, 19, 20–21, 84; invisibility, 96; made unknown, 232; racially differentiated, 45, 61; racially segregated, 49, 231; and social efficacy, 225; transporting home for burial, 126, 138; tropical, 41; and visibility, 4, 18, 226
bodily fluids, 127–28
Bomana Prison, 139
"border crossings", 134
Bosa, Dr., 2, 3–4, 6–7, 100, 112, 147, 155; on control, 106; and Daniel, 89, 97, 101–2; and Dr. Masib, 104, 107; and the glasman, 160; on lack of resources, 103, 153; and Mary, 130; and Michael, 136; and pastors, 161; problems of sole doctor, 98, 150–51; on traditional beliefs, 156–57; and ultrasound scans, 96
Botswana, 16, 24
Bougainville, 80
Bowker, G., 92
Braun, Dr., 71
Brazil, 230
Breinl, Anton, 50–51
Brighenti, A., 26–27
broad-spectrum antibiotics, 101, 102, 103, 106
burial, 117, 126, 138

Burnet, Macfarlane, 198, 199
buttressing coalition, 202, 203

Cameron-Smith, A., 52, 53
cancer, 7, 16, 24, 133
capacity building, 196
Catholic health service, 71
ceftriaxone, 101
Celli, Giorgio, 47
"centers of calculation", 105
CEO, 179, 184, 185, 186, 187–88, 190, 193
ceremonies, public, 174–76, 178
Chambers, Cyril, 70
chemical poisoning, 2, 4
children and malaria, 205, 206, 220
Chinese population, 70, 71
chloramphenicol, 101, 102
cholera, 47
Christianity, 134, 135, 140, 186
Cilento, Raphael, 52, 53–55
Clare, 2–3, 4–6, 7
Cleland, Donald, 72
climate, affect on health, 41–43
clinical gaze, 23, 133, 224, 226
clinical knowledge, 15
clinical trials, 205–9, 211, 220, 230
Clinton, Bill, 181–82
Clinton Foundation, 181
Clinton Global Initiative, 182
coalition, buttressing, 202, 203
colonial hospitals, 19–21, 40–41, 43–44, 47–48, 54–56, 67, 231
colonialism, 19–20, 39–58, 85, 155
colored bodies, 43
colored laborers, 231
Comaroff, J., 24
Commonwealth Laboratory, 53
complaints' ledger, 185–87
consumption, 179–80, 191
containment, 56, 139, 140
control, 24, 55, 106, 158, 207, 211, 223; and Foucault, 23; and Strathern, 26
convalescence, 56
convicts, 140

cooking, 125
cooperation, lack, 105
corruption, 22, 133, 136, 152, 184
"crisis" diseases, 24. *See also* HIV
cryptococcal (fungal) meningitis, 96
Curtin, T., 81

Daniel, 89, 97, 101–2, 110–11, 115, 116
Das, V., 224
death, 111, 114, 115, 116, 125–26, 136–38,
    230; affect of invisibility, 233; doctors
    blamed, 158
death certificates, 138–39, 158–59
decline: of body, 125, 135, 148; of indig-
    enous population, 51; postcolonial,
    51, 62, 77, 78–79, 83, 85; of public
    hospital, 171
decolonization, 66
Decolonization Committee, 146
Deirdre, 184, 185, 186, 187, 188, 190
Dempwolff, Dr., 40
Den, 123–24, 125–26, 134, 137–38
Denoon, D., 44, 46, 53, 54, 55, 199,
    202; on neglect of public health,
    57; on training of doctors, 148
depravation, 77
detachment, 159, 163, 164, 166
diagnoses, 15, 16, 89–90, 105, 107,
    108–11, 116, 211; affect of test
    results, 95, 96; by HEOS, 97–98;
    multiple, 97, 106; preliminary, 93;
    unclear, 106, 116, 117, 232
dilapidation, 22, 68, 77, 79
Dinnen, Sinclair, 79
discharge, 111, 114, 116
disease, 23, 24–25, 103, 108–11; in *Birth
    of the Clinic*, 14; during German colo-
    nization, 39–40, 44; infectious, 17,
    71; visibility, 18. *See also* tuberculosis
disease control, 227–29, 230
disease ecology, 198
distance, social, 163, 164
distinctions, social, 164
"dividuals", 29, 30

diviners, 160
Divine Word University, 172–74, 176–77
doctors, 17–18, 146–66, 211–12, 214;
    and diagnosis, 89–90, 95–96, 97–98,
    100–111; ignoring patients, 133,
    135–36, 139, 141; invisibility, sense
    of, 231; knowledge and authority,
    83, 222; and lack of resources, 232;
    and medical research, attitude to,
    218–19; oncology, 16; and patients,
    mediating between, 33; and the
    state, desire to be seen by, 233
donations, 71, 113, 175, 178, 191, 232
donor funding, 82, 171–72, 173, 175, 177,
    178, 181
donors, 192, 232
DOTS (directly observed treatment
    short course) program, 104, 107,
    113, 215
drinks, branded, 115, 116
drugs, 63, 101, 102, 109, 113, 208, 213;
    lack of, 81, 151–52. *See also* medicine,
    hospital
dysentery, 40, 44

economy, 80–81
effect and visibility, 27
efficacy, 26
Eliza and Walter Research Institute, 198
Elyachar, J., 50
emplacement, 196, 204, 205–6, 208–11,
    220, 221
epidemics, 44–45
epistemic displacement, 206–8, 221
epistemic emplacement, 196, 205–6,
    208, 221
equipment, comparison between
    researchers and hospital, 217
Eric, 98, 108, 109, 110, 130, 157
Errington, F., 164, 166
essentialization, 29
ethical emplacement, 196, 204, 208–11,
    220, 221
ethical protocols, 215–16, 219–20, 221

Euro-America, 25, 28, 29
European doctors, 73, 148, 155, 156
European hospitals, 55, 69, 70, 73–76, 83
Europeans, 42, 75, 231
"Everybody's Business" report, 228
Ewers, W. H., 40
examination, medical, 91–93, 95
exchange object, 189–90
exclusion, 230–31, 232
expert gaze, 43, 96, 233

failure, 31, 135, 142, 191, 226, 232; of
  hospitals, 19, 34, 85, 224; of patients,
  231; of political gifts, 178–79; of the
  state, 77, 78–79, 83, 169–71, 184, 223
family. See relatives
Fassin, Didier, 232
field science, 208–9
Finkler, K., 123
Finschafen, 39–40
Firth, S., 40
Fischer, M., 204
Fischer, M. M. J., 228
fizzy drinks, 115, 116
food, 4–5, 118, 122, 124, 138–39
Fore, 144
Foster, R. J., 180
Foucault, M., 14–15, 20, 23, 25, 26, 27,
  43, 90
fragility of the state, 78, 170, 224
Fran, 91
Frank, 218
Fred Hollows Foundation, 173
Frerichs, A., 71
Frerichs, S., 71
Friedrich Wilhelmshafen (now
  Madang Town), 40, 48–49
frontier hospitals, 57–58
funding, 72, 171–72, 173, 227; donations,
  175, 177, 178; for IMR, 202, 203; for
  infectious diseases, 17; reduction,
  80, 81; for research, 209–10, 231–32;
  for superhospital, 181
fund-raising, 214

Gadjusek, Carleton, 144, 198, 199, 202
Galang, 115
Gambe, Bertha, 2, 3
Gambe, William, 1–2, 3, 4, 5, 6–7
garden food, 121, 122, 124
Gawale, Dr., 163
Gawande, Atul, 16
gaze, 44, 224, 226; authoritative, 15;
  biomedical, 23, 93, 97, 141; clinical,
  133, 224, 226; expert, 43, 96, 233;
  medical, 18, 49; public, 67; state, 40
Geest, S. van der, 123
Geissler et al., 221
Gell, A., 127
generally sick bodies, 16–17, 19, 20–21,
  84, 112, 113, 231; and Dr. Masib, 110;
  and Dr. Wali, 97
German New Guinea, 39–40, 41, 44–49
Gewertz, D., 164, 166
Giemsa stain, 113
gifts, 124–25, 145, 166, 189; to family,
  162, 163; to the hospital, 175–76,
  177–79, 180, 191
glasman, 5, 6, 160, 161
global funding, 113, 227, 228
global science, 155–56, 213, 214, 219–20
God, relationship with, 5, 134, 135, 140
Good et al., 22
Goroka, 201
governing gaze, 224
government: and basic services, inability
  to provide, 148; corruption, 133, 136;
  and disappointment with, 169; and
  rural people, how envisaged by, 234–35
gradualism, 66
graves, mass, 141
guardian, 120, 121, 122
Gunther, Dr. John, 61, 63–65, 72, 198, 199
Guntner, M. W., 72

Hacking, I, 24
Hagahai tribe, 210
Halland, Dr., 195, 205, 206, 207–8,
  212–14, 220–21

Harloe, L., 55
Harrison, Mark, 49
Harry, 91–93
Hasluck, Paul, 59, 66, 147
healers, 160
health activism, 27
health administration, 171–72; Australian, 53, 54, 63; funding, 80, 81. *See also* CEO
health extension officer (HEO), 1, 81, 91, 98, *118*; Eric, 108, 109, 110, 130, 157
Health Management Department, 172
health sector improvement program (HSIP) fund, 173
health systems strengthening, 228–29
hemoglobin levels, 2, 102, 251
herbal remedies, 160
Hillier, K., 55
Hirsch, Eric, 26, 189
HIV, 3, 24, 112–13, 124, 125, 216
Hobbins, P., 55
Hodgkin, David, 68–69
Holbraad, M., 34
homeless people, 115–16, 121
hope, 19, 34, 133, 134, 141, 191
Hornabrook, Richard, 199, 200–201
Hospital Board, 81–82
hospital-building program, 62, 73
Hospital Committee, 63–64, 67, 68, 73–74
hospitals: under Australian administration, 55–56, 57–58, 59–60, 61; colonial, 19–21, 40–41, 43–44; financing, 81–82; as site for research, 203, 204; and the state, 85; and visibility, 23; as waiting places, 140–41. *See also* Madang General Hospital
hospital sickness compared with village sickness, 158
housing, doctors', 154–55
Hughes, H., 78

human biology, 200–201
"human kinds", 27
Human T-Lymphotropic Virus-1, 210

Iliffe, J., 155
imaging technologies, 18, 95–96, 131–32. *See also* X-rays
IMF, 80, 81
immunity, 45, 46
improvement, social, 67
"improvisational medicine," 17
IMR (Institute of Medical Research), Papua New Guinea, 201–4, 208, 210, 214–16, 217, 218, 219
inclusion, 231
independence, 66–67, 79–80, 147
individualism, 29
industrial action, 171, 184–87, 192, 193
inequalities, 69, 77, 79, 82, 155–56, 218, 221, 232
infectious diseases, 17, 47, 48, 71
infrastructure, 63, 79, 81–83, 169–70, 173, 195; gifts, 175–76, 177, 192; hospitals, 48–49; medical, 111; research versus public health, 219, 220, 221; wards, 208; weak state, 22, 30, 225
Institute for Human Biology, Papua New Guinea, 199, 200, 201
Institute of Medical Research, 173, 177
institutional anxiety, 25, 27
Institutional Review Board, 215–16
internal medicine, 89–90
International Council of Scientific Unions, 199
International Geophysical Year, 1959, 199–200
International Human Biology Program (IHB), 199–200
Internet, 143
"interpretive flexibility", 18
invisibility, 19, 21, 31, 35, 67, 191, 224, 232; of nurses, 193; of patients' bodies, 4, 18, 96, 131, 136, 141, 233; of public ward, 231

isolation, 53, 73, 74, 80, 128, 151; of infectious diseases, 47, 48, 71

Jackman, H. H., 47, 49
Jay, Martin, 27
Jenkins, Carol, 210

Kaiser Wilhelmshafen, 39
Kalim, Dr., 89–90, 149
Kanu, Nurse, 5
Karkar, 149, 150, 151, 200
Kelly, A., 46–47
kin. *See* relatives
knowledge, 15, 23, 24–25, 26, 219, 220, 221–22
Knowles, Dr., 68, 72
Koch, Robert, 17, 45–46, 47, 49, 197–98
kuru, 28, 198–99, 201

laboratory, 15, 93–94, 96–97, 113, 207, 208, 211, 217; move to new site, 176–77
laboratory technicians, 7, 96, 105, 212, 213, 214, 222
laborers and malaria, 45–46
Lae hospital, 76–77, 154
larval control, 46, 47
law, using power of, 189
Leach, James, 140
League of Nations Mandate, 49–53
"Leaving hospital at own risk" form, 157, 158
Levin, Adam, 24
Lewis, M., 54, 58
lifestyles, doctors', 154–56
Lima, Dr., 161
Livingstone, D. N., 205, 206
Livingston, J., 16
Lorna, 115
Lowe, C., 112
Lufa, 200
Luluais, 44
Lutheran health service, 71
Lutheran mission hospital, Karkar, 151

MacGregor, William, 50–51
MacLeod, R., 54, 58
Madang General Hospital, *xiii*, 11, 18–19, 22, 169–77, 224, 225; attitude to disease, 16; differences between private and public wards, 15; and "improvisational medicine", 17; lack of resources, 150–51; lack of support from regional and national hospitals, 153–54; opening, 59–60; pediatric ward, 194–95; as research site, 203, 205–8, 211–15, 216–17; site of Institute for Human Biology, 199; strikes, 184–85; uncertainty, 30, 232; and visibility, 27
Madang Nurses Association, 184, 185–88
Madang Town, 71. *See also* Friedrich Wilhelmshafen (now Madang Town)
Mairu, Sister, 160
malaria, 39, 40, 41, 42, 93–94, 97, 113; high rates, 214; research, 17, 45–48, 203, 215; trial, 205, 206–7
malaria microscopy unit, 177
malaria vaccine program, 202
malnutrition, 116
Malu, 116–17, 118
mandate system, 49–53
marginality, 133, 142, 232, 233
Marsland, R., 17
Mary, 119, 122, 130–31, 138
Masib, Dr., 104–5, 106–11, 112, 130–31
mass graves, 141
Mattingly, C., 133–34
May, Dr., 68
medical examination, 1, 2, 89, 91–93, 95, 101, 103, 195
medical gaze, 18, 49
medical history, 91, 95
medical infrastructure, 111. *See also* infrastructure
medical orderlies, 44
medical research, 17, 21, 45–48, 53, 198, 200–211, 212–22, 231–32

medical ward, 2, 15, 31, 89, 93, 94–111, 113; lack of resources, 90; ratio of patients to doctors, 83–84
medicine, hospital, 3, 4, 116, 117, 125; and Michael, 120, 121, 122, 127, 135
Melanesia compared with Euro-America, 25, 26, 28, 29, 33
meningitis, 96, 101, 215
Michael, 118, 119–21, 122, 123–24, 125, 126–27; and invisibility, sense of, 131, 132–33, 135–39, 141; and relationship with doctor, 128–29, 134–35
microscopist, 93–94
Middleton, Mr. H. T. M., 69
Millennium Development Goals, 17, 203
minibus, 174
mining, 80
missionaries, 71
Miyazaki, H., 131, 176
modernization, 63, 64
Mol, A., 34, 95, 103
Mola, G. D. L., 183
money: as gift, 162, 163; lack of, affect, 122–23, 135
morgue, 115–16
mosquito, 46
MRAC (Medical Research Advisory Committee), 210, 216
Munn, N., 180, 197

Nabik, Dr., 149–50, 153, 155
national development, 146, 147, 148
National Health Plan, 79, 81, 172
National Institute of Health in Bethesda, 198, 199
National Nurses Association, 184
National Research Institute, 183
nation-state, 61, 67, 77, 79, 85
native hospitals, 55–56, 57, 67–69, 73–74, 76
neglect, 133, 135, 169–70, 177–78, 192
networking site, 143–44, 164
Neuguinea Compagnie, 39

New Guinea, 41, 44–58, 198
New Guinea Times Courier, 76
New Ireland, 44
New Melanesian Ethnography, 29
nurses: cooperation, lack, 104, 105; and donations, attitude to, 178, 179–80, 192, 193, 232; duties, 98; and invisibility, sense of, 231; shortage, 114; and the state, desire to be seen by, 233; strikes, 171, 184–89, 190–91

Okapa, 199
oncology, 24
oncology doctors, 16
orderlies, medical, 44
otherness, 134

Pacific Medical Center, 181–84
painim nem, 129, 131
Panguna mine, 80
Pan Pacific and Southeast Asian Women's Society, 68
parasites, 46–47, 93–94, 113
partnerships, 172–75, 181–84, 192, 193, 217, 231–32
pastors, 160–61
pathological anatomy, 14–15
pathology laboratory, 176–77, 207. *See also* laboratory
pathology machines, 11
pathology shed, 93–94
patients, 18, 32, 33, 98–100, 107–11, 231, 232, 233; Rose, 129–30; Tutas, 124, 125. *See also* Daniel; Gambe, William; Michael
Paul, 195, 206, 207, 210, 218
pay, 155, 184, 202
Pedersen, M. A., 34
pediatric ward, 194–95
personhood, 18, 23, 24, 28–29, 33, 90, 145, 225, 226, 232, 233; and collaboration, affect, 144; of doctors, 147, 164, 165, 214; and recognition, 145

personification, 25, 26, 28
person-making, 23–24
Petryna, A., 152, 209
pharmaceuticals, lack of, 151–52
Philo, C., 43
pigs, 179, 180–81
plantations, 39, 40, 45–46
poisoning, chemical, 2, 4
politicians and personal gain, 178–79, 183–84. *See also* corruption
politics and role of health professional, 146–47
Pols, H., 147
Poole, D., 224
"poor majority," 231
Porter, D., 44
Port Moresby, 151–52, 155
Port Moresby General Hospital, 77, 149, 153
"postcolonial disorder", 22
postcolonial institutions, 19–21
Post Courier, 170
power, 22, 23, 25, 26, 29, 180–81, 184, 189
power cuts, 3, 11
praying, 5
Prednisone, 135
pregnancy, 24
preventative medicine, 61
primary health care, 61
Prince, R., 17
prison, 139
prisoners on remand, 140
private health sector, 223
private wards, 15, 82, 83, 231
provincial hospital, 151, 154. *See also* Madang General Hospital
public ceremonies, 174–75, 178
public gaze, 44, 67
public health, 21, 43, 44, 46, 61, 221; under Australian administration, 51, 54–55, 57
public hospital, 191, 223–24, 226, 235; design, 19; and research, 209, 217;

and uncertainty, 22. *See also* Madang General Hospital
Public Hospitals Act, 81
publics, 35, 76, 81, 84, 85, 175, 209, 232; and Gunther, 64; and hospital design, 61; invisibility, 232; poor, 170; and the state, 191; white, 70–73
public spaces, 72
public spending cuts, 202
public wards, 15, 82–84, 231

quarantine, 43, 48, 55
quinine, 46, 47

race, 23, 45, 46, 61. *See also* segregation
radiation sickness, 24
Rapp, Rayna, 23–24, 30
reagents, 3, 11, 96, 113, 207
recognition, 134, 140, 145, 189, 233
Redfield, Peter, 197
Reed, Adam, 139, 140, 141
Reeder, John, 202–3
reification, 24, 25–26, 27, 28, 29
Reite, 140
rejection, 116, 135
relational technologies, 118, 132
relationships, 13, 28, 135, 156, 159, 225; gifts of food, affect, 124–25; between medical researcher and hospital, 212–14; mobilizing into a powerful form, 26; of politicians, 178–79, 184; village, 120–22
relatives, 18, 121, 123, 135, 139–40; anger against sick, 126–27; of doctors, 162–64, 165; donating blood, 128
religion, 134, 135, 140, 186
remand prisoners, 140
research governance, 209
research, medical, 17, 21, 53, 198, 200–211, 212–22, 231–32
responsibility, internalized, 233
Riles, Annelise, 190
Rose, 129–30

Rose, N., 25
Ross, Ronald, 45, 46, 50–51
Rotary Club, 164
Royal Australian College of Surgeons, 77
rural areas, 149–50, 151
rural health services, 57, 61, 63, 71, 79
rural hospital, 149, 151
rural population, 11–12
rural tropics, 206, 207

salaries, 155, 184, 202
samples, 127
Schellong, Dr., 39, 40
school fees, 162
School of Medical and Health Sciences, University of Papua New Guinea, 146
science, 146, 196, 197, 200, 204; in the field, 208–9; global, 155–56, 213, 214, 219–20
scientific emplacement, 196
scientists, 144–45, 198, 200, 204, 219, 221–22
Scragg, Roy, 59
segregation, 52, 54–55, 56–57, 69, 71, 73–75, 76, 86; in German New Guinea, 43, 48, 49
self-governance, 146
separation from kin, 139–40
Siba, Peter, 204
sick bodies, generally. See generally sick bodies
sickness: caused by social conflicts, 120–21; reasons for, 32; village and hospital, 156–58
sik bilong marasin, 3, 32, 158
sik bilong ples, 32, 120–21, 127, 128, 129, 156–58
sik i kamap nating, 32
Sinclair, J. P., 40, 48, 74
skin nodules, 1, 2, 5–6
smallpox, 44
soap, 6
social distance, 163, 164
social distinctions, 164

social failure, 135, 231. See also failure
social improvement, 67
social invisibility, 31, 35. See also invisibility
social recognition, 134. See also recognition
social relationships. See relationships
soft drinks, 115, 116
Somare, Michael, 181, 183
sorcery, 5, 117, 120, 127
spaces, 56, 58, 61, 64, 72, 82, 114, 231–32
specimens, 127
spending cuts, public, 202
spirits, 156–57
sputum test, 104, 113, 114
state, the, 77, 78, 176, 179, 181; absence, 232; building, 22, 30, 40, 62, 85; failure, 83, 169–71, 184, 223; neglect, 22, 191, 192
status of doctors, 46, 134, 148, 154, 165
Stephansort, 40, 45
sterilizer, 177
steroids, 135
Strathern, M., 25–26, 27, 28, 29, 145, 189, 225
strikes, 171, 184–87, 192, 193
structural adjustment programs, 80, 81, 202
superhospital, 181–84
suppositories, 205, 208, 213
surgical doctors, 150. See also doctors
surgical ward, 3, 93, 130

tax, 44
TB. See tuberculosis
technicians, laboratory, 96
technologically advanced medicine, 61
technologies, 18, 23–24, 139, 225, 226, 228, 233–34; donated, 177; imaging, 95–96, 131; unstable, 30
technologies of knowledge production, 131–32. See also X-rays
technology of progress, 66
tibi. See tuberculosis

Tolai, 5

town, attitude of wantok, 121, 122, 123, 135

Townsville Institute of Tropical Medicine, 50–51, 52, 53

training, medical, 71, 148–49

transactions, 180, 189

transmission and consumption, 179–80

"trans-temporal comparison", 34

trials, clinical, 205–9, 211, 220, 230

tropical climate, affect on health, 41–43, 45

tropical disease, 44

tropical medicine, 47–48, 49, 50, 51–52, 54, 57–58

trust in doctors, 134

Tscharke, Edwin, 149

tuberculosis, 2, 3, 7, 95, 103, 107, 112, 119; difficult to diagnose, 102; and funding, impact, 113; high rates, 214; research, 215, 231–32; and Rose, 129–30

Tultuls, 44, 54

tuna, 4–5

Tutas, 124, 125

ultrasound scanning, 24, 96, 128–29, 133, 225

UN, 61, 73, 146

uncertainty, 19, 22, 25, 30, 141–42, 189, 224, 225, 226; of diagnosis, 106, 111, 232; and Dr. Masib, 110

unemployment, 80–81

University of Papua New Guinea, 146

urban health infrastructure, 63

USAID, 202

user fees, 81, 82

vaccinations, 44

value creation, 180

village, 120–22, 162–64, 234–35; sickness, 156–58

virus, 210

visibility, 11, 13–14, 24, 224, 225, 226, 232–34; of anthropologist, 32; and Foucault, 15, 27; and gift giving, 178, 179; of hospital, 23; medical, 18, 76; of native hospitals, 67; nurses', 184; patients', 118, 134; and power, 189–90; professional, 222; of public hospital, 191; and recognition, 140; to the state, 22; value, 25

Wagner, R., 33

waiting place, 141, 142

Wali, 234

Wali, Dr., 97, 106

wanbel relationships, 5, 6, 7, 124, 127

Wani, Dr., 156, 162–63

wantok, 121, 122, 123, 135, 155

wards, 3, 82–84, 93, 130, 208, 231. See also medical ward

wasman, 120, 121, 122

water, 6, 44

Wendland, C. L., 16, 105–6

white bodies, 48, 50–51, 52, 56, 83

White Nation policy, 50

Whyte, Susan, 19, 142

William. See Gambe, William

witchcraft, 156, 190, 191

Wokaisor, 234–35

Woods, Dr., 70, 71

World Bank, 80, 81

World Health Organization (WHO), 61, 113, 228

X-rays, 1, 2, 95–96, 118, 128–30, 131–32, 133–34, 225

Yagaum hospital, 71–72

Yarwood, A., 52

Zibe, Sasa, 183